Jaffer A. Ajani, MD, Steven A. Curley, MD,
Nora A. Janjan, MD, and
Patrick M. Lynch, MD, JD
Editors

The University of Texas M. D. Anderson Cancer Center,
Houston, Texas

Gastrointestinal Cancer

Foreword by James L. Abbruzzese, MD,
and Raphael E. Pollock, MD, PhD

With 61 Illustrations

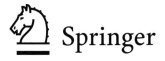 Springer

Jaffer A. Ajani, MD
Department of Gastrointestinal
  Medical Oncology
The University of Texas
  M. D. Anderson Cancer Center
Houston, TX 77030-4009, USA

Steven A. Curley, MD
Department of Surgical Oncology
The University of Texas
  M. D. Anderson Cancer Center
Houston, TX 77030-4009, USA

Nora A. Janjan, MD
Department of Radiation Oncology
The University of Texas
  M. D. Anderson Cancer Center
Houston, TX 77030-4009, USA

Patrick M. Lynch, MD, JD
Department of Gastrointestinal
  Medicine and Nutrition
The University of Texas
  M. D. Anderson Cancer Center
Houston, TX 77030-4009, USA

Series Editors:
Aman U. Buzdar, MD
Department of Breast Medical
  Oncology
The University of Texas
  M. D. Anderson Cancer Center
Houston, TX 77030-4009, USA

Ralph S. Freedman, MD, PhD
Immunology/Molecular Biology
  Laboratory
Department of Gynecologic Oncology
The University of Texas
  M. D. Anderson Cancer Center
Houston, TX 77030-4009, USA

Cover illustration: © Peter Siu/Images.com

Library of Congress Cataloging-in-Publication Data
Gastrointestinal cancer / [edited by] Jaffer A. Ajani . . . [et al.].
        p. ; cm. — (M. D. Anderson cancer care series)
     ISBN 0-387-22090-9 (sc : alk. paper)
     1. Digestive organs—Cancer. I. Title: Gastrointestinal cancer.
II. Ajani, Jaffer A. III. Series.
     [DNLM: 1. Gastrointestinal Neoplasms—therapy. 2. Gastrointestinal
Neoplasms—diagnosis. 3. Risk Factors. WI 149 G2596 2004]
     RC280.D5G386 2004
     616.99′433—dc22   2004050125

ISBN 0-387-22090-9   Printed on acid-free paper.

© 2005 Springer Science+Business Media, Inc.

Printed in the United States of America.   (BS/EB)

9 8 7 6 5 4 3 2 1   SPIN 10984437

springeronline.com

M. D. ANDERSON
CANCER CARE
S E R I E S

Series Editors

Aman U. Buzdar, MD   Ralph S. Freedman, MD, PhD

M. D. ANDERSON CANCER CARE SERIES

Series Editors: Aman U. Buzdar, MD, and
             Ralph S. Freedman, MD, PhD

K.K. Hunt, G.L. Robb, E.A. Strom, and N.T. Ueno, Eds., *Breast Cancer*

F.V. Fossella, R. Komaki, and J.B. Putnam, Jr., Eds., *Lung Cancer*

J.A. Ajani, S.A. Curley, N.A. Janjan, and P.M. Lynch, Eds.,
     Gastrointestinal Cancer

FOREWORD

Cancers of the gastrointestinal tract remain a major challenge for oncologists and other cancer specialists in the United States and worldwide. This volume on the evaluation and treatment of patients with gastrointestinal malignancies represents an important milestone in the M. D. Anderson Cancer Center Series on the multidisciplinary management of cancer. Gastrointestinal cancers exemplify the importance of multidisciplinary management in modern oncologic care. Contributors to the management of patients with the spectrum of diseases that emanate from the gastrointestinal tract include pathologists, radiologists, surgical oncologists, radiation oncologists, medical oncologists, and others. It is the close interaction and interplay between these highly trained specialists that result in the improving care of patients with these challenging diseases. In the following chapters, gastrointestinal oncology specialists at M. D. Anderson Cancer Center describe the state of the art in the multidisciplinary management of diseases developing from all parts of the gastrointestinal tract.

Increasingly, we are recognizing that many gastrointestinal malignancies have a strong inherited component. In many cases, the early recognition of patients at high risk for specific preneoplastic processes involving the gastrointestinal tract—such as Barrett's esophagus and colonic polyposis—represents an important opportunity to prevent the emergence of neoplasia. Optimizing prevention strategies remains our best hope for eradicating gastrointestinal cancers as an important cause of cancer-related deaths in the United States.

Each of the malignancies discussed in the 20 chapters of this monograph has specific highly unique features. Tailored to the unique natural history of each malignancy, the management of these diseases varies considerably. Despite the progress being made, a great deal of work remains to be done to understand the basic molecular biology of gastrointestinal malignancies. It is this knowledge that will be crucial for the development of new therapeutics and new opportunities for screening and early diagnosis for gastrointestinal cancers. We believe that readers of this volume will be impressed at the dramatic improvements that are being made with these difficult cancers.

James L. Abbruzzese, MD
Raphael E. Pollock, MD, PhD

PREFACE

As a group, gastrointestinal-tract cancers are the second most common cancers among males and females in the United States. The most dominant is colorectal cancer; remarkably, only a small proportion of people nationwide receive adequate screening for this malignancy. Patients with gastrointestinal-tract cancers are benefiting from a multidisciplinary treatment approach. For example, multidisciplinary collaboration has enabled sphincter preservation in rectal cancer. The interdisciplinary approach is also yielding favorable results for the more difficult tumors, such as pancreatic cancer and liver cancer. We are seeing the advantages of early systemic therapy as an adjunct to surgery in colorectal cancer, and novel agents are showing improved results in advanced disease. Increased utilization of adjuvant therapy in early disease could very well change the natural history of gastrointestinal-tract malignancies such as colorectal cancer.

Much effort has been put into this 20-chapter volume. We would like to thank the volume editors, Drs. Jaffer Ajani, Steven Curley, Nora Janjan, and Patrick Lynch, for their steadfast efforts in bringing this book to fruition. Also, sincere thanks to Mariann Crapanzano, Stephanie Deming, Ginny Norris, Michael Worley, and Chris Yeager of the Department of Scientific Publications for editing and compiling this volume.

Aman U. Buzdar, MD
Ralph S. Freedman, MD, PhD

CONTENTS

CONTRIBUTORS

Banke Agarwal, MD, Assistant Professor, Department of Gastrointestinal Medicine and Nutrition

Jaffer A. Ajani, MD, Professor, Department of Gastrointestinal Medical Oncology

Christopher I. Amos, PhD, Professor, Department of Epidemiology

Karen A. Beaty, PA-C, Physician Assistant, Department of Surgical Oncology

Annette K. Bisanz, MPH, Advanced Practice Nurse, Department of Nursing Administration

Carol H. Bosken, MD, ScM, Instructor, Department of Epidemiology

Chusilp Charnsangavej, MD, Professor, Department of Diagnostic Radiology

Charles Cleeland, PhD, Professor, Chair, Department of Symptom Research

Christopher Crane, MD, Associate Professor, Department of Radiation Oncology

Steven A. Curley, MD, Professor, Department of Surgical Oncology

Marc E. Delclos, MD, Assistant Professor, Department of Radiation Oncology

Douglas B. Evans, MD, Professor, Department of Surgical Oncology

Barry W. Feig, MD, Associate Professor, Department of Surgical Oncology

Marsha L. Frazier, PhD, Associate Professor, Department of Epidemiology

Nora A. Janjan, MD, Professor, Department of Radiation Oncology

Ishaan S. Kalha, MD, Fellow, Gastroenterology

Ritsuko Komaki, MD, Professor, Department of Radiation Oncology

Edward H. Lin, MD, Assistant Professor, Department of Gastrointestinal Medical Oncology

Patrick M. Lynch, MD, JD, Associate Professor, Department of Gastrointestinal Medicine and Nutrition

Angela J. McIntosh, PA-C, Physician Assistant, Department of Surgical Oncology

Peter W. T. Pisters, MD, Associate Professor, Department of Surgical Oncology

Asif Rashid, MD, PhD, Associate Professor, Department of Pathology

Miguel A. Rodriguez-Bigas, MD, Professor, Department of Surgical Oncology

Frank A. Sinicrope, MD, Associate Professor, Department of Gastrointestinal Medicine and Nutrition

John M. Skibber, MD, Professor, Department of Surgical Oncology

Amr S. Soliman, MD, PhD, Assistant Professor, Department of Epidemiology

Dejka M. Steinert, MD, Fellow, Department of Medical Oncology

Stephen G. Swisher, MD, Associate Professor, Department of Thoracic and Cardiovascular Surgery

Jonathan Trent, MD, PhD, Assistant Professor, Department of Sarcoma Medical Oncology

Jean-Nicolas Vauthey, MD, Professor, Department of Surgical Oncology

Michelle B. Waller, PA-C, Physician Assistant, Department of Surgical Oncology

Robert A. Wolff, MD, Associate Professor, Department of Gastrointestinal Medical Oncology

Henry Q. Xiong, MD, Assistant Professor, Department of Gastrointestinal Medical Oncology

James C. Yao, MD, Assistant Professor, Department of Gastrointestinal Medical Oncology

1   STAGING OF GASTROINTESTINAL MALIGNANCIES

Michelle B. Waller, Karen A. Beaty,
Angela J. McIntosh, and Steven A. Curley

CHAPTER OVERVIEW

Clinical and pathologic staging of gastrointestinal malignancies is critically important in the planning of neoadjuvant, adjuvant, and multidisciplinary treatment programs. This chapter describes the approach at M. D. Anderson Cancer Center to the clinical staging of cancers arising in the stomach, liver, biliary system, pancreas, colon, and rectum. Emphasis is placed on our use of state-of-the-art diagnostic modalities, including endoscopic ultrasonography, computed tomography, and magnetic resonance imaging. Accurate staging in patients with gastrointestinal malignancies assists us in identifying patients who are most likely to benefit from multimodality therapy.

INTRODUCTION

Gastrointestinal (GI) malignancies are a heterogeneous group of diseases that must be segregated by organ of origin, histologic type, and stage at presentation when the clinician considers appropriate treatment modalities. Despite impressive advances in the equipment and software used in diagnostic radiology and the development of improved diagnostic imaging modalities, a complete history and physical examination are still critical in the evaluation and follow-up staging of GI malignancies. Taken as a group, GI malignancies are the most common type of human solid cancer worldwide. However, the incidence varies dramatically from organ to organ within the GI system. Even within a single organ site in the GI system, the incidence can be highly variable because of population, geographic, and environmental differences. Complete clinical staging of GI malignancies is the first important step in assessing new patients, developing a treatment plan, and designing new protocol-based therapies at M. D. Anderson Cancer Center.

GASTRIC CANCER

Gastric adenocarcinoma is one of the most common human solid tumors worldwide. In the United States, approximately 25,000 people are diagnosed annually with gastric adenocarcinoma. We see approximately 300 patients with newly diagnosed gastric cancer yearly at M. D. Anderson.

The symptoms related to gastric cancer are typically vague and long-standing in many patients. Thus, advanced-stage disease is diagnosed in a significant proportion of patients. Esophagogastroduodenoscopy is considered the standard of care in the evaluation of patients with new or worsening symptoms of epigastric pain, gastroesophageal reflux, early satiety, or unremitting nausea and vomiting. A Clo test is performed on gastric aspirates to determine the presence of *Helicobacter pylori* infection. Any suspicious mass lesion, areas of inflammation, or edges of ulcers are biopsied to assess for the presence of malignant disease.

The history obtained from a new gastric cancer patient includes symptoms, risk factors, and family history. During the physical examination, evidence of advanced-stage disease can be found in the form of a palpable epigastric mass or a nodule located in the periumbilical region (Sister Mary Joseph's node) or supraclavicular region (Virchow's node) or on digital rectal examination (Blummer's shelf). Lymphatic regions in the neck, supraclavicular, and infraclavicular regions are thoroughly examined, and suspicious lymph nodes are biopsied by fine-needle aspiration.

At M. D. Anderson, the diagnostic evaluation includes initial laboratory tests, including a complete blood cell count (CBC), liver function studies, and measurement of serum electrolytes. Baseline serum tumor markers, carcinoembryonic antigen and carcinoma antigen 125, are measured and then followed serially during treatment and follow-up. Standard 2-view chest radiographs are evaluated for the presence of pulmonary metastasis. Chest computed tomography (CT) is performed only in patients with abnormal results on standard chest radiography or with gastroesophageal junction tumors to assess extent of disease. Helical CT of the abdomen and pelvis is performed in all patients to evaluate the stomach, regional lymph nodes, liver, and peritoneal cavity.

Esophagogastroduodenoscopy with endoscopic ultrasonography (EUS) is now a routine component of our staging in new patients with gastric cancer. At M. D. Anderson, we follow the American Joint Committee on Cancer (AJCC) staging guidelines (Table 1–1). EUS is extremely useful in determining the T classification of the tumor and may be helpful in assessing the presence of regional lymph node metastases. State-of-the-art EUS endoscopes are equipped with biopsy channels that can be used to perform needle aspiration biopsies of the stomach wall or of lymph nodes adjacent to the stomach.

Subclinical peritoneal spread (carcinomatosis) of gastric adenocarcinoma may not be diagnosed by high-quality CT or EUS. Because of this limitation, surgeons at M. D. Anderson routinely employ staging laparoscopic evaluation in patients with potentially resectable gastric carcinoma. Staging laparoscopy is generally the final staging procedure in gastric cancer patients who are thought to be surgical candidates with stage II or III disease. A finding of peritoneal carcinomatosis diagnoses stage IV disease, and the patient is considered for systemic rather than surgical therapy.

Hepatobiliary Malignancies

Physicians and physician assistants in the GI Tumor Center at M. D. Anderson evaluated more than 900 new patients with primary or metastatic hepatobiliary tumors in 2002. Patients with primary liver cancer include those with hepatocellular carcinoma (HCC), gallbladder cancer, and intrahepatic or extrahepatic cholangiocarcinoma. Patients with liver metastases from other organ sites, most commonly colorectal adenocarcinoma, and with disease confined to the liver may be considered for surgery, tumor ablation, regional chemotherapy, or systemic chemotherapy. The initial screening evaluation of new patients includes a thorough review of outside medical records, pathologic assessment of any surgical or needle-biopsy specimens, and review of prior diagnostic CT scans and plain radiographs. Once again, a thorough history and physical examination are mandatory. In patients with liver metastases, recent assessment of the primary site of disease, such as colonoscopy for colorectal cancer, is critical to exclude local recurrence. The history also includes an evaluation of risk factors, such as chronic hepatitis B or C virus infection in patients with HCC, and a family history. While family history is not a component of staging of malignant disease, it is an important component of the

Table 1–1. Stage Grouping for Gastric Cancer

Stage 0	Tis	N0	M0
Stage 1A	T1	N0	M0
Stage 1B	T1	N1	M0
	T2a/b	N0	M0
Stage II	T1	N2	M0
	T2a/b	N1	M0
	T3	N0	M0
Stage IIIA	T2a/b	N2	M0
	T3	N1	M0
	T4	N0	M0
Stage IIIB	T3	N2	M0
Stage IV	T4	N1–3	M0
	T1–3	N3	M0
	Any T	Any N	M1

Definition of TNM

Primary Tumor (T)

TX   Primary tumor cannot be assessed
T0   No evidence of primary tumor
Tis   Carcinoma *in situ*: intraepithelial tumor without invasion of the lamina propria
T1   Tumor invades lamina propria or submucosa
T2   Tumor invades muscularis propria or subserosa*
T2a   Tumor invades muscularis propria
T2b   Tumor invades subserosa
T3   Tumor penetrates serosa (visceral peritoneum) without invasion of adjacent structures**, ***
T4   Tumor invades adjacent structures**, ***

* *Note:* A tumor may penetrate the muscularis propria with extension into the gastrocolic or gastrohepatic ligaments, or into the greater or lesser omentum, without perforation of the visceral peritoneum covering these structures. In this case, the tumor is classified T2. If there is perforation of the visceral peritoneum covering the gastric ligaments or the omentum, the tumor should be classified T3.

** *Note:* The adjacent structures of the stomach include the spleen, transverse colon, liver, diaphragm, pancreas, abdominal wall, adrenal gland, kidney, small intestine, and retroperitoneum.

*** *Note:* Intramural extension to the duodenum or esophagus is classified by the depth of the greatest invasion in any of these sites, including the stomach.

Regional Lymph Nodes (N)

NX   Regional lymph node(s) cannot be assessed
N0   No regional lymph node metastasis*
N1   Metastasis in 1 to 6 regional lymph nodes
N2   Metastasis in 7 to 15 regional lymph nodes
N3   Metastasis in more than 15 regional lymph nodes

* *Note:* A designation of pN0 should be used if all examined lymph nodes are negative, regardless of the total number removed and examined.

Distant Metastasis (M)

MX   Distant metastasis cannot be assessed
M0   No distant metastasis
M1   Distant metastasis

Used with the permission of the American Joint Committee on Cancer (AJCC), Chicago, Illinois. The original source for this material is the AJCC Cancer Staging Manual, Sixth Edition (2002), published by Springer-Verlag New York, www.springer-ny.com.

mission at M. D. Anderson to evaluate and diagnose early-stage, treatable malignant disease. The physical examination focuses on assessment of accessible lymph node basins, cardiopulmonary examination to determine suitability for surgery and cytotoxic chemotherapy, an abdominal examination to measure palpable organomegaly or extrahepatic masses, a rectal examination for gross or occult blood, and an evaluation for clinical stigmata of chronic liver disease.

Laboratory evaluation includes a CBC, coagulation profile, liver function tests, electrolytes, and serum tumor markers when appropriate. Serum carcinoembryonic antigen levels are measured in patients with colorectal cancer liver metastases, serum alpha fetoprotein levels are measured in HCC patients, carcinoma antigen 19-9 levels are measured in patients with gallbladder cancer and cholangiocarcinoma, and serum hormone or urinary metabolite levels are measured in patients with neuroendocrine-tumor liver metastases. A 2-view chest radiograph is obtained to evaluate for pulmonary metastasis, with chest CT reserved for patients with abnormal findings on chest radiographs. Helical 3-phase liver protocol CT has become our standard to accurately measure the number, size, and intrahepatic site of primary and metastatic hepatic tumors. The advantage of this type of CT is the speed of information acquisition (less than 45 seconds). The 3 phases of the scan are an early arterial phase after a bolus intravenous administration of iodinated contrast, a portal venous phase, and a delayed phase. Hypervascular lesions, such as HCC or neuroendocrine metastases, are demonstrated nicely in the arterial phase because of the vascular enhancement of the tumor with minimal hepatic parenchymal enhancement. Less vascular lesions, such as metastatic adenocarcinoma or cholangiocarcinoma, are more distinct during the portal phase of the CT scan, as the contrast enhancement of the normal hepatic parenchyma is greater than that of the tumor tissue. The high resolution of this helical high-speed scan also permits 3-dimensional reconstruction of intrahepatic biliary and vascular structures, volumetric determination of tumor volume and of the volume of liver that would remain after hepatic resection, and assessment of regional lymph node involvement by tumor.

By definition, patients with liver metastases from other organs have stage IV disease, and their assessment focuses on determining suitability of surgical or regionally directed therapies. Patients with liver metastases and extrahepatic malignant disease are treated with suitable systemic or protocol-based therapy. The AJCC staging system is employed for patients with HCC (Table 1–2), gallbladder cancer (Table 1–3), and bile duct cancer (cholangiocarcinoma, Table 1–4). The sequence and timing of surgical, medical, and radiation treatment modalities are based on the stage of disease and the severity of any coexistent chronic hepatic dysfunction.

Table 1–2. Stage Grouping for Hepatocellular Cancer

Stage I	T1	N0	M0
Stage II	T2	N0	M0
Stage IIIA	T3	N0	M0
IIIB	T4	N0	M0
IIIC	Any T	N1	M0
Stage IV	Any T	Any N	M1

Definition of TNM

Primary Tumor (T)

TX   Primary tumor cannot be assessed
T0   No evidence of primary tumor
T1   Solitary tumor without vascular invasion
T2   Solitary tumor with vascular invasion or multiple tumors none more than 5 cm
T3   Multiple tumors more than 5 cm or tumor involving a major branch of the portal or hepatic vein(s)
T4   Tumor(s) with direct invasion of adjacent organs other than the gallbladder or with perforation of visceral peritoneum

Regional Lymph Node(s)

NX   Regional lymph nodes cannot be assessed
N0   No regional lymph node metastasis
N1   Regional lymph node metastasis

Distant Metastasis (M)

MX   Distant metastasis cannot be assessed
M0   No distant metastasis
M1   Distant metastasis

Pancreatic Cancer

Cancer of the pancreas is the fifth leading cause of cancer death in the United States. Almost 30,000 new patients will be diagnosed with pancreatic cancer in 2003, and at least 28,000 of these individuals will die of the disease. Because there are no proven or standardized laboratory or radiologic diagnostic tests for pancreatic carcinoma, most patients present with locally advanced or metastatic disease. The patients with the highest probability of long-term survival are those who present with AJCC early-stage disease (Table 1–5). This translates into cancer localized to the pancreas that can be resected completely, with no regional nodal, peritoneal, or liver metastases. Unfortunately, fewer than 10% of patients diagnosed with pancreatic adenocarcinoma present with surgically treatable disease.

The rapid onset of jaundice is the most frequent complaint of patients with pancreatic-head cancers. Patients with tumors originating in the body or tail of the pancreas may present with abdominal or back pain or with upper GI bleeding from splenic vein thrombosis and resultant gastric

Table 1–3. Stage Grouping for Gallbladder Cancer

Stage 0	Tis	N0	M0
Stage 1A	T1	N0	M0
Stage 1B	T2	N0	M0
Stage IIA	T3	N0	M0
Stage IIB	T1	N1	M0
	T2	N1	M0
	T3	N1	M0
Stage III	T4	Any N	M0
Stage IV	Any T	Any N	M1

Definition of TNM

Primary Tumor (T)

TX   Primary tumor cannot be assessed
T0   No evidence of primary tumor
Tis   Carcinoma *in situ*
T1   Tumor invades lamina propria or muscle layer
T1a   Tumor invades lamina propria
T1b   Tumor invades muscle layer
T2   Tumor invades perimuscular connective tissue; no extension beyond serosa or into liver
T3   Tumor perforates the serosa (visceral peritoneum) and/or directly invades the liver and/or one other adjacent organ or structure, such as the stomach, duodenum, colon, or pancreas, omentum or extrahepatic bile ducts
T4   Tumor invades main portal vein or hepatic artery or invades multiple extrahepatic organs or structures

Regional Lymph Nodes (N)

NX   Regional lymph nodes cannot be assessed
N0   No regional lymph node metastasis
N1   Regional lymph node metastasis

Distant Metastasis (M)

MX   Distant metastasis cannot be assessed
M0   No distant metastasis
M1   Distant metastasis

varices. Patients with locally advanced pancreatic-head tumors may also present with symptoms of gastric outlet obstruction or upper GI bleeding from tumor invasion into the duodenum. Once again, clinical staging at M. D. Anderson begins with a thorough history and physical examination. A routine 2-view chest radiograph and laboratory tests including a CBC, coagulation profile, liver function tests, and serum electrolytes are obtained. A helical, thin-section CT scan is obtained; a multiphase study is performed to obtain arterial contrast phase, venous contrast phase, and delayed-phase images. Pancreatic adenocarcinoma appears as a hypo-dense mass within the pancreas compared with the normally perfused pancreatic parenchyma. The more uncommon pancreatic islet cell tumors

Table 1–4.   Stage Grouping for Extrahepatic Bile Duct Cancer

Stage 0	Tis	N0	M0
Stage 1A	T1	N0	M0
Stage 1B	T2	N0	M0
Stage IIA	T3	N0	M0
Stage IIB	T1	N1	M0
	T2	N1	M0
	T3	N1	M0
Stage IIII	T4	Any N	M0
Stage IV	Any T	Any N	M1
	T4	N0	M0

Definition of TNM

Primary Tumor (T)

TX	Primary tumor cannot be assessed
T0	No evidence of primary tumor
Tis	Carcinoma *in situ*
T1	Tumor confined to the bile duct histologically
T2	Tumor invades beyond the wall of the bile duct
T3	Tumor invades the liver, gallbladder, pancreas, and/or unilateral branches of the portal vein (right or left) or hepatic artery (right or left)
T4	Tumor invades any of the following: main portal vein or its branches bilaterally, common hepatic artery, or other adjacent structures, such as the colon, stomach, duodenum, or abdominal wall

Regional Lymph Nodes (N)

NX	Regional lymph nodes cannot be assessed
N0	No regional lymph node metastasis
N1	Regional lymph node metastasis

Distant Metastasis (M)

MX	Distant metastasis cannot be assessed
M0	No distant metastasis
M1	Distant metastasis

Used with the permission of the American Joint Committee on Cancer (AJCC), Chicago, Illinois. The original source for this material is the AJCC Cancer Staging Manual, Sixth Edition (2002), published by Springer-Verlag New York, www.springer-ny.com.

are hypervascular lesions that appear as enhancing tumors within the pancreas on the initial arterial phase that is obtained immediately after bolus intravenous administration of iodinated contrast. The high-resolution CT scan is critical for evaluating the local extent of tumor with invasion into the superior mesenteric or portal vein, the superior mesenteric artery, the base of the mesentery, or the duodenum and for evaluating evidence of lymph node, peritoneal, or liver metastases.

EUS has become a standard part of our staging evaluation in patients who are considered possible surgical candidates. Pancreatic adenocarcinomas and islet cell tumors can be visualized ultrasonographically in most patients, and the tumor association with the common bile duct, portal

Table 1–5. Stage Grouping for Exocrine Pancreatic Cancer

Stage 0	Tis	N0	M0
Stage 1A	T1	N0	M0
Stage IB	T2	N0	M0
Stage IIA	T3	N0	M0
Stage IIB	T1	N1	M0
	T2	N1	M0
	T3	N1	M0
Stage III	T4	Any N	M0
Stage IV	Any T	Any N	M1

Definition of TNM

Primary Tumor (T)

TX   Primary tumor cannot be assessed
T0   No evidence of primary tumor
Tis   Carcinoma *in situ**
T1   Tumor limited to the pancreas, 2 cm or less in greatest dimension
T2   Tumor limited to the pancreas, more than 2 cm in greatest dimension
T3   Tumor extends beyond the pancreas but without involvement of the celiac axis or the superior mesenteric artery
T4   Tumor involves the celiac axis or the superior mesenteric artery (unresectable primary tumor)

Regional Lymph Nodes (N)

NX   Regional lymph nodes cannot be assessed
N0   No regional lymph node metastasis
N1   Regional lymph node metastasis

Distant Metastasis (M)

MX   Distant metastasis cannot be assessed
M0   No distant metastasis
M1   Distant metastasis

Used with the permission of the American Joint Committee on Cancer (AJCC), Chicago, Illinois. The original source for this material is the AJCC Cancer Staging Manual, Sixth Edition (2002), published by Springer-Verlag New York, www.springer-ny.com.

vein, and superior mesenteric artery can be assessed. As in cases of gastric cancer, suspicious peripancreatic lymph nodes can be visualized with EUS and biopsied under ultrasonographic guidance using the fine-needle aspiration biopsy channel of the endoscope.

In the past at M. D. Anderson, patients who were considered candidates for resection had their disease staged laparoscopically prior to initiation of neoadjuvant chemoradiation therapy. This served to exclude the presence of subclinical carcinomatosis and to stage the liver with laparoscopic ultrasonography. It was also possible to place a feeding jejunostomy tube with laparoscopic guidance to provide nutritional support for patients during chemoradiation therapy. However, current protocols for neoadjuvant chemoradiation therapy for potentially resectable pancreatic adenocarcinoma at M. D. Anderson use a shorter course of 2–3 weeks of treatment, and laparoscopy is reserved for selected patients with suspicious findings on CT scans. The Pancreatic Cancer Treatment Group at M. D. Anderson has demonstrated that state-of-the-art preoperative imaging studies can accurately predict the local extent of disease and identify patients who will be candidates for a margin-negative resection.

Patients with pancreatic islet cell tumors have their disease staged with helical pancreas protocol CT scans and EUS. CT- or EUS-guided biopsy of the pancreatic tumor is critical in distinguishing a neuroendocrine from a pancreatic exocrine tumor. A thorough clinical history is obtained to determine symptoms possibly related to excess hormone secretion, and the physical examination focuses on signs related to endocrine syndromes. A family history to detect familial neuroendocrine tumor syndromes, such as multiple endocrine neoplasia or Von Hippel-Lindau syndrome, is obtained. Serum levels of pancreatic peptides, including glucagon, insulin, gastrin, vasoactive intestinal peptide, and somatostatin, may be obtained as baseline measurements in these patients. A helical 3-phase liver protocol CT scan may also be obtained, as the liver is the most common site of distant organ metastasis.

Colorectal Cancer

Colorectal adenocarcinoma is the second most common cause of cancer death in the United States, and patients with colon and rectal cancer form the largest single group of GI cancer patients seen at M. D. Anderson.

Presenting complaints in patients with colorectal cancer may include rectal bleeding, fatigue related to anemia, change in bowel habits, or the development of abdominal pain. A significant number of patients referred to M. D. Anderson are asymptomatic but have positive findings on a Hemoccult test on stool specimens. Complete colonoscopy is essential during the staging process to document the location of the primary tumor and to exclude the presence of synchronous premalignant polyps or additional malignant lesions. Physical examination consists of an assessment of lymph node basins, particularly the inguinal lymph nodes in patients with rectal tumors; assessment of cardiopulmonary findings; abdominal examination; and digital rectal examination. Patients with rectal tumors may also undergo rigid proctoscopy at the initial evaluation to determine the location and extent of tumor within the rectum, degree of luminal compromise by the tumor, and evidence of tumor invasion or fixation to pelvic structures.

Most patients referred to M. D. Anderson with colorectal cancer have already undergone CT of the abdomen and pelvis or magnetic resonance (MR) imaging after the diagnosis. Patients with colon cancer may not require a preoperative CT scan, although it can be useful in demonstrating a locally advanced (T4) tumor in the ascending, transverse, or sigmoid colon that involves adjacent structures or organs (Table 1–6). Patients with

Table 1–6. Stage Grouping for Colon and Rectal Cancer

Stage	T	N	M	Dukes*
Stage 0	Tis	N0	M0	—
Stage I	T1	N0	M0	A
	T2	N0	M0	A
Stage IIA	T3	N0	M0	B
Stage IIB	T4	N0	M0	B
Stage IIIA	T1–T2	N1	M0	C
Stage IIIB	T3–T4	N1	M0	C
Stage IIIC	Any T	N2	M0	C
Stage IV	Any T	Any N	M1	—

* Dukes B is a composite of better (T3 N0 M0) and worse (T4 N0 M0) prognostic groups, as is Dukes C (Any T N1 M0 and Any T N2 M0).

Definition of TNM

Primary Tumor (T)

TX   Primary tumor cannot be assessed
T0   No evidence of primary tumor
Tis   Carcinoma *in situ*: intraepithelial or invasion of lamina propria*
T1   Tumor invades submucosa
T2   Tumor invades muscularis propria
T3   Tumor invades through the muscularis propria into the subserosa, or into non-peritonealized pericolic or perirectal tissues
T4   Tumor directly invades other organs or structures, and/or perforates visceral peritoneum**, ***

* *Note:* Tis includes cancer cells confined within the glandular basement membrane (intraepithelial) or lamina propria (intramucosal) with no extension through the muscularis mucosae into the submucosa.

** *Note:* Direct invasion in T4 includes invasion of other segments of the colorectum by way of the serosa; for example, invasion of the sigmoid colon by a carcinoma of the cecum.

*** Tumor that is adherent to other organs or structures, macroscopically, is classified T4. However, if no tumor is present in the adhesion, microscopically, the classification should be pT3. The V and L substaging should be used to identify the presence or absence of vascular or lymphatic invasion.

Regional Lymph Nodes (N)

NX   Regional lymph nodes cannot be assessed
N0   No regional lymph node metastasis
N1   Metastasis in 1 to 3 regional lymph nodes
N2   Metastasis in 4 or more regional lymph nodes

Note: A tumor nodule in the pericolorectal adipose tissue of a primary carcinoma without histologic evidence of residual lymph node in the nodule is classified in the pN category as a regional lymph node metastasis if the nodule has the form and smooth contour of a lymph node. If the nodule has an irregular contour, it should be classified in the T category and also coded as V1 (microscopic venous invasion) or as V2 (if it was grossly evident), because there is a strong likelihood that it represents venous invasion.

Distant Metastasis (M)

MX   Distant metastasis cannot be assessed
M0   No distant metastasis
M1   Distant metastasis

Used with the permission of the American Joint Committee on Cancer (AJCC), Chicago, Illinois. The original source for this material is the AJCC Cancer Staging Manual, Sixth Edition (2002), published by Springer-Verlag New York, www.springer-ny.com.

KEY PRACTICE POINTS

- Esophagogastroduodenoscopy is considered the standard of care in the evaluation of patients with new or worsening symptoms of epigastric pain, gastroesophageal reflux, early satiety, or unremitting nausea and vomiting.

- In patients with gastric cancer, EUS is extremely useful in determining the T classification of the tumor and may be helpful in assessing the presence of regional lymph node metastases.

- Subclinical peritoneal spread of gastric adenocarcinoma may not be diagnosed by high-quality CT or EUS. Because of this limitation, surgeons at M. D. Anderson routinely employ staging laparoscopic evaluation in patients with potentially resectable gastric carcinoma.

- In patients with liver metastases from other organ sites, assessment of the primary tumor site—such as colonoscopy for colorectal cancer—is critical to exclude local recurrence prior to any liver-directed therapy.

- In patients with pancreatic cancer, high-resolution CT is critical for evaluating the local extent of tumor with invasion into the superior mesenteric or portal vein, the superior mesenteric artery, the base of the mesentery, or the duodenum and for evaluating evidence of lymph node, peritoneal, or liver metastases.

- In patients with colorectal cancer, complete colonoscopy is essential during the staging process to document the location of the primary tumor and to exclude the presence of synchronous premalignant polyps or additional malignant lesions.

- Evaluation of the local extent of disease is particularly important in rectal cancer patients as local disease extent is one of the factors that determines whether sphincter-preserving surgery may be possible.

locally advanced colon cancer at these sites can still be treated with curative surgical intent if an en bloc resection of the primary tumor and involved organs can be performed. Patients with rectal cancer routinely undergo CT of the abdomen and pelvis to assess local extent of tumor and to check for extension of tumor into adjacent pelvic structures. The abdominal CT scan in colorectal cancer patients can also help detect liver and regional lymph node metastases and occasionally provides evidence of peritoneal spread of disease. A 2-view chest radiograph is standard, with a CT of the chest limited to those patients with abnormal findings on the standard chest x-ray. Patients undergo routine laboratory evaluation with a CBC, liver function tests, serum electrolytes, and serum carcinoembryonic antigen measurement; a urinalysis is added in patients with rectosigmoid tumors.

EUS is a standard component of staging in rectal cancer patients treated at M. D. Anderson. With EUS, the ultrasonographic T classification of the tumor and extent of local invasion into the perirectal fat or adjacent structures can be assessed. Enlarged or suspicious-appearing lymph nodes (N classification) can be identified in the mesorectum and biopsied through the biopsy channel of the EUS scope. The evaluation of local extent of disease (T and N classifications) is particularly important in rectal cancer patients. A significant proportion of rectal cancer patients evaluated at M. D. Anderson undergo preoperative chemoradiation therapy. Thus, presenting T classification and tumor location within the rectum are crucial factors in decisions regarding the appropriate definitive surgical procedure, including sphincter-preserving operations, in patients who may achieve marked local tumor downsizing following pelvic chemoradiation therapy.

Patients referred to M. D. Anderson for evaluation and treatment of a pelvic recurrence of rectal adenocarcinoma undergo MR imaging of the pelvis in addition to CT and laboratory assessment to exclude distant metastatic disease. MR imaging permits detailed axial, sagittal, and coronal views of pelvic organs in relation to recurrent tumor and more accurately delineates postsurgical and postirradiation scarring from local tumor recurrence. Emphasis is placed on MR-imaging-based evidence of contiguous organ, sciatic nerve, blood vessel, and sacral involvement in order to assess resectability and to inform the patient of the nature of a potential resection.

2 RECENT ADVANCES IN HISTOPATHOLOGY OF GASTROINTESTINAL CANCERS: PROGNOSTIC AND THERAPEUTIC ASSESSMENT OF COLORECTAL CANCERS

Asif Rashid

CHAPTER OVERVIEW

The genetics and molecular biology, precursor lesions and predisposing conditions, and hereditary syndromes of gastrointestinal cancers, especially colorectal cancers, are well characterized. Fifteen to twenty percent of sporadic colorectal carcinomas have microsatellite instability (MSI; replication-error phenotype), characterized by defective DNA repair resulting in alterations of short tandem repeat sequences, including mononucleotide, dinucleotide, and tetranucleotide repeats. This is due to alteration of mismatch repair enzymes. Patients with colorectal cancers with MSI have a better prognosis than do those without. In contrast, about 50% to 60% of colorectal cancers have loss of the long arm (q) of chromosome 18, the chromosomal location of the *deleted in colorectal cancer*, *SMAD4*, and *SMAD2* genes. Chromosome 18q loss has been associated with poor outcome in patients with colorectal cancer. Growth factors and growth factor receptors play a major role in the development and progression of cancer. Gastrointestinal cancers express epidermal growth factor receptor (EGFR) and related receptors that activate intrinsic tyrosine kinase activity and result in signals of cell proliferation. This activity can be modulated by a variety of therapeutic options, including monoclonal antibody against EGFR or related receptors and selective inhibition of tyrosine kinase activity. Immunohistochemical analysis for EGFR can select patients who have EGFR-overexpressing gastrointestinal cancer and thus are potential candidates for anti-EGFR therapy.

INTRODUCTION

Among the most important recent advances in the field of gastrointestinal cancer are elucidation of the genetics of these cancers and characterization of the molecular pathways utilized by these neoplasms. This work has revolutionized many aspects of patient care, including prevention, screening, and treatment. The goal now is to identify new therapeutic targets that can be utilized for therapy and for increasing our understanding of prognosis. In cases of gastrointestinal cancer, histopathologic analysis typically provides diagnosis of predisposing conditions, information necessary for the surveillance of such conditions, and diagnosis of the type, grade, and stage of cancer. The evaluation of molecular predictors of prognosis and therapeutic response is a recent development in histopathology.

HISTOPATHOLOGIC FEATURES OF GASTROINTESTINAL CANCERS

Malignancies of the gastrointestinal tract can be classified histopathologically as epithelial tumors, endocrine or mesenchymal tumors, or lymphomas (Table 2–1; Hamilton and Aaltonen, 2001). Epithelial tumors can be subclassified as adenocarcinoma, squamous cell carcinoma, adenosquamous carcinoma, small cell carcinoma, carcinoid tumor, or other.

Table 2–1. Histopathologic Classification of Primary Malignant Neoplasms of the Esophagus, Stomach, and Colon and Rectum

Histopathologic Classification	Histopathologic Subtype by Anatomic Location			
	Esophagus	Stomach	Small Intestine	Colon and Rectum
Epithelial	Squamous cell carcinoma	Adenocarcinoma	Adenocarcinoma	Adenocarcinoma
	Verrucous (squamous) carcinoma	Intestinal type	Mucinous adenocarcinoma	Mucinous adenocarcinoma
	Basaloid squamous carcinoma	Diffuse type	Signet-ring-cell adenocarcinoma	Signet-ring-cell adenocarcinoma
	Spindle cell (squamous) carcinoma	Papillary adenocarcinoma	Adenosquamous carcinoma	Adenosquamous carcinoma
	Adenocarcinoma	Tubular adenocarcinoma	Squamous cell carcinoma	Squamous cell carcinoma
	Adenosquamous carcinoma	Mucinous adenocarcinoma	Small cell carcinoma	Small cell carcinoma
	Mucoepidermoid carcinoma	Signet-ring-cell adenocarcinoma	Medullary carcinoma	Medullary carcinoma
	Adenoid cystic carcinoma	Adenosquamous carcinoma	Undifferentiated carcinoma	Undifferentiated carcinoma
	Small cell carcinoma	Squamous cell carcinoma	Other	Other
	Undifferentiated carcinoma	Small cell carcinoma		
	Other	Undifferentiated carcinoma		
		Other		
Endocrine	Carcinoid tumor (well-differentiated endocrine neoplasm)	Carcinoid tumor (well-differentiated endocrine neoplasm)	Carcinoid tumor (well-differentiated endocrine neoplasm)	Carcinoid tumor (well-differentiated endocrine neoplasm)
		Mixed carcinoid-adenocarcinoma	Mixed carcinoid-adenocarcinoma	Mixed carcinoid-adenocarcinoma

Nonepithelial Mesenchymal	Gastrointestinal stromal tumor Leiomyosarcoma Rhabdomyosarcoma Kaposi's sarcoma Malignant melanoma Other	Gastrointestinal stromal tumor Leiomyosarcoma Kaposi's sarcoma Other	Gastrointestinal stromal tumor Leiomyosarcoma Angiosarcoma Kaposi's sarcoma Other	Gastrointestinal stromal tumor Leiomyosarcoma Angiosarcoma Kaposi's sarcoma Other
Malignant Lymphomas	Marginal zone B-cell lymphoma of MALT type Mantle cell lymphoma Diffuse large B-cell lymphoma	Immunoproliferative small intestinal disease (includes α-heavy-chain disease) Marginal zone B-cell lymphoma of MALT type Mantle cell lymphoma Diffuse large B-cell lymphoma Burkitt's lymphoma Burkitt's-like/atypical Burkitt's lymphoma Enteropathy-associated T-cell lymphoma Other	Marginal zone B-cell lymphoma of MALT type Mantle cell lymphoma Diffuse large B-cell lymphoma Burkitt's lymphoma Burkitt's-like/atypical Burkitt's lymphoma Other	Marginal zone B-cell lymphoma of MALT type Mantle cell lymphoma Diffuse large B-cell lymphoma Burkitt's lymphoma Burkitt's-like/atypical Burkitt's lymphoma Other

Adenocarcinoma can be further subclassified as adenocarcinoma, not otherwise specified, or intestinal, signet-ring-cell, or mucinous (colloid) adenocarcinoma.

Tumor stage at the time of diagnosis is the most important factor in determining prognosis. Current TNM staging systems for gastrointestinal cancer are shown in chapter 1 (Tables 1–1 through 1–6) and chapter 15 (Tables 15–1 and 15–2). The 5-year survival rates for patients with gastrointestinal cancer differ by anatomic site and histologic subtype of cancer.

Metastatic Carcinoma of Unknown Primary Origin

In most patients, the site of origin of a metastatic carcinoma of unknown primary origin cannot be reliably determined by light microscopy (Hammar, 1998). Almost 60% of metastatic carcinomas of unknown primary origin are adenocarcinomas. Some metastatic adenocarcinomas (e.g., colonic adenocarcinomas) have distinctive histologic features that allow for determination of their site of origin. For most other metastatic adenocarcinomas of unknown primary origin, immunohistochemical analysis can help to identify the primary site. Immunophenotyping for cytokeratin 7, cytokeratin 20 (Chu et al, 2000), and other antigens used in conjunction with histologic analysis is effective in narrowing the potential primary site of origin of adenocarcinomas (Table 2–2), although these and other antigens are not absolutely site specific and cannot be reliably used to determine the site of origin. Other antigens that help determine the site of origin are thyroglobulin for thyroid, prostate-specific antigen and prostatic alkaline phosphatase for prostate, estrogen receptor for breast, and thyroid transcription factor 1 for lung and thyroid. Thyroglobulin, prostate-specific antigen, and prostatic alkaline phosphatase are site specific. Ultrastructural details of neoplastic cells can be studied by electron microscopy and may help determine the tumor type and site of origin of poorly differentiated cancers.

Genetic Alterations of Colorectal Cancer

The molecular genetic alterations in colorectal carcinoma are among the best understood in human cancer and involve abnormalities in multiple dominant-acting oncogenes and tumor-suppressor genes (Kinzler and Vogelstein, 1996; Fearon and Dang, 1999). Various pathways of colorectal carcinogenesis are evident in sporadic, familial, and inflammatory bowel disease–associated neoplasms. The somatic alterations in sporadic colo-

Table 2–2. Immunophenotype of Various Adenocarcinomas

Immunophenotype		
Cytokeratin 7	*Cytokeratin 20*	*Tumors by Site and Type*
Positive	Positive	93% of ovarian mucinous carcinomas
		62% of pancreatic adenocarcinomas
		43% of cholangiocarcinomas
		25% of bladder transitional cell carcinomas
		13% of gastric adenocarcinomas
Positive	Negative	100% of salivary gland carcinomas
		98% of thyroid carcinomas
		96% of breast carcinomas
		96% of ovarian endometrioid, serous, and clear cell carcinomas
		80% of endometrial endometrioid carcinomas
		72% of lung carcinomas
		65% of malignant mesotheliomas
Negative	Positive	95% of colorectal carcinomas
		78% of Merkel cell tumors of skin
		37% of gastric carcinomas
Negative	Negative	100% of prostatic carcinomas
		89% of renal cell carcinomas
		81% of hepatocellular carcinomas
		79% of pulmonary and gastrointestinal carcinoid tumors

rectal carcinoma include truncating mutations or deletions of the *adenomatous polyposis coli* (*APC*) gene on chromosome 5q and mutations of the *β-catenin* gene. Point mutations of the K-*ras* proto-oncogene, loss of the *deleted in colorectal cancer* gene and nearby *SMAD2* and *SMAD4* genes on chromosome 18q, and mutations and deletions of the *p53* gene on chromosome 17p are also common. Familial adenomatous polyposis is an autosomal-dominant inherited syndrome characterized morphologically by more than 100 colorectal adenomas and is due to a germline mutation in the *APC* gene. The tumors have somatic alterations similar to those of sporadic cancers.

In a second pathway to colorectal neoplasia, microsatellite instability (MSI; also termed DNA replication errors and ubiquitous somatic mutations) is caused by the alteration of a nucleotide mismatch repair gene, including *hMSH2*, *hMLH1*, *PMS1*, *PMS2*, or *GTBP*. MSI is characterized by additions and deletions of nucleotides in numerous repeated nucleotide sequences (microsatellites). Germline mutation of a mismatch repair gene causes hereditary nonpolyposis colorectal cancer (HNPCC), an autosomal-dominant syndrome characterized by early-onset, right-sided, familial colorectal cancer. Affected individuals have a tendency to develop synchronous and metachronous lesions and have an increased incidence of endometrial, ovarian, gastric, small bowel, and renal pelvic cancer. Silencing of the *hMLH1* gene by methylation is common in sporadic MSI-positive cancers. Alterations of mononucleotide tracts that are present in *transforming growth factor β type II receptor* and *BAX* are commonly found in MSI-positive carcinomas. MSI-positive colorectal carcinomas are more commonly right-sided with diploid total DNA content and are associated with slightly better patient survival than are MSI-negative cancers. Sporadic gastric and endometrial cancers also commonly are MSI positive.

Recently, a distinct pathway of colorectal carcinogenesis, termed CpG island methylator phenotype (CIMP), was described (Toyota et al, 2000). CIMP-positive colorectal cancers are characterized by a high degree of concordant CpG island methylation of multiple genes and loci in the tumor that are not methylated in normal colorectal mucosa (Baylin et al, 1998). CpG islands are 0.5- to 2.0-kilobase regions rich in the cytosine-guanine dinucleotides and are present in the 5′ region of about half of all human genes. The methylation of cytosines within CpG islands is associated with loss of gene expression by repression of transcription and is observed not only in physiologic conditions such as X chromosome inactivation and aging but also in neoplasia. Examples of this process in colorectal cancer include inactivation of the *p16* cell-cycle regulator, the *THBS1* angiogenesis inhibitor, the *TIMP3* metastasis suppressor, the O^6-*methylguanine DNA methyltransferase* DNA repair gene, and the *hMLH1* nucleotide mismatch repair gene. Most sporadic MSI-high colorectal cancers (tumors in which 2 or more defined markers show instability) are due to methylation of the *hMLH1* mismatch repair gene.

HISTOPATHOLOGIC FEATURES OF COLORECTAL CANCERS WITH MSI

MSI-high colorectal cancers have a distinct clinicopathologic phenotype (Kim et al, 1994; Jass et al, 1998; Alexander et al, 2001). MSI-high colorectal cancers are more frequent in younger patients. Most are right-sided (proximal to the splenic flexure), bulky (large) tumors, with an exophytic growth pattern; are poorly differentiated, with signet-ring-cell, mucinous, medullary, or variegated (mixed) histologic subtypes; have an intense lymphocytic response with Crohn's-like lymphoid reaction (lymphoid follicles with germinal centers at the tumor edge) and peritumoral and intratumoral lymphocytosis; and show an expanding (pushing) invasive pattern at the margins. However, one third of colorectal carcinomas with MSI do not have these histologic characteristics.

Prognostic Significance of Chromosome 18q Loss and MSI

Chromosome 18q loss (Jen et al, 1994) and MSI (Gryfe et al, 2000) are prognostic factors for sporadic colorectal cancer. In a study of 319 patients with stage III colon cancer, chromosome 18q loss was associated with a worse prognosis after chemotherapy (Watanabe et al, 2001). Patients with tumors that retained chromosome 18q had a 5-year overall survival rate of 69%, compared with 50% for patients with loss of heterozygosity at chromosome 18q. Similarly, patients with sporadic MSI-positive colorectal cancers had a better prognosis. In a population-based study of 587 patients 50 years of age or younger, MSI-high cancers were associated with better survival and decreased likelihood of metastasis to regional lymph nodes or distant organs (Gryfe et al, 2000). The 5-year survival rate was 76% for patients with MSI-high colorectal cancers but 64% for those with microsatellite-stable cancers. The MSI-high phenotype is less frequent in metastatic colorectal cancers. MSI is also a prognostic factor for gastric cancers: MSI-high gastric cancers are associated with a better survival than are microsatellite-stable gastric cancers.

Chromosome 18q Loss and MSI Assay in Surgical Pathology Practice

Chromosome 18q loss and MSI can be assessed by using archival blocks of surgically resected tumors that have been fixed in formalin and embedded in paraffin. At M. D. Anderson Cancer Center, these assays are performed by the Diagnostic Molecular Laboratory. The tumor and normal tissue are microdissected, and DNA is extracted by proteinase K digestion. Genomic DNA is used to amplify sequences by polymerase chain reaction (PCR) using 5 markers (oligonucleotides that can amplify microsatellite repeats) present on chromosome 18q for chromosome 18q loss analysis, and 5 markers recommended by the National Cancer Institute workshop for MSI assay (Boland et al, 1998). The markers for MSI assay include 2 mononucleotide markers, BAT-25 and BAT-26, and 3 dinucleotide markers, D2S123, D5S346, and D17S250. The PCR products are electrophoresed on an automated sequencer. Chromosome 18q loss is assessed by allelic loss of a polymorphic (with 2 alleles) marker indicating loss of 1 copy of chromosome 18q. The presence of an additional band in the PCR product from tumor DNA, not observed in DNA from normal tissue from the same patient, is scored as an allelic shift (instability) at that locus. In accordance with the National Cancer Institute consensus on MSI, any pair of samples of normal DNA and tumor DNA that displays instability at 2 or more of 5 loci is scored as MSI high; any pair that displays instability at 1 locus is scored as MSI low; and any pair that displays no instability at 5 loci is scored as microsatellite stable.

IMMUNOHISTOCHEMISTRY FOR MISMATCH REPAIR GENES

Mismatch repair genes are tumor-suppressor genes, and loss or inactivation of both alleles is required in tumors. Detection of loss of expression of *hMLH1*, *hMSH2*, or *hMSH6* by immunohistochemical analysis (Figure 2–1) can help to identify MSI-high cancers. Most sporadic MSI-high cancers have loss of expression of *hMLH1* due to hypermethylation of the gene (Thibodeau et al, 1998). The detection of the loss of a mismatch repair gene, in conjunction with the age and family history of the patient, can help determine appropriate management. Patients who are young at the onset of colorectal cancer or who have a family history of colorectal cancer may be tested for a germline mutation and undergo genetic counseling. On the other hand, colorectal cancer in patients who are older at the onset of disease, have no family history of colorectal cancer, and demonstrate loss of *hMLH1* by immunohistochemical analysis is probably due to hypermethylation of the *hMLH1* promoter site, and testing for a germline mutation is not indicated.

INDICATIONS FOR MSI ASSAY

The indications for an MSI assay are listed in chapter 10 (Table 10–1). The primary reason to perform an MSI assay is to rule out HNPCC. HNPCC kindreds may develop multiple cancers of the colorectum or other sites, and the operation of choice in affected individuals is pancolectomy. Surveillance for cancers of other sites should be considered. Family members of patients with HNPCC are at risk, and genetic counseling for these individuals is recommended. The second reason to perform an MSI assay is that the MSI phenotype in colorectal cancer has prognostic significance.

The International Collaborative Group on HNPCC has established minimal criteria for identifying patients with HNPCC. These criteria are known as the Amsterdam criteria and are as follows: (1) at least 3 relatives with histologically verified colorectal cancer, 1 of them a first-degree relative of the other 2; (2) at least 2 successive generations affected; and (3) in 1 of the individuals, colorectal cancer should have been diagnosed before the age of 50 years.

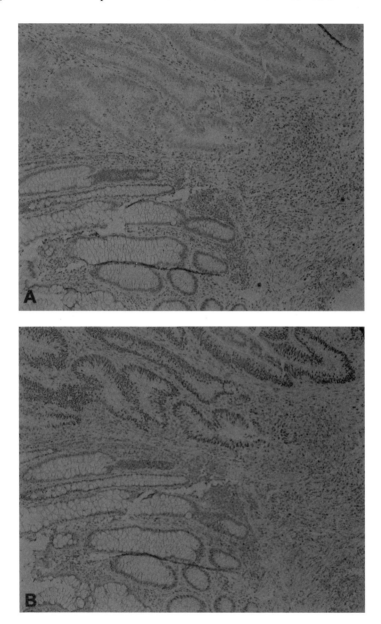

Figure 2–1. Immunohistochemical analysis for hMLH1 (*A*) and hMSH2 (*B*). There is nuclear staining of the epithelium of normal mucosa (lower half of both panels) and lymphocytes and stromal cells. Colon carcinoma (upper half of both panels) has loss of expression of hMLH1, but hMSH2 is expressed. Loss of a mismatch repair gene is invariably associated with microsatellite instability in tumors.

Therapeutic Importance of Overexpression of Epidermal Growth Factor Receptor and Related Receptors

The epidermal growth factor and related polypeptides, including transforming growth factor α, amphiregulin, heparin-binding epidermal growth factor–like growth factor, betacellulin, and epiregulin, are synthesized as propeptides containing a cytoplasmic domain, a transmembrane domain, and an extracellular domain. Metalloproteases proteolytically release mature peptides from the extracellular domain. These peptides bind epidermal growth factor receptor (EGFR) and related receptors. There are 4 members of the human EGFR family: human epidermal growth factor receptor 1 (HER1, also known as ErbB1), ErbB2 (HER2 or neu), ErbB3 (HER3), and ErbB4 (HER4). These proteins are membrane-associated receptor tyrosine kinases with an extracellular ligand-binding domain, a transmembrane domain, and an intracellular domain that has intrinsic tyrosine kinase activity. The tyrosine kinase activity is activated by ligand-induced receptor homodimerization and heterodimerization. No ligand has been shown to bind directly to ErbB2. Instead, ErbB2 functions as a coreceptor, forms heterodimers with other members of the EGFR family, and increases the affinity of ligands for the receptor complex. Activated homodimeric or heterodimeric receptors recruit proteins with *Src* homology 2 domains. Ras and phospholipase C-γ signaling pathways are activated by the activation of the EGFR. The end result of signaling by these pathways is stimulation of cellular proliferation, enhancement of cell survival, modulation of cell migration, and adhesion.

ErbB1, ErbB2, and ErbB3 are overexpressed in gastrointestinal malignancies, including colorectal, esophageal, gastric, pancreatic, and hepatocellular cancers. Overexpression or amplification of these receptors in gastrointestinal cancers correlates with a poor prognosis and aggressive disease.

Blockage of epidermal growth factor signaling may reduce the growth of malignant cells. A variety of agents—including transforming growth factor-α and EGFR-neutralizing antibodies, epidermal growth factor–related peptide antisense constructs, ADAM metalloprotease inhibitors, and epidermal growth factor tyrosine kinase inhibitors—have been utilized to block the epidermal growth factor pathway (Barnard, 2001). Human clinical trials using anti-ErbB2 monoclonal antibody (trastuzumab, Herceptin; Genentech, Inc., South San Francisco, CA), anti-human EGFR antibody (ICM-C225), and EGFR tyrosine kinase inhibitor (OSI-774) have been reported.

Immunohistochemistry for EGFR
and Related Receptors

Overexpression of EGFR and related receptors can be assessed by immunohistochemical analysis using formalin-fixed, paraffin-embedded tissue (Figure 2–2). At M. D. Anderson, EGFR expression is assayed using mouse monoclonal antibody 31G7 (Zymed Laboratories, San Francisco, CA), and ErbB2 expression is assayed using AD8 monoclonal antibody (NeoMarkers, Lab Vision Corporation, Fremont, CA). The intensity of EGFR reactivity is scored as follows: 0, no reactivity or cytoplasmic staining of neoplastic cells; 1+, weak or faint, discontinuous, membranous staining of neoplastic cells; 2+, intermediate, incomplete, membranous staining of neoplastic cells; and 3+, intense, continuous membranous staining (Goldstein and Armin, 2001). The percentage of immunoreactive cells also is reported. In a study of EGFR immunohistochemical reactivity in colon cancer, 31.4% of neoplastic cells had 3+ reactivity in more than 10% to 50% of the neoplastic cells, and 3.9% of neoplastic cells had 3+ reactivity in more than 50% of the neoplastic cells (Goldstein and Armin, 2001). Overexpression of ErbB2 is due to amplification of the *ErbB2* gene. This can be corroborated by fluorescence in situ hybridization analysis.

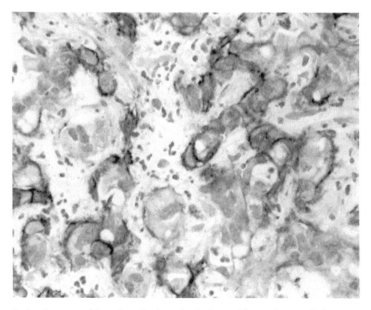

Figure 2–2.   Immunohistochemical analysis for epidermal growth factor receptor. Metastatic colon cancer has an intense, continuous, membranous staining (3+) for epidermal growth factor receptor.

KEY PRACTICE POINTS

- Chromosome 18q loss and MSI are prognostic factors for patients with colorectal cancer.

- MSI assay and immunohistochemical analysis for mismatch repair genes, in conjunction with the age and family history of the patient, can help to differentiate sporadic from HNPCC-associated colorectal carcinomas.

- Overexpression of EGFR can be assessed by immunohistochemical analysis and can help select patients who will benefit from therapy against EGFR.

SUGGESTED READINGS

Alexander J, Watanabe T, Wu T-T, Rashid A, Li S, Hamilton SR. Histopathological identification of colon cancer with DNA replication errors (RER). *Am J Pathol* 2001;158:527–542.

Barnard J. Epidermal growth factor receptor blockage: an emerging therapeutic modality in gastroenterology. *Gastroenterology* 2001;120:1872–1874.

Baylin SB, Herman JG, Graff JR, Vertino PM, Issa JPJ. Alterations in DNA methylation: a fundamental aspect of neoplasia. *Adv Cancer Res* 1998;72:141–196.

Boland CR, Thibodeau SN, Hamilton SR, et al. A National Cancer Institute workshop on microsatellite instability for cancer detection and familial predisposition: development of international criteria for the determination of microsatellite instability in colorectal cancer. *Cancer Res* 1998;58:5248–5257.

Chu P, Wu E, Weiss LM. Cytokeratin 7 and cytokeratin 20 expression in epithelial neoplasms: a survey of 435 cases. *Mod Pathol* 2000;13:962–972.

Fearon ER, Dang CV. Cancer genetics: tumor suppressor meets oncogene. *Curr Biol* 1999;9:R62–R65.

Goldstein NS, Armin M. Epidermal growth factor immunohistochemical reactivity in patients with American Joint Committee on Cancer stage IV colon adenocarcinoma: implications for a standardized scoring system. *Cancer* 2001;92:1331–1346.

Gryfe R, Kim H, Hsieh ETK, et al. Tumor microsatellite instability and clinical outcome in young patients with colorectal cancer. *N Engl J Med* 2000;342:66–77.

Hamilton SR, Aaltonen LA, eds. *World Health Organization Classification of Tumors: Pathology and Genetics of Tumors of the Digestive System.* Lyon, France: IARC Press; 2001.

Hammar SP. Metastatic adenocarcinoma of unknown origin. *Hum Pathol* 1998; 29:1393–1402.

Jass JR, Do K-A, Simms LA, et al. Morphology of sporadic colorectal cancer with DNA replication error. *Gut* 1998;42:673–679.

Jen J, Kim H, Piantadosi S, et al. Allelic loss of chromosome 18q and prognosis in colorectal cancer. *N Engl J Med* 1994;331:213–221.

Kim H, Jen J, Vogelstein B, Hamilton SR. Clinical and pathological characteristics of sporadic colorectal carcinomas with DNA replication errors in microsatellite sequences. *Am J Pathol* 1994;45:148–156.

Kinzler KW, Vogelstein B. Lessons from hereditary colorectal cancer. *Cell* 1996;87:159–170.

Thibodeau S, French AJ, Cunningham JM, et al. Microsatellite instability in colorectal cancer: different mutator phenotypes and the principal involvement of hMLH1. *Cancer Res* 1998;58:1713–1718.

Toyota M, Ohe-Toyota M, Ahuja N, Issa J-PJ. Distinct genetic profiles in colorectal tumors with or without the CpG island methylator phenotype. *Proc Natl Acad Sci U S A* 2000;97:710–715.

Watanabe T, Wu T-T, Catalano PJ, et al. Molecular predictors of survival after adjuvant chemotherapy for colon cancer. *N Engl J Med* 2001;344:1196–1206.

3 CURRENT STATUS OF IMAGING TECHNIQUES IN GASTROINTESTINAL CANCERS

Chusilp Charnsangavej

CHAPTER OVERVIEW

Diagnostic imaging studies provide important information in the diagnostic and staging evaluation of patients with gastrointestinal malignancies. Advances in imaging techniques, contrast development, and image-processing techniques continue to improve our ability to display images, make a correct diagnosis, and accurately stage disease. To maximize the potential of advanced imaging techniques, imaging protocols must be designed properly. Proper interpretation is also critical to maximizing the clinical benefit of imaging studies.

INTRODUCTION

Advances in imaging technology since the early 1970s have improved the ability of diagnostic radiologists to detect, diagnose, and stage malignant tumors of the abdominal organs. During the past few years, new developments in hardware, software, and image-processing techniques have further advanced our ability to image the liver, bile duct, pancreas, and gastrointestinal (GI) tract and to display images in the planes that are familiar to clinicians. Better spatial resolution and rapid data acquisition provided by new imaging technology have improved our understanding of tumor morphology and physiology and provided detailed anatomic information about how tumors spread. Ultrasonography (US), computed tomography (CT), and magnetic resonance imaging (MRI) have emerged as important and necessary modalities in diagnosing disease in the GI tract and in treatment-planning algorithms for tumors of the GI tract. In addition, the recent approval of positron emission tomography (PET) for evaluation of various GI cancers has made this imaging technique another powerful tool for the management of GI cancers. The purpose of this chapter is to describe how we use current imaging techniques for the diagnosis and staging of malignant disease in the GI tract at M. D. Anderson Cancer Center.

ULTRASONOGRAPHY

US is universally the most widely available imaging modality for screening of liver masses or obstructive jaundice. It is noninvasive, quick, portable, and relatively inexpensive, and it uses no ionizing radiation. The most significant advances in abdominal US are harmonic imaging and the use of intravenous contrast agents to characterize and detect lesions in the liver (Leifer et al, 2000). Analysis of image quality has shown that sonograms obtained with the harmonic imaging technique are significantly better than those obtained with the conventional B-mode technique, and most investigators have recommended routine use of harmonic imaging for abdominal US studies, especially in adult patients. In experienced hands, US can accurately distinguish a benign or insignificant lesion, such as a cyst or cavernous hemangioma, from a malignant lesion, such as a hepatic metastasis or a hepatocellular carcinoma (Wilson et al, 2000). Harmonic imaging has significantly enhanced the uses of sonographic contrast agents in hepatic imaging, and the combination has improved lesion detection and lesion characterization (Yasuda et al, 1995; Tanaka et al, 2001).

Another significant technical development in US is the application of endoscopic US in the evaluation of GI malignancies. Endoscopic US has become a primary imaging modality for determining the depth of bowel-wall invasion by many GI malignancies, such as those of the esophagus, stomach, and rectum. The combination of fine-needle aspiration and endoscopic US is currently used to diagnose pancreatic masses, define regional nodal metastasis of these malignancies, and define local vascular involvement from pancreatic masses (Chang et al, 1994; Gress et al, 1999).

The disadvantages of US are the limited field of view, the relative insensitivity and nonspecificity compared with CT and MRI, and the limited utility of the technique in patients with a large body habitus. These limitations make US not practical for the initial staging of malignancies of the GI tract. Moreover, US is also very operator dependent and may be difficult to reproduce when follow-up is required.

COMPUTED TOMOGRAPHY

The effect of helical CT and the recently developed multidetector helical CT on abdominal and pelvic imaging has been substantial. The advantage of helical CT over conventional CT is the speed at which imaging can be acquired. The organs in the upper abdomen, including the liver, spleen, and pancreas, can be imaged within a single breath-hold, and therefore, respiratory misregistration and motion artifacts can be minimized. The speed at which images are acquired also allows multiphasic imaging of the liver, spleen, and pancreas after intravenous contrast administration, and this imaging technique often improves lesion detection and characterization and provides information about vascular anatomy and the extent of tumor involvement of adjacent vessels for planning treatment (Foley et al, 2000; Ji et al, 2001).

An important advantage of helical CT is the ability to reconstruct the image data acquired on the initial scan at intervals as small as 1 mm. Such reconstruction can improve lesion conspicuity by placing the lesion directly within the image plane rather than volume-averaging it between 2 contiguous reconstructed images. Smaller lesions can therefore be detected with helical CT. In addition, the reconstructed images can be stacked to form a volume of image data so that they can be displayed in multiple planes or in a 3-dimensional format. This image processing technique forms the basis for CT colonography, CT angiography, and CT cholangiography.

MAGNETIC RESONANCE IMAGING

The advantages of MRI include the lack of ionizing radiation and the ability to scan without an iodinated contrast agent. Inherent tissue contrast on T1- and T2-weighted images and the use of proper imaging pulse sequences often allow lesion detection and characterization without the use of contrast agent. However, gadolinium chelates and new tissue-specific contrast agents further improve lesion detection and characterization (Semelka and Helmberger, 2001). The major limitations of abdominal MRI have been motion artifacts, particularly those related to respiration, the heart, and the aorta, and limited temporal and spatial resolution. Recent developments in MRI hardware and software have solved or minimized these problems. The current state-of-the-art scanner can perform fast imaging pulse sequences with high spatial and temporal resolution, and the technique has become widely available in clinical practice (Keogan and Edelman, 2001).

Multiphasic, contrast-enhanced T1-weighted 3-dimensional or 2-dimensional spoiled gradient-echo sequences are now routinely performed to characterize lesions in the liver and pancreas. The 3-dimensional image data acquired during the arterial phase can display angiographic images for planning treatment. Furthermore, a specialized pulse sequence with heavily T2-weighted images can provide additional data to evaluate the bile duct and pancreatic duct.

POSITRON EMISSION TOMOGRAPHY

The basic principle of PET imaging is the detection of coincidence photons at 511 keV that are generated as a result of the positron-electron annihilation after positron emission (Ak et al, 2000; Delbeke and Martin, 2001; Mankoff and Bellon, 2001). Currently, clinical PET has very high sensitivity in the detection of these coincidence photons. PET can detect radiopharmaceuticals in the femtomolar to picomolar range, compared with the millimolar range of contrast materials used in CT or MRI. This sensitivity makes it possible to detect metabolic activity at the cellular and molecular level and overcomes the relatively low spatial resolution of 5 to 10 mm in clinical practice. Although several isotopes, such as ^{11}C and ^{15}O, have been used in clinical PET imaging, ^{18}F is the most commonly used positron-emitting isotope because it has a half-life of 110 minutes, which makes it commercially accessible. ^{18}F fluoro-2-deoxy-D-glucose (FDG) is the most commonly used radiopharmaceutical for PET imaging in clinical oncology.

The increased uptake of ^{18}F-FDG in tumor cells is based on the upregulation of glucose transporter and hexokinase activity of the tumor. ^{18}F-FDG is transported into tumor cells and phosphorylated into ^{18}F-FDG-6-P by hexokinase. However, ^{18}F-FDG-6-P cannot be rapidly cleared from cells because of its low membrane permeability. Accumulation of ^{18}F-FDG-6-P in tumor cells is therefore the basis for ^{18}F-FDG PET imaging in clinical oncology (Reske and Kotzerke, 2001). In GI malignancies, ^{18}F-FDG PET imaging is currently approved for diagnosis, staging, and restaging of colorectal and esophageal cancers (Figures 3–1 and 3–2).

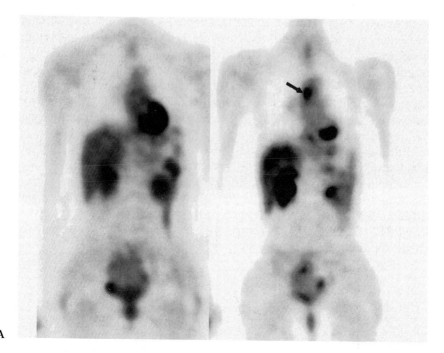

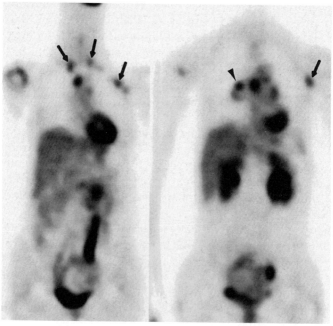

Figure 3–1. (*A*) Whole body ^{18}F-FDG PET images of a patient with metastatic carcinoma of the esophagogastric junction show an area of increased uptake at the right paratracheal region (arrow). (*B*) Follow-up PET images obtained 3 months later show progression of the disease with increased FDG uptake at multiple supraclavicular lymph nodes, axillary lymph nodes (arrows), and hilar lymph nodes (arrowhead). Also note hydronephrosis of the left ureter due to pelvic metastasis.

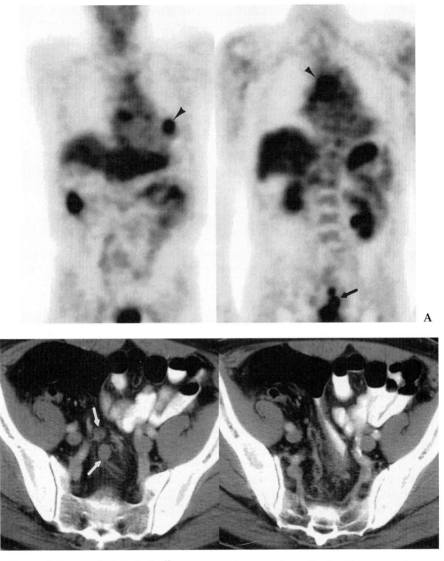

Figure 3–2. (*A*) Whole-body ^{18}F-FDG PET images of a patient with recurrent carcinoma of the rectum in the pelvis (arrow) and mediastinal nodes (arrowheads). (*B*) CT scans of the pelvis show enlarged nodes (arrows) in the mesorectum and sigmoid mesocolon.

CLINICAL APPLICATIONS

Imaging protocols need to be carefully designed to answer the clinical question. Screening examinations to look for a disease process are different from "tailored" examinations to define the extent of disease or to determine if a lesion can be cured by surgical resection. For example, designing an examination to look for the cause of obstructive jaundice is different from designing an examination to determine whether a patient with a mass in the pancreas is a candidate for surgery. Transabdominal US or MR cholangiopancreatography may be adequate for the former circumstance. However, the latter requires a thin-section, multiphasic helical CT to characterize the lesion and to determine whether the major vessels near the pancreas—such as the superior mesenteric artery, the celiac axis, the superior mesenteric vein, and the portal vein—are involved. This protocol design provides the pancreatic surgeons with anatomic information and the extent of the disease so that they can plan proper treatment. At M. D. Anderson, we design our imaging studies on the basis of the clinical objective.

Lesion Detection

In most general practices, the use of imaging studies to screen for a disease process depends on clinical presentation. For example, US is used to evaluate a liver mass, obstructive jaundice, or flank pain, while CT is used to evaluate an abdominal mass or abdominal pain. At M. D. Anderson, most patients are referred to us with a known or potential diagnosis, and screening examinations are performed to look for metastatic disease or new disease. For patients with GI malignancies, CT is the most practical technique for this purpose because the entire abdominal cavity can be examined. We emphasize the proper technique of intravenous contrast enhancement to optimize the enhancement of the liver and the abdominal vessels, and we routinely use oral and rectal contrast material to opacify the bowel. The imaging protocol is adjusted according to the individual patient. For patients with a primary tumor that is hypervascular, such as a hepatocellular carcinoma or a neuroendocrine tumor, we use a multiphasic scanning technique that includes the arterial phase, late arterial phase, and venous phase to detect hepatic metastases. For patients with metastatic adenocarcinoma, such as colorectal cancer, scanning during the portal venous phase is adequate.

We use MRI in selected patients, including those who are allergic to iodinated intravenous contrast material, those with renal failure, and those with fatty liver. However, new and advanced MRI techniques continue to expand the applications of MRI, particularly in hepatic imaging.

Lesion Characterization

We use various imaging studies to characterize lesions, with particular emphasis on distinguishing benign lesions from malignant lesions. US is an excellent modality for distinguishing a benign cavernous hemangioma from a malignant lesion. A small, well-defined, hyperechoic lesion with posterior acoustic shadow and without a hypoechoic rim is characteristic of a cavernous hemangioma.

Multiphasic, contrast-enhanced CT or MRI of the liver is now widely used for characterization of hepatic masses, such as focal nodular hyperplasia, cavernous hemangioma, hepatocellular carcinoma, and intrahepatic cholangiocarcinoma (Paulson et al, 1994; Loyer et al, 1999; Charnsangavej et al, 2000; Brancatelli et al, 2001; Ruppert-Kohlmayr et al, 2001). These lesions have different patterns of enhancement and can be distinguished from each other with high accuracy. Proper contrast enhancement techniques are essential. For CT, we inject 150 mL of non-ionic contrast material at 5 mL/sec and scan the liver at 20 to 30 seconds for the early arterial phase, 40 to 50 seconds for the late arterial phase, and 60 to 70 seconds for the venous phase. For MRI, a similar principle is used, but the rate and volume of contrast material are lower.

Using our contrast-enhanced CT technique, focal nodular hyperplasia shows a uniform enhancement pattern during the early phase and becomes isodense or slightly hypodense to the surrounding liver, with no definable capsule. Cavernous hemangioma shows a globular enhancement in the lesion during the arterial phases and slowly diffuses throughout the lesion during the later phase. Hepatocellular carcinoma shows nodular enhancement within the mass that is nonuniform in density because of areas of necrosis. The tumor nodule becomes relatively hypodense to the surrounding parenchyma during the later phase, and the capsule of the tumor is usually identified. The enhancement patterns of intrahepatic cholangiocarcinoma are different from those of the previously described lesions but not from the enhancement patterns of metastases from adenocarcinoma of other organs. Cholangiocarcinoma shows various patterns of enhancement, from early enhancement at the periphery of the lesion and slow enhancement toward the center to lack of enhancement.

MRI provides more information than CT does owing to the use of certain imaging pulse sequences and liver-specific contrast agents that can characterize the lesion better. For example, the use of in-phase and out-of-phase gradient T1-weighted images can detect fat in the lesion to diagnose fatty liver or to distinguish liver cell adenoma from focal nodular hyperplasia. Enhancement of the lesion after intravenous contrast administration of mangafodipir trisodium, a hepatocyte-specific agent, can distinguish focal nodular hyperplasia from hemangioma or hepatic metastasis (Keogan and Edelman, 2001).

Staging Evaluation

Imaging studies have become essential in staging evaluation and treatment planning for patients with GI malignancies. Our approach in designing the imaging study is not only to screen for distant metastases but also to use the imaging study to define the extent of local involvement for planning treatment. Screening for distant metastases requires an imaging study that is sensitive in the detection of abnormalities over large anatomic areas, such as the entire abdomen and pelvis and the chest. However, to determine the extent of local involvement, the imaging study must have a high spatial resolution to demonstrate the anatomy and define the anatomic relationship between the tumor and the adjacent structures. Moreover, interpretation of the studies requires knowledge of how tumors spread and anatomic patterns of tumor spread and an understanding of the anatomic information the clinician will need to plan treatment. Therefore, proper interpretation requires good collaboration and a multidisciplinary approach among radiologists and clinicians.

Staging evaluation of pancreatic tumors is an excellent example of how a multidisciplinary approach works at M. D. Anderson. It was well recognized in the late 1980s that diagnostic and staging evaluations of pancreatic carcinoma using conventional CT underestimated the extent of local tumor involvement and adjacent vascular involvement (Megibow et al, 1995; Freeny et al, 1998). Our group, working in collaboration with Douglas Evans, MD, a surgical oncologist at M. D. Anderson, proposed the new technique of scanning the pancreas with thin scanning collimation (1.5 mm or 3 mm) at the period that produced maximum contrast enhancement. The approach increased lesion conspicuity and clearly demonstrated the anatomic relationship between the tumor and the adjacent vessel, which is important for planning surgery. The results of that study showed an improvement in the ability to predict surgical resectability, from 55% in the historical data to 83% (Fuhrman et al, 1994). Moreover, the criteria of vascular involvement were defined and are now commonly used in clinical practice (Loyer et al, 1996). This approach is now widely applied in pancreatic imaging, and advanced imaging techniques, such as multidetector, multiphasic helical CT, continue to improve the results of staging of pancreatic cancer (Figure 3–3).

Collaboration between diagnostic radiologists and surgeons also led to a new approach—the use of vascular anatomic landmarks in the mesocolon in defining the pathways of lymphatic spread in colorectal cancer. We were the first to report this approach to define the pathways of nodal metastasis in colorectal cancer (Figures 3–4 and 3–5) (Charnsangavej et al, 1993a and 1993b; McDaniel et al, 1993). We now apply a similar approach to define lymphatic spread in most GI malignancies in the abdomen and pelvis.

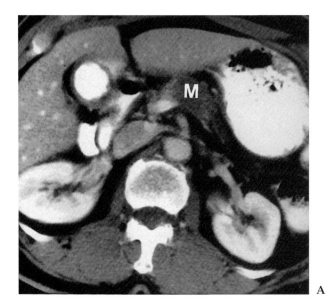

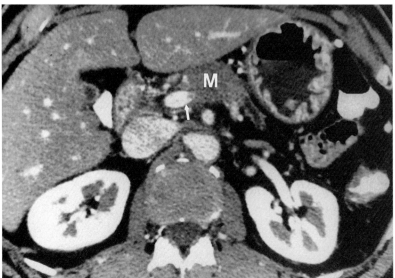

Figure 3–3. A patient with carcinoma of the pancreas. (*A*) Screening CT scan of the pancreas shows a hypodense mass (M) at the body of the pancreas. It is not clear whether the superior mesenteric artery or vein is involved. (*B*) Multiphasic helical CT scan obtained at 2.5-mm slice thickness shows the mass (M) involving the superior mesenteric vein (arrow).

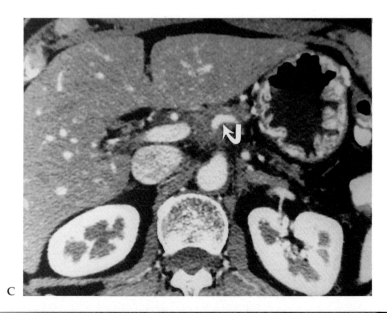

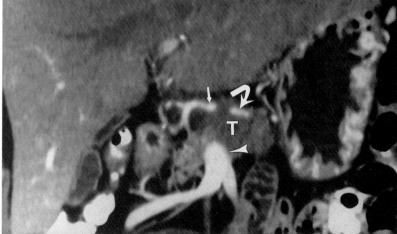

Figure 3–3. *(continued)* (C) CT scan 1 cm above the level in *B* shows involvement of the splenic artery (curved arrow). (*D*) Image display in the coronal oblique plane shows tumor (T) involvement of the hepatic artery (arrow), splenic artery (curved arrow), and superior mesenteric vein (arrowhead), making the tumor unresectable.

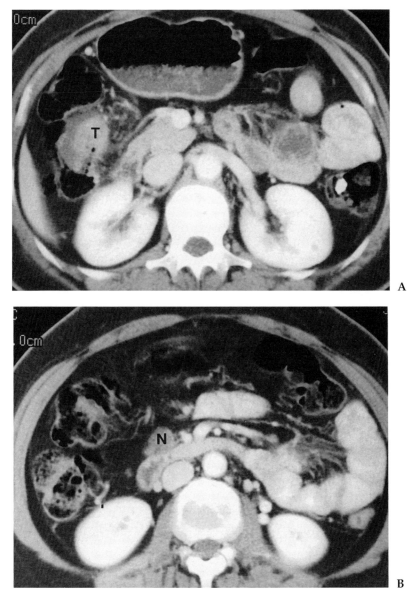

Figure 3–4.   A patient with carcinoma of the hepatic flexure of the colon. (*A*) CT scan shows the tumor (T) at the hepatic flexure of the colon. (*B*) CT scan 2 cm below the level in *A* shows a metastatic lymph node (N) in the mesocolon.

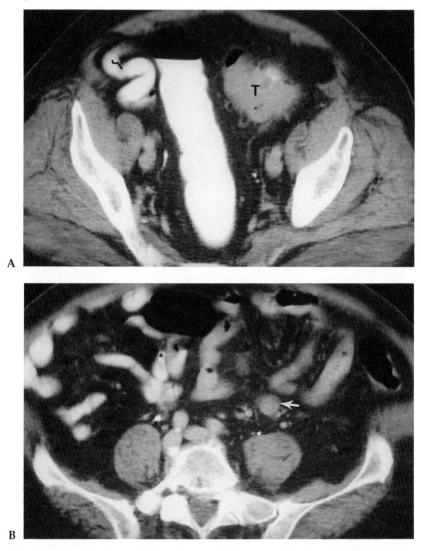

Figure 3–5. A patient with carcinoma of the sigmoid colon. (*A*) CT scan shows the tumor (T) at the sigmoid colon. (*B*) CT scan 4 cm above the level in *A* shows a metastatic node (arrow) at the root of the sigmoid mesocolon.

KEY PRACTICE POINTS

- The purpose of screening studies is to detect lesions over an entire anatomic range. In contrast, the purpose of staging studies is to determine local involvement of organs or vascular structures.

- PET is an excellent modality for screening of lesions that have high metabolic activity, such as metastatic tumors, but cannot provide anatomic detail.

- Imaging studies such as thin-section, multiphasic CT are excellent for defining tumor involvement of adjacent organs or vascular structures.

- MRI is excellent for tissue characterization.

SUGGESTED READINGS

Ak I, Stokkel MP, Pauwels EK. Positron emission tomography with 2-[^{18}F]fluoro-2-deoxy-D-glucose in oncology. Part II. The clinical value in detecting and staging primary tumors. *J Cancer Res Clin Oncol* 2000;126:560–574.

Brancatelli G, Federle MP, Grazioli L, et al. Focal nodular hyperplasia: CT findings with emphasis on multiphasic helical CT in 78 patients. *Radiology* 2001;219:61–68.

Chang KJ, Albers CG, Erickson RA, et al. Endoscopic ultrasound guided fine needle aspiration of pancreatic carcinoma. *Am J Gastroenterol* 1994;89:263–266.

Charnsangavej C, Cinqualbre A, Herron DH, et al. Diagnosis of pancreatic masses: evaluation with CT at 1.5-mm slice thickness and bolus IV contrast enhancement. *Postgrad Radiol* 1992;12:270–287.

Charnsangavej C, DuBrow RA, Varma DGK, et al. Computed tomography of the mesocolon: anatomic considerations. *Radiographics* 1993a;13:1035–1045.

Charnsangavej C, DuBrow RA, Varma DGK, et al. Computed tomography of the mesocolon: pathologic considerations. *Radiographics* 1993b;13:1309–1322.

Charnsangavej C, Loyer EM, Iyer RB, et al. Tumors of the liver, bile duct, and pancreas. *Curr Probl Diagn Radiol* 2000;29:69–107.

Choudhry S, Gorman B, Charboneau JW, et al. Comparison of tissue harmonic imaging with conventional US in abdominal disease. *Radiographics* 2000;20:1127–1135.

Delbeke D, Martin WH. Positron emission tomography imaging in oncology. *Radiol Clin North Am* 2001;39:883–917.

Foley WD, Mallisee TA, Hohenwalter MD, et al. Multiphase hepatic CT with a multirow detector CT scanner. *AJR Am J Roentgenol* 2000;175:679–685.

Freeny PC, Marks WM, Ryan JA, et al. Pancreatic ductal adenocarcinoma: diagnosis and staging with dynamic CT. *Radiology* 1988;166:125–133.

Fuhrman GM, Charnsangavej C, Abbruzzese JL, et al. Thin-section contrast-enhanced computed tomography accurately predicts resectability of malignant pancreatic neoplasms. *Am J Surg* 1994;167:104–113.

Gress FG, Hawes RH, Savides TJ, et al. Role of EUS in the preoperative staging of pancreatic cancer: a large single-center experience. *Gastrointest Endosc* 1999;50:786–791.

Ji H, McTavish JD, Mortele KJ, et al. Hepatic imaging with multidetector CT. *Radiographics* 2001;21:S71-S80.

Keogan MT, Edelman RR. Technologic advances in abdominal MR imaging. *Radiology* 2001;220:310–320.

Leifer DM, Middleton WD, Teefey SA, et al. Follow-up of patients at low risk for hepatic malignancy with a characteristic hemangioma at US. *Radiology* 2000; 214:167–172.

Loyer EM, Chin H, DuBrow RA, et al. Hepatocellular carcinoma and intrahepatic peripheral cholangiocarcinoma: enhancement patterns with quadruple phase helical CT—a comparative study. *Radiology* 1999;212:866–875.

Loyer EM, David C, Dubrow RA, et al. Vascular involvement in pancreatic adenocarcinoma: reassessment by thin-section CT. *Abdom Imaging* 1996;21:202–206.

Mankoff DA, Bellon JR. Positron-emission tomographic imaging of cancer: glucose metabolism and beyond. *Semin Radiat Oncol* 2001;11:16–27.

McDaniel KP, Charnsangavej C, DuBrow RA, et al. Pathways of nodal metastasis in carcinomas of the cecum, ascending colon, and transverse colon: CT demonstration. *AJR Am J Roentgenol* 1993;161:61–64.

Megibow AJ, Zhou XH, Rotterdam H, et al. Pancreatic adenocarcinoma: CT versus MR imaging in the evaluation of resectability—Report of the Radiology Diagnostic Oncology Group. *Radiology* 1995;195:327–332.

Paulson EK, McClellan JS, Washington K, et al. Hepatic adenoma: MR characteristics and correlation with pathologic findings. *AJR Am J Roentgenol* 1994;163: 113–116.

Reske SN, Kotzerke J. FDG-PET for clinical use. *Eur J Nucl Med Mol Imaging* 2001; 28:1707–1723.

Ruppert-Kohlmayr AJ, Uggowitzer MM, Kugler C, et al. Focal nodular hyperplasia and hepatocellular adenoma of the liver: differentiation with multiphasic helical CT. *AJR Am J Roentgenol* 2001;176:1493–1498.

Semelka RC, Helmberger TK. Contrast agents for MR imaging of the liver. *Radiology* 2001;218:27–38.

Tanaka S, Ioka T, Oshikawa O, et al. Dynamic sonography of hepatic tumors. *AJR Am J Roentgenol* 2001;177:799–805.

Wilson SR, Burns PN, Muradali D, et al. Harmonic hepatic US with microbubble contrast agent: initial experience showing improved characterization of hemangioma, hepatocellular carcinoma, and metastasis. *Radiology* 2000;215:153–161.

Yasuda K, Mukai H, Nakajima M. Endoscopic ultrasonography diagnosis of pancreatic cancer. *Gastrointest Endosc Clin N Am* 1995;5:699–712.

4 ENDOSCOPY IN THE MANAGEMENT OF GASTROINTESTINAL MALIGNANCIES

Banke Agarwal

CHAPTER OVERVIEW

Gastrointestinal endoscopy has an important role in the diagnosis, tumor staging, and treatment of patients with known or suspected gastrointestinal cancers and in patients with involvement of the gastrointestinal tract due to extragastrointestinal cancers. Endoscopic ultrasonography (EUS) has emerged as the most accurate method for regional staging (T and N classification) of esophageal, gastric, and rectal tumors and is a useful adjunct to computed tomography scanning for pretreatment staging in these patients. Endoscopic retrograde cholangiopancreatography and EUS with fine-needle aspiration (EUS-FNA) are invaluable in the diagnostic evaluation of patients with suspected pancreatic cancer. EUS-FNA can detect small pancreatic tumors, which frequently are missed with conventional imaging methods, including computed tomography and magnetic resonance imaging, and can provide a cytologic diagnosis in the vast majority of patients with suspected pancreatic cancer. Early definitive diagnosis of pancreatic tumors by EUS-FNA and their timely treatment can potentially improve outcomes in patients with pancreatic cancer. Endoscopic placement of self-expandable metal stents provides effective palliation in patients with unresectable esophageal, gastric, duodenal, pancreatobiliary, and colorectal cancers and can obviate surgery in these patients.

INTRODUCTION

As a part of the truly multidisciplinary care of patients at M. D. Anderson Cancer Center, the gastroenterologists work closely with the medical oncologists and the surgeons. Most patients who come to M. D. Anderson have cancer that is proven or suspected on the basis of clinical presentation or tests performed at referring institutions. The endoscopists at M. D. Anderson participate in confirmation of the cancer diagnosis, staging, palliation, and endoscopic follow-up, if required. Patients who have undergone endoscopies at other hospitals are strongly encouraged to bring with them the pathology slides and diagnostic specimens so that these can be reviewed by the pathologists at M. D. Anderson. When the pathologists at M. D. Anderson are not satisfied that a confident diagnosis of cancer can be made on the basis of the specimens provided, endoscopic examination is repeated to provide adequate specimens.

The endoscopy unit at M. D. Anderson provides a complete array of endoscopic services, ranging from basic endoscopic procedures, including esophagogastroduodenoscopy (EGD), colonoscopy, and percutaneous endoscopic gastrostomy (PEG), to advanced endoscopic procedures, including endoscopic ultrasonography (EUS), EUS-guided fine-needle aspiration (EUS-FNA), endoscopic retrograde cholangiopancreatography (ERCP), and endoscopic stenting for palliation of malignant obstruction of the esophagus, small bowel, or colon.

BASIC ENDOSCOPIC PROCEDURES

Because of our patient mix, the usual indications for EGD and colonoscopy in our endoscopy unit are cancer diagnosis, follow-up, or management of complications of cancer therapy. Patients with primary luminal gastrointestinal cancers undergo appropriate endoscopic procedures to document the extent of tumor involvement and undergo biopsies. EGD or colonoscopy is also performed to look for gastrointestinal involvement by extragastrointestinal cancers such as lymphoma and leukemia. Patients who have had bone marrow transplantation undergo EGD and sigmoidoscopy for diagnosis of graft-versus-host reaction. Endoscopy is also used to diagnose and treat complications of cancer treatment, such as gastrointestinal bleeding and strictures, including anastomotic strictures. A small number of patients undergo endoscopic evaluation for incidental or coexisting gastrointestinal problems, either at the time of presentation to M. D. Anderson or during follow-up after cancer treatment.

Esophageal Stricture Dilation

Most esophageal strictures in our patients are due to esophageal cancer or are secondary to its treatment. The posttreatment strictures include postirradiation strictures and anastomotic strictures. We do not dilate malignant esophageal strictures in previously untreated patients, as the benefit (dysphagia relief) tends to be very brief. Rather, the majority of these patients undergo chemoradiation, definitive or preoperative, which results in substantial and often complete resolution of the esophageal stricture. The significant risk (1% to 5%) of perforation associated with dilation of malignant esophageal strictures does not seem to be justified in this setting. For a complete evaluation of the distal esophagus, stomach, and duodenum, a 6-mm ultrathin endoscope (Pentax, Orangeburg, NY) is used to go past the stricture. We prefer PEG for nutritional supplementation in these patients.

The majority of posttreatment esophageal strictures in our patients are secondary to radiation or due to scarring of the surgical anastomosis. Every effort is made to rule out residual or recurrent tumor at the site of stricture prior to embarking on stricture dilation. We dilate strictures only if the patient has significant dysphagia that prevents adequate nutrition and the stricture is less than 10 mm in diameter. Both bougies (Savary-Guillard dilators) and "through-the-scope" balloons are used for stricture dilation. The through-the-scope balloons are more convenient because they do not require fluoroscopic guidance. However, in patients with long strictures that cannot be traversed by endoscope or with tight strictures in which the lumen cannot be seen, a guidewire is used with fluoroscopic assistance. Balloon or Savary dilation over the guidewire is performed with fluoroscopic guidance. Dilation is usually limited to no more than 3 sizes in a single session, and patients are brought back for repeat sessions as indicated by their symptoms. After dilation, patients are observed for at least 1 hour in the recovery area. If a patient has no neck pain or crepitus, a trial of clear liquids is given before the patient is discharged home. Patients are usually advised to eat soft foods for 2 days before resuming a regular diet as tolerated. Refractory strictures may occur despite frequent and progressively aggressive dilation. Adjuncts to dilation in such cases include injection of steroids, use of a "needle knife" for stricture plasty, and—in carefully selected candidates—the use of (blind) self-dilation. Because of a long-term risk of complications, the use of expandable metallic stents for relief of benign strictures is rarely considered.

Percutaneous Endoscopic Gastrostomy

Most patients requiring nutritional supplementation undergo PEG. Feeding through a PEG tube is the preferred method of nutrition in patients with esophageal cancer who have dysphagia prior to starting chemoradiation. Esophageal stents are placed only when chemoradiation has been unsuccessful and patients are being considered for palliative care. Patients with tight strictures that cannot be traversed with a regular upper endoscope are referred to interventional radiology for gastrostomy. Patients receive an intravenous dose of prophylactic antibiotic (ampicillin and gentamicin or vancomycin and gentamicin if the patient is allergic to penicillin) before PEG tube insertion.

There are few contraindications to PEG. These include gastric outlet obstruction and extensive scarring of the anterior abdominal wall. Relative contraindications include ascites with portal hypertensive gastropathy, morbid obesity, significant bleeding diathesis, gastric cancer, and partial gastrectomy. PEG should be deferred and performed only after treatment of sepsis and correction of bleeding diathesis. Some surgeons believe that mobilization of the stomach is more difficult if the patient has a gastrostomy tube, so it is important to establish the subject's candidacy for later surgery as well as the surgeon's preferences.

Percutaneous endoscopic jejunostomy (PEJ) involves passing a PEJ tube through a PEG tube and advancing it over a wire to beyond the ligament of Trietz. The procedure is performed by passing a wire through the PEG tube, grasping it with a biopsy forceps or snare passed through an endoscope introduced from the mouth. The wire is then advanced beyond the ligament of Trietz. A PEJ tube is then carefully advanced over the wire. The PEJ tube may be anchored by use of a jejunal clip. The main indication for PEG/PEJ is treatment of patients with recurrent aspiration pneumonia. Though the use of PEG/PEJ seems logical, there is no good clinical evidence clearly demonstrating that the incidence of aspiration pneumonia is significantly lower in patients with PEG/PEJ than in those with PEG. We use PEG/PEJ sparingly and favor PEG. Patients with advanced gastric or pancreatic cancer sometimes have placement of a jejunal feeding tube at the time of staging laparoscopy (performed for some patients as part of experimental protocols) to supplement nutrition when the patients receive chemoradiation prior to surgery.

Advanced Endoscopic Procedures

The advanced endoscopic procedures performed at M. D. Anderson include ERCP, EUS with or without FNA, and placement of esophageal and enteral stents.

Endoscopic Retrograde Cholangiopancreatography

Most patients who present to M. D. Anderson with pancreatic and biliary malignancies have undergone ERCP prior to presentation. Some patients present after an unsuccessful attempt at ERCP at another hospital. ERCP is also performed to rule out pancreatobiliary disease in a small group of patients being treated at M. D. Anderson for other cancers. We prefer ERCP over magnetic resonance (MR) cholangiopancreatography in most of these patients. We use MR cholangiopancreatography largely for patients with a low index of suspicion for pancreatobiliary disease, particularly in seriously ill patients who might not be able to withstand the risks of sedation. Patients with acute cholangitis, usually due to occlusion of a previously placed biliary stent, undergo emergent ERCP. All ERCPs at M. D. Anderson are performed with monitored anesthesia employing propofol and other conscious-sedation agents.

Unless the disease has been deemed inoperable on the basis of staging evaluation prior to ERCP, we invariably place a plastic biliary stent in patients with biliary obstruction due to pancreatic cancer or cholangiocarcinoma. Stents are placed only in patients with biliary strictures with obstructive jaundice. We do not recommend biliary stents in patients with biliary stricture on ERCP who have abnormal findings on liver function tests (alkaline phosphatase and transaminases) but do not have conjugated bilirubinemia. Biliary stents with a diameter less than 10 French are not used for biliary drainage, largely because the stent occlusion rates with 7- and 8.5-French stents are unacceptably high. We do not routinely perform sphincterotomy prior to placement of biliary stents. In our experience, the concern about an increased incidence of acute pancreatitis associated with placement of plastic biliary stents without sphincterotomy is more theoretical than real. This could be because the subset of patients who present to M. D. Anderson are least prone to acute pancreatitis, due to underlying pancreatic cancer. We believe that the risks of bleeding and perforation, though small, outweigh the risk of acute pancreatitis in our patients. We perform sphincterotomy in patients with papillary stenosis to facilitate passage of a stent beyond the papilla.

We proceed to placement of self-expandable metal stents in patients with pancreatic cancer involving the superior mesenteric artery or the celiac axis on spiral computed tomography (CT) examination and in patients with metastatic cancer. Before we place metal stents, we obtain a definitive cytologic diagnosis of pancreatobiliary cancer and metastatic disease by FNA. We usually deploy metal stents extending from above the level of the stricture to the ampulla. Sphincterotomy is rarely needed for deployment of metal stents except in patients with stenotic papilla. In patients with tight strictures due to fibrotic tumors, we sometimes dilate the stricture with "stepped" dilators or balloon dilators to facilitate placement of the stent.

For patients with single or multiple strictures at the hilum (bifurcation of the common hepatic duct) or higher due to cholangiocarcinoma, patients with metastases in the porta hepatis or the liver, and patients with stricture following injection of 5-fluorouracil into the hepatic artery, multiple metal stents are often required. When bilateral hilar stents are placed, we ensure that the ductal systems drained by each stent can be accessed from the ampulla. This ensures that when these stents become occluded (which almost invariably happens with sufficient passage of time), they can be cleaned endoscopically without the need for percutaneous drainage. It is important to note, however, that in the vast majority of patients with malignant hilar obstruction involving both left and right hepatic ducts, drainage of one of the ducts is sufficient for palliation.

Patients undergo repeat ERCP as needed for maintaining stent patency. In patients with resectable cancers who have plastic biliary stents when they are undergoing preoperative chemoradiation, biliary stents are exchanged when the patient has clinical evidence of stent obstruction (dark urine, pale stool, elevated findings on liver function tests) or suspicion of cholangitis. In these patients, we replace the stent with another plastic stent. In patients with metal biliary stents, the usual causes of biliary occlusion are stent occlusion due to tumor ingrowth or deposition of amorphous debris from biliary precipitate. Some patients may have progression of tumor above the level of the stent, necessitating a second, overlapping stent above the first. We try to clear the previously placed metal stents of debris with repeated balloon sweeps. If we are unable to clean the occluded stent, typically because of tumor ingrowth, we sometimes put another metal stent or a plastic stent inside the previously placed stent. The availability of plastic-coated metal stents has improved the patency rates of metal biliary stents, largely by decreasing the chances of tumor ingrowth. However, coated wallstents can be used only in patients who have had prior cholecystectomy. Coated wallstents are also contraindicated for malignant strictures extending to the hilum. In our experience, coated wallstents carry a higher risk of migration and should therefore be used only in a carefully selected group of patients. We have used ursodiol in patients in whom the stents are occluded with debris at frequent intervals, but the benefit has been marginal.

Procedures in Patients with Acute Cholangitis

In patients with acute cholangitis, we take care to aspirate 10 to 20 ml of bile before injecting contrast into the bile ducts at the time of ERCP. This reduces the risk of further bacteremia. Patients usually recover very rapidly after stent exchange and biliary decompression. Antibiotics are continued for 5 to 7 days, and patients can usually be discharged 1 to 2 days after biliary decompression.

Endoscopic Ultrasonography

EUS is becoming invaluable in the management of patients with gastrointestinal cancers. EUS is performed with specialized endoscopes, called echoendoscopes, that have ultrasound transducers incorporated into their tips in addition to the video camera. Because these echoendoscopes can be positioned very close to the site of cancer, EUS allows the use of high ultrasound frequencies (7.5 to 20 MHz). High ultrasound frequencies are preferred, as imaging resolution is directly related to the frequency used. EUS allows clear visualization of individual layers of the gut wall and therefore can help determine the wall layers involved by the tumor for accurate T classification of luminal tumors. For nodal staging, EUS can identify enlarged lymph nodes that may be infiltrated by tumor. Several criteria have been developed to differentiate malignant lymph nodes from lymph nodes enlarged owing to inflammation. EUS is also emerging as an invaluable tool for the diagnosis of pancreatic cancer. EUS provides high-resolution imaging of the pancreas with placement of the echoendoscope in the stomach and duodenum and can identify small tumors that are frequently missed by other imaging modalities.

At M. D. Anderson, EUS has become an integral part of the diagnosis and management of most gastrointestinal cancers. Both radial and linear echoendoscopes are used, and FNA of the lesions is performed whenever indicated. The availability of a team of highly qualified cytopathologists at M. D. Anderson is of tremendous help to the endosonographers, since a confident cytologic interpretation of the EUS-FNA specimens is critical if EUS is to significantly affect patient management. EUS is particularly useful in the management of esophageal, pancreatic, and rectal cancers. It is sometimes useful in the management of gastric cancer and of rare duodenal neoplasms.

Esophageal Cancers

EUS is highly accurate and is superior to CT for the preoperative T and N classification of esophageal carcinoma. However, EUS is not useful for M classification and therefore is not a substitute for CT. EUS is best used to complement CT in the staging of esophageal cancer.

At M. D. Anderson, all patients with esophageal cancer undergo EUS for the staging of esophageal cancer. Complete endoscopic evaluation includes EGD with biopsies of the suspected malignant lesion. EUS is performed using a radial echoendoscope (EUM-30, Olympus, Melville, NY). We do not dilate strictures that cannot be traversed with a regular EGD endoscope simply to allow passage of an echoendoscope. In such cases, it is usually possible to complete the endoscopic assessment by using ultra-thin 6-mm endoscopes to define the length of the stricture and its distance from the gastroesophageal junction. EUS examination is then performed using a thin echoendoscope (MH-908, Olympus) that can be passed over a guidewire (such as a superstiff Jagwire, Boston Scientific, Natick, MA) through most strictures under ultrasound guidance without a significant risk of perforation. The MH-908 echoendoscope is limited by a lack of optics and has only a single frequency (7.5 MHz). However, its depth of penetration and its image quality are similar to those of a regular echoendoscope and allow complete EUS staging of esophageal cancer in patients with tight esophageal strictures. We prefer the use of the MH-908 over the alternative—i.e., balloon dilation of stricture at the time of EUS examination—because balloon dilation is associated with a significant risk of perforation (approaching 25% in some studies). The image quality and depth of imaging with "through-the-scope" ultrasound probes are much inferior to those of the MH-908 echoendoscope and not to our satisfaction.

For the staging of esophageal cancers, we begin by passing the echoen-doscope beyond the esophageal tumor and all the way to the gastric body. The scope is then gradually withdrawn to evaluate the tumor, with atten-tion to the esophageal wall layers involved by the tumor; extension beyond the esophagus; and involvement of the surrounding organs, including the aorta, azygos vein, diaphragm, pleura, pericardium, trachea, and bronchi.

We then search for any enlarged celiac and mediastinal lymph nodes. Suspicious lymph nodes may be sampled by EUS-FNA. In patients with multiple enlarged paraesophageal lymph nodes, we sample nodes in each lymph node group until 1 of the lymph nodes in that group is positive for malignancy or all the nodes in that group are negative for malignancy. We have gradually moved away from exclusive reliance on morphologic criteria for lymph node staging of esophageal cancers. The specificity of the morphologic criteria is not adequate, and lymph node staging can be vastly improved by the use of EUS-FNA. We have encountered several small paraesophageal mucinous cysts that are morphologically indistin-guishable from malignant lymph nodes. These benign cysts, if mistaken for malignant lymph nodes, can significantly influence treatment, partic-ularly in patients with T1 or T2 tumors, which may be considered for sur-gical resection without preoperative chemoradiation in the absence of identifiable malignant lymphadenopathy.

We restage esophageal cancers after preoperative chemoradiation. Repeat biopsies are obtained from the tumor site for completeness. In our analysis, biopsies of the tumor site are only 27% sensitive for diagnosing residual tumor. Tumor stage is reevaluated using EUS. Although T classi-fication of the tumor with EUS is inaccurate owing to the inability of EUS to reliably distinguish inflammation and scar tissue from tumor, it is possible to identify patients with tumor extending into important para-esophageal structures, such as the aorta, and thereby prevent surgical mishaps. Celiac and mediastinal lymph nodes are reevaluated, and all enlarged lymph nodes are sampled with EUS-FNA.

Gastric Cancers

The principles of staging gastric cancer with EUS are the same as for esophageal cancers. The depth of tumor invasion into the gastric wall layers is determined, as is the involvement of paragastric and celiac lymph nodes. At M. D. Anderson, we still have not been convinced about the adequacy of saline-assisted endoscopic mucosal resections of (rarely encountered) early gastric cancers, and we still prefer surgical resection of these tumors. EUS can help by identifying T1N0 lesions that may be surgically resected without preoperative chemoradiation. All lymph nodes that are suspected of having malignant infiltration are sampled with EUS-FNA.

EUS or EUS-FNA is also helpful in the workup of patients with thickened gastric folds seen on endoscopy or sometimes on abdominal CT. The presence of thickened third and fourth echolayers on EUS in patients with normal gastric mucosa on endoscopy is highly suspicious for malignant infiltration. In patients with such findings, EUS-FNA of the thickened layers is often helpful in diagnosing lymphoma or linitis plastica adenocarcinoma. EUS is also helpful for staging gastric lymphoma and linitis plastica. Patients with these conditions have a markedly thickened gastric wall (normal, 3 to 5 mm), often with destruction of the wall architecture. EUS can identify the wall layers involved by the neoplastic process and detect enlarged perigastric and celiac lymph nodes and the presence of any malignant ascites or peritoneal tumor nodules.

Ultrasonography is also helpful in patients with benign gastric polyps who are being evaluated for endoscopic mucosal resection. EUS is performed in these patients to ascertain that the polyp is confined to the mucosa or submucosa and does not involve the muscularis propria and that the polyp can thereby be separated from the muscularis propria by saline injection. EUS also helps to exclude vascular etiology of the polypoid lesion or the presence of large vessels inside the polyp.

Pancreatic Cancers

EUS-FNA is emerging as an invaluable tool in the diagnosis of patients with suspected pancreatic cancers. At M. D. Anderson, all patients referred with suspicion of pancreatic cancer without tissue or cytologic diagnosis undergo EUS-FNA for their initial evaluation. FNA of all suspicious lesions identified by EUS is attempted. The accuracy of EUS-FNA in the diagnosis of pancreatic cancer is 90% in our experience. Since the surgeons and oncologists at M. D. Anderson are proponents of preoperative chemo-radiation for pancreatic cancer, EUS-FNA has become critical in managing pancreatic cancer at M. D. Anderson.

No special patient preparation is required for EUS-FNA of the pancreas. Patients need to fast overnight prior to the test. We perform EUS-FNA only in patients with a normal international normalized ratio value (less than 1.3), a platelet count greater than 75,000 (preferably more than 100,000), and no evidence of platelet dysfunction. We usually ask patients not to use aspirin and other nonsteroidal anti-inflammatory drugs (NSAIDs) for 5 to 7 days prior to EUS-FNA, although there are no clinical data regarding the influence of NSAIDs on postprocedure bleeding after EUS-FNA. The risk of clinically significant bleeding after EUS-FNA of the pancreas is very low in patients with normal coagulation values. The risk of complications with EUS-FNA is low at M. D. Anderson, and my patients have had a complication rate of less than 0.5%. Minor complications, such as abdominal pain lasting less than 24 hours, are managed readily with analgesics.

The accuracy of EUS-FNA is very high in patients with suspected pancreatic cancer without obstructive jaundice as the presenting feature. In patients with a suspicious pancreatic mass lesion on CT or MR imaging, with or without associated symptoms such as weight loss, abdominal pain, or recurrent acute pancreatitis, EUS is the most definitive test for diagnosing pancreatic cancer. If no malignancy is identified in these patients by EUS or EUS-FNA, further investigation for pancreatic cancer is unlikely to be helpful. These patients undergo follow-up EUS in 3 months.

EUS-FNA is less accurate in patients with suspected pancreatic cancer with obstructive jaundice at presentation. At M. D. Anderson, these patients usually present after placement of biliary stents. Cytologic assessment of EUS-FNA specimens from these patients is challenging because of the presence of inflammation induced by biliary stents. It is often impossible to identify well-differentiated cancers in patients with biliary stents in place, since cellular atypia can also be caused by inflammation. As a result, the negative predictive value of EUS-FNA is low in these patients.

EUS or EUS-FNA can detect small pancreatic cancers that are missed by other currently available imaging modalities, including multidetector spiral CT. In our experience, EUS-FNA can provide a definite cytologic diagnosis in 75% of patients with tumors less than 20 mm in diameter and is about 90% accurate in the diagnosis of pancreatic cancer in patients with suspected pancreatic cancer with no mass or a doubtful mass on spiral CT.

At M. D. Anderson, we do not routinely attempt to stage pancreatic cancers with EUS. With recent improvements in the resolution of spiral CT scanners and with the ability to reconstruct the CT images and generate angiograms, spiral CT is emerging as a better staging modality for pancreatic cancers. At M. D. Anderson, tumor encasement of the superior mesenteric artery or the celiac trunk, but not involvement of the portal vein, are considered contraindications to surgery. Spiral CT is superior to EUS in the identification of arterial encasement by tumor. The practical advantage of CT angiograms is that they are more visually appealing than EUS images and allow surgeons to more easily appreciate the anatomy.

Cystic Neoplasms of the Pancreas

All patients presenting with a cystic lesion of the pancreas undergo EUS-guided cyst aspiration. Complete drainage of the cyst is attempted in most patients. The cyst fluid is sent for cytologic examination and also tested for carcinoembryonic antigen and mucin. We also routinely perform EUS-FNA of the wall of the cyst after cyst aspiration. In cysts with septations or with focal thickening of the wall, FNA of the septa or the thickened part of the cyst wall is performed. The material is submitted for cytologic assessment to rule out malignancy. However, preoperative identification of malignancy is often difficult in cystic lesions of the pancreas. Because of their malignant potential, we recommend surgical resection for all mucinous cystic lesions identified by mucin staining and high carcinoembryonic antigen levels in cyst fluid. Broad-spectrum antibiotics (e.g., levofloxacin) are prescribed for 3 to 5 days after cyst aspiration.

Celiac Plexus Neurolysis

Celiac plexus neurolysis (CPN) is chemical neurolysis of the celiac plexus, resulting in ablation of the afferent nerve fibers that transmit pain from abdominal viscera. In patients with unresectable pancreatic cancers and intractable abdominal pain, CPN can often significantly reduce the amount of narcotics required and improve the patient's quality of life. We usually perform CPN in 2 sessions. In the first, bupivacaine with epinephrine is injected around the celiac axis. This relieves pain in 70% to 80% of patients, and the pain relief lasts 4 to 24 weeks. Patients who have significant pain relief after injection of bupivacaine are brought back for CPN when the pain reappears. During the second session, bupivacaine with epinephrine and then absolute alcohol are injected around the celiac trunk. To prevent orthostatic hypotension due to pooling of blood in the dependent part of the body after celiac block, patients receive 1 liter of normal saline prior to CPN. Major reported complications of CPN are uncommon and occur in approximately 1% of patients. These include lower-extremity weakness and paresthesia, paraplegia, pneumothorax, impotence, loss of bladder control, and prolonged gastroparesis or diarrhea. The anterior approach to CPN with EUS potentially has a lower risk of neurologic complications, because the needle does not traverse the perispinal region or somatic nerves.

Gastropancreatic Neuroendocrine Tumors

M. D. Anderson is a major referral center for management of gastropancreatic neuroendocrine tumors. EUS is emerging as a useful tool in localization of functioning neuroendocrine tumors, both insulinomas and
gastrinomas. FNA for cytologic diagnosis is not critical in patients with
neuroendocrine tumors suspected on the basis of abnormal findings on
endocrine workup. In patients with suspected gastrinomas (Proye et al,
1998), including patients with Zollinger-Ellison syndrome, EUS has use-
fulness comparable to that of somatostatin receptor scintigraphy (SRS),
with sensitivities of 73% for EUS and 75% for SRS. The combined sensitivity of EUS and SRS in the detection and localization of tumors is 93%.
In patients with suspected insulinomas, EUS localized 93% of insulinomas, compared to 29% with the use of a combination of CT, ultrasonography, and MR imaging (Zimmer et al, 1996). Use of EUS has been shown
to be cost-effective in the preoperative localization of functioning neuroendocrine tumors.

Nonfunctioning neuroendocrine tumors have a presentation similar to
that of pancreatic tumors. They often present with obstructive jaundice
when they are located in the pancreatic head. They are commonly detected
incidentally on CT or MR imaging of the abdomen in patients being investigated for unrelated symptoms. EUS-FNA can provide definite cytologic
diagnosis of malignancy in these patients and can preoperatively identify
these lesions as neuroendocrine tumors on the basis of special stains performed on EUS-FNA specimens. This is valuable in treatment planning,
as the natural history of nonfunctioning pancreatic neuroendocrine
tumors is significantly different from that of pancreatic adenocarcinoma.

Rectal Tumors

EUS staging is also helpful in the management of rectal cancer. We pass
the echoendoscope beyond the lesion to about 30 cm from the anal verge.
The echoendoscope is then gradually withdrawn, and we carefully search
for any enlarged lymph nodes. EUS-FNA is performed for enlarged
pararectal or pericolic lymph nodes. We determine the extent of tumor
(length of rectum involved, circumferential extent, and depth of infiltration of rectal wall by the tumor), and we ascertain involvement of surrounding organs, including the bladder, prostate, and seminal vesicles in
men and the bladder, uterus, and vagina in women. Involvement by the
tumor of internal and external anal sphincters and the pelvic diaphragm
is routinely assessed.

Indeterminate Mediastinal, Upper Abdominal, and Pararectal Masses

Patients are often seen at M. D. Anderson with abnormal CT scans or MR
images showing mass lesions in the mediastinum, upper abdomen, or
pararectal area, the etiology of which is not known. We perform EUS-FNA

of these masses for cytologic assessment. Special stains are used as needed to determine the origin of these lesions. EUS-FNA has proven to be very safe and effective in these patients.

Esophageal and Enteral Stent Placement

Self-expandable metal stents (SEMS) are frequently used in patients requiring palliation for advanced cancer of the gastrointestinal tract. We normally place metal stents only after patients have received chemotherapy or radiation therapy or both, since chemoradiation frequently reduces tumor size markedly and can obviate stent placement. Furthermore, a reduction in tumor size after chemoradiation can potentially remove the anchor for the stent and can result in stent displacement and migration. We use SEMS in patients with significant dysphagia caused by advanced esophageal cancers; symptomatic gastric outlet obstruction due to distal gastric, duodenal, or pancreatic cancers; and colonic obstruction due to metastatic or unresectable colorectal tumors. Because of a significant risk of complications associated with SEMS, including stent occlusion and stent migration, we try to time stent placement so that the benefit-risk ratio is favorable.

For esophageal cancers, we consider stent placement in patients who have significant dysphagia that interferes with adequate nutrition. In patients with tracheoesophageal fistula, stent placement is considered the palliation of choice. Before insertion of SEMS for high esophageal strictures, it is important to ensure that the tumor does not significantly compress the airway, since airway obstruction may be precipitated by placement of the esophageal stent. In patients with compromised airways, we recommend placement of tracheobronchial stents prior to or along with placement of the esophageal stent. While placing the esophageal stent, we define the extent of the stricture by performing an endoscopy with a 6-mm endoscope or injecting iodine contrast agent through a double-lumen plastic cannula that is passed through the stricture over a guidewire. We do not routinely dilate the stricture prior to the placement of esophageal stents.

In patients with gastric outlet obstruction due to distal gastric cancer, duodenal cancer, or pancreatic cancer, we use SEMS to restore the lumen. Stents are deployed only when the patient has overt signs and symptoms of gastric outlet obstruction with marked proximal dilation of the stomach. Prophylactic placement of stents in patients without overt gastric outlet obstruction is not helpful and currently not recommended. We use a through-the-scope enteral stent in these patients. In patients with concomitant biliary obstruction, we place a metal stent in the bile duct before placement of the duodenal stent, since it is virtually impossible to access the ampulla after placement of the duodenal stent.

Colorectal stents are placed in patients with colonic obstruction due to unresectable or metastatic colon cancer. Because of significant risks asso-

KEY PRACTICE POINTS

- Feeding through a PEG tube is the preferred method of nutrition in esophageal cancer patients with dysphagia prior to starting chemoradiation. Esophageal stents should be placed when chemoradiation has been unsuccessful and patients are being considered for palliative care.

- In patients with acute cholangitis, it is helpful to aspirate 10 to 20 ml of bile before injecting contrast agent into the bile duct at the time of ERCP.

- In the vast majority of patients with malignant hilar obstruction involving both left and right hepatic ducts, drainage of 1 of the ducts is sufficient for palliation.

- EUS should always be used in conjunction with CT for staging of gastrointestinal tumors.

- EUS-FNA is invaluable in the diagnostic workup of patients with suspected pancreatic cancer and can often diagnose pancreatic tumors that are missed by other imaging modalities.

- Significant compromise of airway by esophageal tumor should be excluded prior to placement of an esophageal stent.

- Because of the significant risk of complications associated with SEMS, enteral stents should be placed only in symptomatic patients, and prophylactic stent placement should be avoided.

ciated with colonic stents, including stent occlusion and stent migration, prophylactic placement of colonic stents is not currently recommended. We use both through-the-scope enteral stents and uncoated large-diameter (30-mm) colonic stents for colonic obstruction. In our experience, the latter have a lower risk of migration, but we have encountered problems with deployment of these stents in more proximal lesions of the colon. Patients are prescribed stool softeners after colonic stent placement and instructed to maintain a semisolid consistency of their stools.

Suggested Readings

Adler DG, Baron TH. Endoscopic palliation of malignant dysphagia. *Mayo Clin Proc* 2001;76:731–738.

Adler DG, Baron TH. Endoscopic palliation of malignant gastric outlet obstruction using self-expanding metal stents: experience in 36 patients. *Am J Gastroenterol* 2002;97:72–78.

Ballinger AB, McHugh M, Catnach SM, et al. Symptom relief and quality of life after stenting for malignant bile duct obstruction. *Gut* 1994;35:467–470.

Freeman ML. Sedation and monitoring for gastrointestinal endoscopy. *Gastrointest Endosc Clin N Am* 1994;4:475–499.

Freeman ML, DiSario JA, Nelson DB, et al. Risk factors for post-ERCP pancreatitis: a prospective, multicenter study. *Gastrointest Endosc* 2001;54:425–434.

Harris GJ, Senagore AJ, Lavery IC, Fazio VW. The management of neoplastic colorectal obstruction with colonic endoluminal stenting devices. *Am J Surg* 2001;181:499–506.

Kochman ML. EUS in pancreatic cancer. *Gastrointest Endosc* 2002;56(suppl):S6–S12.

Lai ECS, Mok FPT, Tan ESY, et al. Endoscopic biliary drainage for severe acute cholangitis. *N Engl J Med* 1992;326:1582–1586.

Mendis RE, Gerdes H, Lightdale CJ, Botet JF. Large gastric folds: a diagnostic approach using endoscopic ultrasonography. *Gastrointest Endosc* 1994;40: 437–441.

Pasricha PJ, Fleischer DE, Kalloo AN. Endoscopic perforations of the upper digestive tract: a review of their pathogenesis, prevention and management. *Gastroenterology* 1994;106:787–802.

Penman ID, Shen EF. EUS in advanced esophageal cancer. *Gastrointest Endosc* 2002; 56(suppl):S2–S6.

Proye C, Malvaux P, Pattou F, et al. Noninvasive imaging of insulinomas and gastrinomas with endoscopic ultrasonography and somatostatin receptor scintigraphy. *Surgery* 1998;124:1134–1143.

Safadi BY, Marks JM, Ponsky JL. Percutaneous endoscopic gastrostomy. *Gastrointest Endosc Clin N Am* 1998;8:551–568.

Savides TJ, Master SS. EUS in rectal cancer. *Gastrointest Endosc* 2002;56(suppl): S12–S18.

Shirai M, Nakamura T, Matsuura A. Safer colonoscopic polypectomy with local submucosal injection of hypertonic saline-epinephrine solution. *Am J Gastroenterol* 1994;89:334–338.

Smith AC, Dowsett JF, Russell RCG, Hatfield ARW, Cotton PB. Randomized trial of endoscopic stenting versus surgical bypass in malignant low bile duct obstruction. *Lancet* 1994;344:1655–1660.

Van Dam J. EUS in cystic lesions of the pancreas. *Gastrointest Endosc* 2002; 56(suppl):S91–S93.

Vermeijden JR, Bartelsman JFWM, Fockens P, et al. Self-expanding metal stents for palliation of esophagocardial malignancies. *Gastrointest Endosc* 1995;41:58–63.

Wiersema M, Harada N, Wiersema L. Endosonography guided celiac plexus neurolysis (EUS-CPN) for abdominal pain: efficacy in chronic pancreatitis and malignant disease. *Acta Endoscopia* 1998;28:67–79.

Yasuda K. EUS in detection of early gastric cancer. *Gastrointest Endosc* 2002; 56(suppl):S68–S75.

Zimmer T, Stolzel U, Bader M, et al. Endoscopic ultrasonography and somatostatin receptor scintigraphy in the preoperative localisation of insulinomas and gastrinomas. *Gut* 1996;39:562–568.

5 ROLE OF LAPAROSCOPY IN GASTROINTESTINAL MALIGNANCIES

Barry W. Feig

CHAPTER OVERVIEW

The introduction of laparoscopy into the armamentarium of the general surgeon in the late 1980s resulted in a revolution of new technology and procedures. Despite this meteoric application in general surgery, there has been only a slow and cautious application of laparoscopic procedures in surgical oncology. This has been due in large part to concerns about peritoneal dissemination and port-site implantation raised by a number of reports that appeared early in the process of evaluating laparoscopic procedures in patients with intra-abdominal malignancies. At M. D. Anderson Cancer Center, we began evaluating the role of laparoscopy in surgical oncology in the early 1990s. Since that time, we have used laparoscopy in a wide variety of disease processes. Our use of laparoscopy in gastrointestinal malignancies has evolved over the last 10 years; this chapter will present some of the original applications and their evolution to our present surgical practice. Additionally, the available data as they pertain to the controversy regarding tumor dissemination and port-site implantation will be presented.

INTRODUCTION

With many new techniques, there is an initial period of exuberance regarding possible additional applications that often leads to unrealistic expectations on the part of both physicians and patients. This was clearly the case with laparoscopy. The successful application of laparoscopy to procedures such as cholecystectomy led to the hope that similar benefits could be realized in patients with cancer. These benefits, which were believed to include faster recovery, shorter hospital stay, decreased pain, and earlier return to normal activity, would clearly benefit the oncology patient. Patients undergoing palliative procedures would potentially benefit by spending less time in the hospital and by requiring less pain medicine. In patients undergoing diagnostic and therapeutic procedures, a faster recovery time after surgery would potentially allow patients to begin definitive treatment regimens sooner than they could after conventional open surgical techniques. Because of this early exuberance, a large variety of procedures were initially attempted laparoscopically at M. D. Anderson. Palliative procedures performed included cholecystojejunostomy for biliary obstruction, gastrojejunostomy for gastric outlet obstruction, and small bowel bypass and colostomy for intestinal obstruction. The main therapeutic procedures performed laparoscopically for tumors of the gastrointestinal tract were in patients with colorectal cancer. The most widely applied use of laparoscopy in patients with gastrointestinal malignancies at M. D. Anderson has been for staging procedures in patients with gastric, hepatobiliary, and pancreatic cancers.

In this chapter, we discuss the role of laparoscopy in palliation, staging, and therapeutic procedures in patients with gastrointestinal malignancies. We also address the concern regarding tumor implantation in cases of laparoscopy.

PALLIATION

Many factors were involved in getting to our current standard of application for laparoscopy. Over the past 12 years, there have been significant technologic advances not only in the laparoscopic field but also in competing fields such as radiology and endoscopy. In many cases, procedures that previously required an operation can now be performed via radiologically guided percutaneous procedures or endoscopic techniques. For example, a patient with an obstructing lesion of the upper rectum would previously have been treated with a diverting colostomy. Traditionally this was an open surgical procedure; in the mid-1990s, this procedure was frequently performed with a laparoscopic-assisted technique. However, it is now often possible to palliate the obstruction without having to use general anesthesia, using endoscopically placed stents or laser ablation of the tumor mass to prevent complete obstruction. Another procedure that has become less commonly performed laparoscopically is biliary bypass. Again, initially it was believed that a laparoscopic cholecystojejunostomy would be a desirable alternative to an open surgical bypass. However, the development of endoscopically placed biliary stents has made the former procedure nearly obsolete.

Because of these nonoperative alternative techniques, we have seen a decrease in enthusiasm for some of the initial laparoscopic applications of palliative procedures, and several palliative techniques for which there was initially great enthusiasm for laparoscopic applications are now only rarely used in our practice.

Despite this change, laparoscopy remains a significant treatment option for patients with gastrointestinal malignancies who are not candidates for percutaneous procedures. In other cases, however, it has clearly become our preference to perform percutaneous procedures as the primary treatment option whenever available in the palliative setting. This avoids the need for a general anesthetic and frequently allows these procedures to be performed on an outpatient basis, minimizing the disruption of the normal daily routine for patients with advanced disease. Additionally, it allows patients to proceed to their next phase of treatment in a more expeditious manner. Just as the recovery from laparoscopic procedures has been quicker and less stressful for the patient than the recovery from open surgical procedures, percutaneous procedures that avoid general anesthesia result in even less trauma to the patient and thus an even shorter recovery period. Furthermore, although many colonic obstructions can be treated with endoscopic techniques, many malignant intestinal obstructions still are not amenable to endoscopic palliation. For these patients, laparoscopic colostomies and bypasses are still frequently employed in our practice.

STAGING

In a similar fashion, the use of laparoscopy in the staging of disease in patients with gastrointestinal malignancies has been dramatically affected by improvements in technology and refinements of radiologic techniques. Initially, there were believed to be multiple benefits of laparoscopic staging related to early recovery, as mentioned above for palliative procedures. Clearly, if adequate staging information could be obtained using minimally invasive techniques, patients could recover faster and proceed with their definitive treatment plans more expeditiously. Additionally, enteral feeding tubes could be placed to allow for enteral feeding during neoadjuvant treatments, as many patients with gastrointestinal malignancies have already lost substantial amounts of weight at the time of diagnosis of malignant disease. For these reasons, staging laparoscopy was initially used in patients with gastric, hepatobiliary, and pancreatic cancers.

The advent of laparoscopic ultrasound probes made evaluation of the liver for metastases much more accurate. Initially, this was perceived as a substantial benefit, especially in patients with pancreatic and hepatobiliary cancer, as well as in patients with liver metastases that were being evaluated for potential resection. Several studies just prior to this time had shown that intraoperative ultrasonography was the most accurate method of determining unrecognized liver metastases (more accurate than liver palpation at the time of surgery or preoperative computed tomography [CT]). Therefore, it was assumed that the introduction of laparoscopic ultrasonography would result in similar benefits.

Although there was initial evidence to support this hypothesis, several changes occurred that challenged the validity of this theory. A problem immediately identified was the learning curve required to perform accurate laparoscopic ultrasonography of the liver. Aside from the technical challenges associated with the first-generation ultrasound probes, most surgeons were not facile in sonogram interpretation, resulting in significant false-negative and false-positive rates. As the technology of the probes improved and as surgeons became more experienced in reading liver sonograms, there was a simultaneous improvement in the technology and technique employed in performing CT of the liver. Initially, preoperative CT of the abdomen was believed to miss liver metastases in 20% to 40% of patients. In patients undergoing surgical exploration for resection of liver metastases, a similar incidence of additional lesions missed by routine CT had been observed. However, the introduction of the helical CT scan, the timing of contrast injection to correlate with the venous, arterial, and portal phases of blood flow (triphasic CT), and the use of thinly spaced (3.5 mm) cuts has resulted in a significantly lower incidence of missed hepatic metastases on CT. More contemporary radiologic studies have found the incidence of missed hepatic metastases in patients with hepatobiliary and pancreatic malignancies to be less than 10% when these radiologic techniques are employed. Therefore, the cost-benefit ratio of performing laparoscopic staging has been questioned in these patients.

In general, in our practice, we have not found routine laparoscopic staging to be of significant benefit in patients with pancreatic and hepatobiliary malignancies, as the incidence of missed hepatic metastases in these patients is less than 10%. Laparoscopy is used selectively in patients with equivocal CT scans or in patients in whom CT shows a questionable lesion. In these patients, the laparoscopic staging procedure is performed just prior to the planned surgical resection so as to avoid an extra induction of anesthesia for the patient.

For patients with gastric adenocarcinoma, our policy has been substantially different for several reasons. In these patients, the incidence of metastatic disease missed on preoperative CT is higher (approximately

20%) because of the increased incidence of peritoneal dissemination in these patients. These small peritoneal deposits are difficult to identify on CT scans, and staging laparoscopy is therefore ideal for both identifying peritoneal spread and providing the opportunity for biopsy of this tissue for histologic confirmation. Additionally, at M. D. Anderson, a large percentage of patients with resectable gastric cancer are entered into treatment protocols that employ preoperative chemotherapy and/or radiation therapy. As mentioned above, the majority of patients with gastric cancer present with substantial weight loss and malnutrition. The placement of enteral feeding tubes allows these patients to improve and then maintain their nutritional status before and during their neoadjuvant treatment, resulting in a larger proportion of patients being able to complete their preoperative treatment plan. For all of these reasons, staging laparoscopy has continued to be performed on a routine basis in patients who present with gastric cancer at M. D. Anderson.

THERAPEUTIC PROCEDURES

As mentioned previously, the most commonly performed therapeutic laparoscopic procedure at M. D. Anderson has been laparoscopic colon resection. There has been considerable controversy surrounding the oncologic safety as well as the quality-of-life benefits of laparoscopic colon resection. We began a prospective, nonrandomized trial of laparoscopic colon resection in 1992. This trial was open to any patient with colorectal carcinoma. At the time of evaluation for publication, laparoscopic colon resection had been completed successfully in 53 (58%) of the 91 enrolled patients. The most common reasons for having to convert from a laparoscopic to an open procedure were adhesions from prior surgery and poor exposure. When characteristics were compared for patients successfully treated laparoscopically and those who required conversion to an open procedure, patients who required conversion to an open procedure had a significantly higher body weight. This suggests that the laparoscopic procedure is more difficult in larger patients, a finding consistent with our clinical impression. Operative parameters were compared for patients successfully treated laparoscopically, those who required conversion to an open operation, and a matched group of patients undergoing a planned open surgical procedure. Patients undergoing a planned open procedure had a significantly shorter operative time than did the laparoscopic and the converted-procedure groups (2.5 hours vs 4.0 and 4.5 hours, respectively; $P < .01$). The hospital stay was significantly shorter in the patients who had the procedure completed laparoscopically (6 days vs 8 days in the converted-procedure group and 7 days in the open-procedure group; $P < .01$). However, cost was significantly increased only in those patients who required conversion from a laparoscopic to an open procedure. Most significantly, the overall and disease-free survivals did not differ significantly between the 3 groups. Additionally, there were no observed instances of port-site tumor implantation in patients who underwent a laparoscopic procedure. Despite these apparently successful initial results with laparoscopic colon resection, there has not been a rapid acceptance of this procedure as standard of care, for a variety of reasons.

It is difficult to justify the increased operative time required to perform the laparoscopic procedure when there are questions as to whether there truly is a quality-of-life benefit associated with the procedure. These questions have become even more prominent following the publication of the National Cancer Institute–sponsored COST trial (Weeks et al, 2002). In this prospective, randomized, multi-institutional study, only minimal quality-of-life benefits could be identified for laparoscopic colon resection. Therefore, based on this information, it becomes difficult to justify the increased operative time and increased cost of a laparoscopic procedure. In contrast to these data, a prospective randomized trial comparing laparoscopic versus open colon resection from Barcelona, Spain (Lacy et al, 2002) reported not only a benefit in morbidity and hospital stay for laparoscopic-assisted colon resection but also improved cancer-related survival and decreased tumor recurrence in patients undergoing the laparoscopic procedure. The improvement in survival was due to differences observed in patients with stage III disease. It is difficult to postulate a scientific explanation for the oncologic benefit that was observed in this study. Clearly, further investigation and experience will be required to resolve the questions that remain regarding the value of laparoscopic-assisted colon resection for malignancy.

TUMOR IMPLANTATION

As mentioned previously, the widespread application of laparoscopic techniques to oncologic procedures has been significantly slowed by concern about tumor implantation at the trocar insertion sites (port sites). The first reported port-site recurrence after a laparoscopic procedure was described in 1978, in a patient with malignant ascites who developed detectable disease at a trocar site 2 weeks after laparoscopy. Subsequent reports surfaced that described port-site recurrences in patients undergoing laparoscopy for widespread ovarian carcinoma. Over the next 20 years, case reports describing port-site recurrences from a variety of histologic subtypes of tumors appeared in the literature. Unfortunately, the anecdotal nature of these case reports made it impossible to determine the true incidence of port-site metastasis. Additionally, the significance of a port-site recurrence also needed to be addressed. The majority of patients in these early reports had widespread disease, including carcinomatosis, at the time of the laparoscopic procedure. Given a clinical scenario with widespread local, regional, or metastatic disease, it was difficult to ascertain the significance of these findings.

A variety of experimental systems have been set up in an attempt to address the question of whether laparoscopy increases the risk of tumor cell dissemination and implantation. A variety of hypotheses have been proposed to explain this phenomenon, including direct wound implantation, "chimney effect," aerosolization of tumor cells, pressure of pneumoperitoneum, effect of CO_2, and a decrease in the local immune response. Despite these various theories, no experimental model has provided consistent evidence to support the contention that there is an increased risk of tumor cell dissemination with laparoscopy.

Two large clinical studies have retrospectively attempted to determine the true incidence of port-site implantation. In the initial study (Pearlstone et al, 1999), we evaluated 533 patients at M. D. Anderson with intra-abdominal malignancies who underwent laparoscopic procedures. In that study, there were 4 port-site recurrences, for an incidence of 0.75%. Most significantly, 3 of these port-site recurrences were in patients with carcinomatosis already present at the time of laparoscopy, suggesting that the finding of a port-site implant is more likely a reflection of the natural biology of disease progression. The incidence of a port-site recurrence was significantly greater in patients with carcinomatosis present at the time of laparoscopy than in patients who did not have carcinomatosis (4% vs 0.2%; $P < .0003$). A subsequent study from Memorial Sloan-Kettering Cancer Center confirmed our findings (Shoup et al, 2002). This study reviewed 1,650 diagnostic laparoscopic procedures for upper gastrointestinal malignancy. In this series, the incidence of port-site implantation was 0.79%, very similar to that in the original study from M. D. Anderson. It was also similar to the incidence of incisional recurrence in patients who went on to have an open surgical procedure (0.86%). Additionally, of the 830 patients undergoing curative resection, 5 (0.60%) developed port-site recurrences and 7 (0.84%) developed a recurrence at the open incision site. All 5 of the patients with a port-site recurrence and 5 of the 7 patients with an open incisional recurrence had additional tumor detected either locally or diffusely at the time the port-site implantation was noted. These results are remarkably similar to those in the review by Hughes et al (1983), which is one of the few studies to look at the incidence of incisional recurrence after open colon resection. In this evaluation of a registry of patients undergoing colon resections in New Zealand, 13 (0.81%) of 1,600 patients developed incisional recurrences.

Conclusion

Our use of laparoscopic procedures in patients with gastrointestinal malignancies has been a continually evolving process. Despite initial enthusiasm, there has been a decline in our use of laparoscopy over the last decade for a variety of reasons, including the increased operative time required

KEY PRACTICE POINTS

- Because of advances in radiologic and endoscopically guided percutaneous techniques, enthusiasm for some laparoscopic palliative procedures has diminished. However, laparoscopic colostomies and bypasses are an important option for palliation of malignant intestinal obstructions that are not amenable to percutaneous or endoscopic approaches.

- Laparoscopic staging is not of significant benefit in patients with pancreatic and hepatobiliary malignancies. In contrast, in patients with gastric cancer, in whom the incidence of missed metastatic disease on preoperative CT is about 20%, laparoscopic staging is ideal for identifying peritoneal spread as well as for providing enteral access in patients who are to undergo neoadjuvant therapy.

- Results to date with laparoscopic colon resection have been promising, but because of the technical expertise required to perform the procedure and demonstration of only minimal quality-of-life benefits, further study of laparoscopic colon resection is required.

- Large retrospective studies of the risk of port-site implantation after laparoscopic procedures in patients with intra-abdominal and upper gastrointestinal malignancies have shown a risk of less than 1%, similar to the risk of incisional recurrence in patients undergoing open colon resection.

for laparoscopy and the increased cost associated with the procedure. Additionally, the concomitant improvements in percutaneous techniques have diminished the need for palliative laparoscopic procedures. We still believe that laparoscopic interventions can be of benefit, most notably for staging of disease in patients with gastric cancer and for performing colostomies in patients with malignant large bowel obstruction. On the basis of our series and other available data, we do not believe that tumor implantation at port sites is a significant risk for patients with gastrointestinal malignancies.

Suggested Readings

Bouvet M, Mansfield PF, Skibber JM, et al. Clinical, pathologic, and economic parameters of laparoscopic colon resection for cancer. *Am J Surg* 1998;176:554–558.

Hughes ES, McDermott FT, Polglase AI, et al. Tumor recurrence in the abdominal wall scar tissue after large-bowel cancer surgery. *Dis Colon Rectum* 1983;26: 571–572.

Lacy AM, Garcia-Valdecasas JC, Delgado S, et al. Laparoscopy-assisted colectomy versus open colectomy for treatment of non-metastatic colon cancer: a randomised trial. *Lancet* 2002;359:2224–2229.

Pearlstone DB, Mansfield PF, Curley SA, et al. Laparoscopy in 533 patients with abdominal malignancy. *Surgery* 1999;125:67–72.

Shoup M, Brennan MF, Karpeh MS, et al. Port site metastasis after diagnostic laparoscopy for upper gastrointestinal tract malignancies: an uncommon entity. *Ann Surg Oncol* 2002;9:632–636.

Weeks JC, Nelson H, Gelber S, et al. Short-term quality-of-life outcomes following laparoscopic-assisted colectomy vs open colectomy for colon cancer: a randomized trial. *JAMA* 2002;287:321–328.

6   RISK FACTORS FOR COLORECTAL CANCER SUSCEPTIBILITY

Christopher I. Amos, Carol H. Bosken,
Amr S. Soliman, and Marsha L. Frazier

CHAPTER OVERVIEW

A wide range of environmental factors influence risks for colorectal cancer. Patterns of food consumption, exercise, and the use of nonsteroidal anti-inflammatory drugs (NSAIDs) affect risk for colorectal cancer. The strong risk reduction for colorectal cancer associated with NSAID use provides a strong rationale for chemoprevention studies. However, in considering the application of any chemopreventive agent, the risk and impact of side effects must be considered. Other possible interventions, such as behavioral modification to increase exercise, would most likely reduce the risk for colorectal cancer, but effecting this type of change may be difficult.

Genetic studies can provide novel insights into the etiology of colorectal cancer. Case-control studies may be readily conducted and have provided novel insights into the role of DNA repair and metabolic genes in colorectal cancer causation. Cohort studies may avoid some biases associated with selection into case-control studies but are often complex and costly to conduct. In this chapter, we describe and compare these approaches.

At M. D. Anderson Cancer Center, we have focused primarily on the study of individuals at genetically high risk for colorectal cancer. Subjects at high risk for cancer are most likely to benefit from chemopreventive strategies and can provide the greatest information about novel screening modalities. However, findings from high-risk subjects may not generalize to a broader population, and large studies are needed to evaluate the role of genetic and environmental factors in lower-risk populations.

INTRODUCTION

Colorectal cancer is the second leading cause of death from cancer at all sites in both sexes; an estimated 148,300 new cases of colorectal cancer and 56,600 deaths from the disease occurred in 2002 in the United States (American Cancer Society, 2003). Incidence rates vary significantly around the world. The highest age-adjusted rates (25 to 35 per 100,000) occur in North America, Western Europe, and Australia. Rates in Asia and Africa are low but are increasing with migration and westernization, largely because of dietary and environmental changes.

The colorectal cancer incidence in the United States and western countries is high among people older than 60 years of age but much lower in people under age 30 (0.86% to 3.2% of cases) and people under age 40 (2% to 6% of cases). The age distribution for colon cancer fits well with the multistage theory of tumorigenesis. This theory predicts an exponential time to onset for cancer, with the age-dependent slope depending on the number of events that are required for tumor development. For colon cancer, the model indicates that for most people, 4 to 6 events are needed for transformation of cells from normal colonic mucosa to carcinoma. Modeling of the different regions of the bowel indicates differences by site, with fewer events needed in models that include younger patients with cancer of the proximal colon (Dubrow et al, 1994).

One approach to identifying novel factors that predispose to colorectal cancer is the search for factors that decrease the age of onset of colorectal cancer. Genetic factors can have a profound effect in decreasing the age of onset of colorectal cancer. In addition, colorectal cancer trends show marked differences by country of origin. Our ongoing international studies have found a high incidence of very early onset colorectal cancer in Egypt not associated with familial or genetic factors (Soliman et al, 2001), suggesting that unique environmental factors predispose this population to colorectal cancer (Soliman et al, 1997). Early-onset cases throughout the world are more likely to show less favorable histologic subtypes, such as mucinous or signet ring cell, suggesting differences in etiology between early-onset cancers and cancers occurring at later ages. Individuals who have carcinomas with an unusual histologic subtype may receive better care in a tertiary care environment, where more of these cancers are treated.

A wide range of environmental and familial risk factors have been implicated as modifying the risk for colorectal cancer (Potter, 1999). In this chapter, we first provide a brief description of the epidemiologic methods used to characterize risk factors. We then summarize data concerning major epidemiologic and genetic risk factors for colorectal cancer. We also provide information about gene-gene and gene-environment interactions in the etiology of colorectal cancer.

IDENTIFYING EPIDEMIOLOGIC AND GENETIC RISK FACTORS FOR COLORECTAL CANCER

Most epidemiologic studies cannot be designed as controlled experiments. Therefore, epidemiologic studies identify associations between risk factors and disease outcomes. Associations can be useful for classifying individuals into risk sets, whether or not a causal relationship between the disease and its correlate can be established. Typical measures of risk include the absolute risk, relative risk, and odds ratio. Here we briefly describe the main risk measures; much more detail can be found in standard epidemiologic reference texts such as those by Selvin (2001) and Rothman (2002).

Absolute risk is the most easily interpreted risk measure and is often specified in terms of risk per time unit per individual. Using the definitions in Table 6–1, the absolute risk among exposed individuals (e.g., individuals exposed to an environmental carcinogen or with a disease-causing genotype) per unit time is $a/(a + c)$. The relative risk is the risk for disease among individuals who have been exposed to a risk factor divided by the risk for disease among individuals who have not been exposed to that risk factor: $[a/(a + c)]/[b/(b + d)]$. Finally, the odds ratio is the ratio of the exposed individuals among the diseased to the exposed individuals among the nondiseased, divided by the ratio of the nonexposed individuals among the diseased to the nonexposed individuals among the

Table 6–1. Parameters for Calculating Risk in Epidemiologic Studies

Disease Condition	Exposed	Not Exposed	Total
Diseased	a	b	a + b
Not diseased	c	d	c + d
Total	a + c	b + d	

nondiseased: $(a/c)/(b/d)$. When the proportion of cases in a population is low, the odds ratio nearly equals the relative risk (i.e., $a + c \approx c$ and $b + d \approx d$). For relative risks greater than 1, the odds ratio overestimates the relative risk; however, the odds ratio is nearly unbiased in studies of uncommon events such as the risk for developing specific cancers. Odds ratios can be obtained directly from case-control studies, while cohort studies can give all 3 risks.

Cohort Studies

Prospective cohort studies are performed by identifying a group of subjects, collecting samples and/or data from them at baseline, and then following them forward over time. The advantage of this design is that one can establish temporal relationships between events and causes, and biases related to incomplete recall of exposures are minimized. The disadvantages of the prospective cohort design include difficulty maintaining follow-up with the study subjects and potential inefficiency if the disease outcome of interest is infrequent. One approach to limit the cost of prospective cohort studies is to establish the cohort and then conduct laboratory analyses only for study subjects who become affected along with a matched set of study subjects who do not become affected. This type of design is called a nested case-control design because it is a case-control study nested within a cohort (Wacholder et al, 1992)

Retrospective cohort studies are conducted by identifying a set of study subjects at present and then tracing their histories. This type of study provides estimates of absolute and relative risk, and it is often easier to conduct than the prospective cohort study. However, the retrospective design may accrue biases if the study subjects are required to recall exposures (such as intake of foods) that occurred in the past. Results from cohort studies may be hard to generalize to any other population, depending on how the cohort is established.

Assessing Familiality and Segregation Analysis

The historical cohort design is often used for family studies (Amos and Rubin, 1995). In this type of study, families are selected through an index case or proband. Information is then collected from the proband about his or her relatives' current age, age at onset of cancer(s), and age at death. The historical cohort design has the advantages of other cohort designs, while minimizing study costs. Data from many cancers are reliably collected for first-degree relatives (King et al, 2002).

The kin-cohort study (Wacholder et al, 1998) is a version of the historical cohort method in which mutation data from probands are used to construct penetrance estimates for the mutations. Penetrance is the probability that an individual with an at-risk genotype will get a disease. In the kin-cohort approach, the age at onset among first-degree relatives of mutation-positive probands is compared with the age at onset among first-degree relatives of mutation-negative probands.

Segregation analysis is an alternative approach for estimating the penetrance of genetic factors predisposing for cancer. Segregation analyses seek to identify the relationship between an individual's genotype and the resulting phenotype. Inheritance of genetic factors results in a specific form of dependence among family members. When the genotypes at a disease locus cannot be directly measured, the inheritance of disease within families can still be compared with that expected under specific genetic models. The models to evaluate include effects from a single genetic factor that substantially affects the penetrance; environmental effects that may be correlated among family members; and residual familial correlations (Lalouel et al, 1983; Demenais, 1991). Segregation analytical methods have been adapted to model penetrance from *BRCA1* and *BRCA2* mutations while allowing for ascertainment (Antoniou et al, 2002), but models to predict genetic risks for colorectal cancer susceptibility remain poorly developed.

FACTORS ASSOCIATED WITH RISK FOR COLORECTAL CANCER

Colorectal cancer is common in the western world, with an estimated 6% lifetime risk for people living in the United States. However, this summary figure obscures significant differences in risk associated with exposure to endogenous and exogenous risk factors (Potter, 1999). A sedentary lifestyle (Le Marchand et al, 1999), a "western diet" (Slattery et al, 2000), and diets low in certain nutrients (Fuchs et al, 2002) are much more highly associated with colorectal cancer in patients with a positive family history than in patients with a negative family history. Moreover, the use of hormone replacement therapy (HRT) may be more protective in women with a negative family history (Kampman et al, 1997).

Inflammatory Bowel Disease

Another endogenous factor associated with an increased risk of colorectal cancer is inflammatory bowel disease. Early studies of patients with

Crohn's disease or ulcerative colitis demonstrated a risk of 20 to 30 times the average population risk. The risk was highest in patients who had been diagnosed with inflammatory bowel disease early in life and those with extensive, active disease. Recent studies from both the United States and Europe have shown decreasing risks over time for colorectal cancer from inflammatory bowel disease. Treatment with sulfasalazine and newer drugs, intense surveillance, and colectomy for intractable disease have all contributed to the decreased incidence of colorectal cancer.

Factors Related to a Western Lifestyle

Many other factors that increase the risk of colorectal cancer are related to a western lifestyle. These include obesity, inactivity, and various dietary elements. Obesity and inactivity are independently associated with an increased risk of colorectal cancer, although the association with obesity is most marked in inactive individuals, and conversely, the effects of inactivity are most prominent in obese individuals. In men, there is a linear relationship between body mass index (weight in kilograms divided by the square of the height in meters) and risk of colorectal cancer, while in women the association is less consistent and is only apparent in younger women. In both sexes, the effects are most marked in frankly obese individuals (body mass index >30 kg/m^2). Long-term, vigorous physical activity is associated with a decreased risk of colorectal cancer. Again, the association is most marked in men, but this conclusion is somewhat uncertain since few of the women in most of the observational studies have been included in the groups that exercised vigorously. At least several hours a week of vigorous, sweat-producing exercise is probably required before a protective effect can be demonstrated.

While consuming a "Western diet" high in saturated fats and red meat and low in fiber has long been suspected to be a risk factor for the development of several cancers, uncertainty remains about which factors are the most important. A high intake of fruits and vegetables exerts a modest protective effect in most studies; however, an adverse effect from a high intake of saturated fat has been difficult to prove. Many investigators think that consumption of red meat, which is also high in saturated fat, is a more important risk factor for the development of colorectal cancer than saturated fat intake. A recent meta-analysis of 13 observational studies estimated a relative risk of only 1.3 (with a 95% confidence interval of 1.13 to 1.49) per 100 grams per day for red meat consumption (Sandhu et al, 2001). A diet high in fiber was suspected to be protective on the basis of the difference in cancer incidence between people living in the United States and those living in Africa, who have high fiber consumption. Although early observational studies supported the association, later, larger trials did not (Potter and Hunter, 2002). A weak but consistent increase in risk has been found with excessive alcohol consumption (Potter, 1999). A meta-analysis of 27 studies found a 10% increased risk in people who had 2 drinks a day (Longnecker et al, 1990).

Calcium and Folate Supplementation

Calcium and folate supplementation have been the subject of intense investigation in recent years. Folate, measured either as dietary folate or as a supplement in vitamin pills, has been shown to be protective in several large observational studies (Giovannucci et al, 1998). The protection increases with duration of therapy and is greatest in people on a low-methionine, high-alcohol diet. In addition, in 1 large cohort, the protection afforded by high folate intake was seen only in women with a positive family history for colorectal cancer (Fuchs et al, 2002). Population studies with long follow-up periods also show a protective effect of calcium intake.

Cigarette Smoking

An association has also been found between cigarette smoking and colorectal cancer, but the smoking pattern appears to be an important co-determinant of risk. An early age of smoking initiation and higher number of pack-years smoked before age 30 appear to be the most important determinants of colorectal cancer risk. These findings may be due to either stronger effects of smoking on tumor initiation than on progression or a higher risk from cigarette formulations of the 1950s and 1960s. Support for the role of cigarette smoke in the development of colorectal cancer comes from the clear-cut association of smoking with the development and progression of colorectal adenomas, which are precursor lesions for colorectal cancer.

Nonsteroidal Anti-inflammatory Drugs

Recent studies showed that several pharmacologic interventions prevent the development of colorectal cancer. On the basis of the observation that patients with rheumatoid arthritis and other diseases that are usually treated with aspirin have a lower-than-average risk for colorectal cancer, cohort and case-control studies were initiated to investigate the therapeutic properties of nonsteroidal anti-inflammatory drugs (NSAIDs) in protecting individuals from malignancies. At least 5 cohort and 6 case-control studies provide evidence of protection from NSAIDs (Thun et al, 2002). In most studies, NSAIDs were taken at least weekly for 5 to 10 years before the effect was found, but the protective effect may be lost a year after discontinuation of NSAID use. Prospective trials of NSAIDs to prevent the recurrence of colorectal adenomas have been successful in patients with familial adenomatous polyposis (FAP) (Steinbach et al, 2000). On the other hand, 1 controlled trial of aspirin to prevent colorectal cancer found no protective effect (Sturmer et al, 1998). However, the 7 years of follow-up in this study may not have been sufficient to detect NSAIDs' effects. Observational studies of NSAID use may be particularly prone to biases in subject selection since healthier subjects may be more likely to report use of NSAIDs. Therefore, well-controlled trials are particularly important to assess the importance of these drugs in colorectal cancer prevention.

Hormone Replacement Therapy

In women, HRT has been shown to protect against colorectal cancer. Numerous observational studies have shown an association between recent and prolonged use of HRT in postmenopausal women and decreased incidence of colorectal cancer. Recently, a controlled trial of HRT conducted by the Women's Health Initiative showed a 38% decrease in the incidence of colorectal cancer after 5 years of HRT use. Before HRT can be considered indicated for colorectal chemoprevention, its protective effect against colorectal cancer must be weighed against the increased risk of breast cancer and thromboembolism.

Screening

Regardless of the genetic or lifestyle risk factors, the incidence of colorectal cancer can be decreased through the use of medical surveillance. Either annual fecal occult blood testing with follow-up endoscopy or endoscopy at 5- to 10-year intervals substantially decreases the risk of developing and dying of colorectal cancer.

Genetic Factors

Aside from age, familial and genetic factors are the most consistently associated with increased risk for colorectal cancer. Numerous studies have assessed the increased risk associated with being a close relative of an individual who develops colon or rectal cancer. Increased risks have been found in all epidemiologic studies of familial risk (Johns and Houlston, 2001). The pooled relative risk across 27 studies for development of colorectal cancer in a first-degree relative of a colorectal cancer patient was 2.25, and this relative risk increased to 4.25 if 2 first-degree relatives had colorectal cancer (Johns and Houlston, 2001).

Hereditary conditions that greatly increase the risk for colorectal cancer include FAP, Peutz-Jeghers syndrome, and hereditary nonpolyposis colorectal cancer (HNPCC). The frequency of FAP is estimated to be 2 cases per 10,000 (Burn et al, 1991), while Peutz-Jeghers syndrome is perhaps 4 times rarer. HNPCC is far more common than other forms of inherited susceptibility to colorectal cancer, but even its frequency has not been well estimated. Aaltonen et al (1998) found that 2% of patients with colorectal cancer had mutations in DNA mismatch repair genes. Worldwide, hereditary bowel cancer usually occurs at a relatively young age but accounts for no more than 5% of all large-bowel malignancies (Longnecker et al, 1990). Individuals in families with a tendency to develop colorectal cancer have a 50% chance of inheriting the cancer gene and a high probability of developing the disease thereafter, depending upon the familial syndrome. The risk for developing colorectal cancer among individuals with FAP approaches 100%. Surgical intervention is indicated for individuals with FAP (see chapter 7), but chemopreventive agents that inhibit cyclooxygenase-2 (COX-2), such as celecoxib, have decreased the number of polyps in subjects with FAP (Steinbach et al, 2000). Rarer mutations of the adenomatous polyposis coli (APC) gene underlying FAP yield lower risks for colorectal cancer (Su et al, 2000). A subset of these mutations that show variable expression in the numbers of polyps result from exonic deletions and would not be identified by direct sequencing of the APC gene (Su et al, 2002). Finally, the I1307K variant form of the APC gene confers a slightly less than 2-fold increased risk of colorectal cancer through unfaithful replication of the APC gene (Woodage et al, 1998). This variant is predominantly found in Ashkenazi Jews and is rare in other populations.

Peutz-Jeghers syndrome is a rare autosomal condition in which carriers often show hyperpigmented mucocutaneous macules and develop hamartomas of the small intestine. Individuals with the syndrome have an estimated 11-fold increased relative risk for colorectal cancer (Boardman et al, 1998). Peutz-Jeghers syndrome predisposes for an increased risk of cancer at numerous sites, including the colon, breast, stomach, small intestine, pancreas, and gonads (Giardiello et al, 2000). Recent studies have shown that COX-2 is overexpressed in polyps from patients with Peutz-Jeghers syndrome (Rossi et al, 2002; McGarrity et al, 2003), suggesting that COX-2 inhibition might be an effective chemopreventive strategy for these individuals.

HNPCC is the most common form of hereditary colorectal cancer. Most cases of HNPCC are due to germline mutations in DNA mismatch repair genes. Germline mutations have been identified in the mismatch repair genes hMSH2, hMLH1, hPMS2, and hMSH6 (Peltomaki, 2003). Colorectal and endometrial carcinomas are the 2 most common cancers in family members with HNPCC (Vasen et al, 2001). Other organs affected are the stomach, pancreas, biliary tract, ovaries, and urinary tract.

The Amsterdam criteria were established to provide a means of identifying subjects at very high risk for inherited susceptibility to colorectal cancer who did not have syndromic forms, such as FAP and Peutz-Jeghers syndrome. A family meets the Amsterdam criteria if it includes 3 individuals affected with colorectal cancer, 1 cancer occurred in a person younger than age 50 years, colorectal cancer occurred in 2 generations, and 1 of the affected individuals is a first-degree relative of the other 2. In 1997, a panel of experts in the field of colorectal cancer suggested modified criteria, referred to as the Bethesda Guidelines, for identifying HNPCC families (Rodriguez-Bigas et al, 1997). Pursuant to these criteria, an HNPCC family is one that has any of the following characteristics: (a) family fulfills Amsterdam criteria; (b) individuals with 2 HNPCC-related cancers, including synchronous and metachronous colorectal cancers or associated extra-colonic cancers; (c) individuals with colorectal cancer and a first-degree relative with colorectal cancer and/or HNPCC-related extracolonic cancer and/or colorectal adenoma; 1 of the cancers diagnosed before age 45 years and the adenoma diagnosed before age 40 years; (d) individuals with colorectal cancer or endometrial cancer diagnosed before age 45 years; (e) individuals with right-sided colorectal cancer with an undifferentiated pattern (solid or cribriform) on histopathologic examination diagnosed before age 45 years; (f) individuals with signet-ring-cell-type colorectal cancer diagnosed before age 45 years; and (g) individuals with adenomas diagnosed before age 40 years. This complex set of criteria has been intro-duced to capture a larger collection of families at high risk for carrying mutations in DNA mismatch repair genes.

In recognition of the elevated risks associated with inherited forms of cancer, we have developed questionnaires and software to collect family information from individuals who are seen at M. D. Anderson Cancer Center. Individuals seen at M. D. Anderson are sent a family history ques-tionnaire. Patients enrolled in epidemiologic studies are also sent a detailed questionnaire that solicits information about the major risk factors described above. Completing these questionnaires prior to their visit pro-vides patients with time to complete all the requested information and to solicit additional input from relatives if needed. A sample page from the family history questionnaire for patients in whom hereditary colorectal cancer is suspected is presented in Figure 6–1. To assist patients in com-pleting the questionnaire, we provide them with a sample pedigree on the first page and then depict a small part of the pedigree on each subsequent page that they are asked to complete. Data are subsequently entered into a secure SQL/server database. This database is linked to Progeny Any-where, a program that allows us to draw the pedigree and depict cancers and other information. A copy of the pedigree is relayed to the patient for confirmation.

To obtain accurate risk information about the relatives of a patient, one must collect the date of birth, current age (if alive) or age at death, and ages at cancer onset for all relatives with cancers. Generally, only cancer information from the patient's first-degree relatives is deemed reliable without additional confirmation from other sources such as other rela-tives. In addition, patients often confuse primary and metastatic forms of cancer for certain sites (e.g., brain and bone). They are also often confused about the site of primary internal-organ cancers, but patients report breast, prostate, and colon cancers rather reliably (King et al, 2002). Cervical, endometrial, and ovarian cancers are often reported with the term "female organs." The cancers in sites that are often misreported should be con-firmed, when possible, by ascertainment of pathologic diagnoses or medical records, before additional analyses (such as genetic testing) are conducted. Confirmation of putative cancers in relatives is complex in the

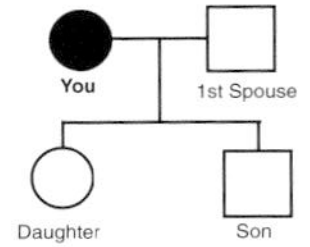

OFFICE USE ONLY
Medical Record No. ________
Study No. ________
DID No. ________

CHILDREN FROM YOUR FIRST SPOUSE OR PARTNER

Please read across the page for each person.

Your Full Name:	Sex	Date of birth	Have you ever had cancer?	First type of cancer	Age at diagnosis or year	Second type of cancer	Age at diagnosis or year	Other major medical conditions?
________ First Middle Last (Maiden)	☐ M ☐ F	________ mo/day/yr	☐ Yes ☐ No		____Age Yr. ____		____Age Yr. ____	

YOUR CHILDREN AND THEIR PARENT (only partnerships with children):

Full Name First Middle Last (Maiden)	Sex	Date of birth mo/day/yr	Alive or dead?	Date of death mo/day/yr	Age at death	Ever had cancer?	First type of cancer	Age at diagnosis or year	Second type of cancer	Age at diagnosis or year	Other major medical conditions?
Spouse/Partner	☐ M ☐ F		☐ Alive ☐ Dead ☐ Unknown			☐ Yes ☐ No ☐ Unknown		____Age Yr. ____		____Age Yr. ____	
Children 1.	☐ M ☐ F		☐ Alive ☐ Dead ☐ Unknown			☐ Yes ☐ No ☐ Unknown		____Age Yr. ____		____Age Yr. ____	
2.	☐ M ☐ F		☐ Alive ☐ Dead ☐ Unknown			☐ Yes ☐ No ☐ Unknown		____Age Yr. ____		____Age Yr. ____	
3.	☐ M ☐ F		☐ Alive ☐ Dead ☐ Unknown			☐ Yes ☐ No ☐ Unknown		____Age Yr. ____		____Age Yr. ____	
4.	☐ M ☐ F		☐ Alive ☐ Dead ☐ Unknown			☐ Yes ☐ No ☐ Unknown		____Age Yr. ____		____Age Yr. ____	

If you need space for more children with the same partner continue on next page. If you had more children with an additional partner, complete that information on **Another Partner Page**.
If you did not have an additional partner and children, go to **Your Parents, Siblings** page to complete the next section.

Figure 6–1. Sample page from the family history questionnaire given to patients with suspected hereditary colorectal cancer at M. D. Anderson Cancer Center. Copyright 1998 The University of Texas M. D. Anderson Cancer Center. Reprinted with permission.

United States and becoming ever more difficult. The new privacy rule implemented as part of the Health Insurance Portability and Accountability Act precludes getting information on decedent individuals without informed consent from a next of kin. Pathologic findings from tumors are also covered by the privacy rule, so informed consent may be required for relatives from whom one would like to obtain confirmatory information about tumor diagnoses, depending upon the ruling of each center's privacy board or Institutional Review Board. An example of a request for release of medical records that could be used for obtaining information from relatives is provided on our Web site, www.epigenetic.org. The barriers to access to information from relatives caused by Health Insurance Portability and Accountability Act regulations is likely to impede accurate diagnosis of HNPCC. Genetic counseling, which may be indicated if there is a strong family history or if syndromic forms are identified, is further discussed in chapter 8.

HYPERMETHYLATION AND COLORECTAL CANCER

Tumor suppressor genes, such as *p16* and *hMLH1*, are inactivated in colorectal cancers by mutation, deletion, or methylation (Kane et al, 1997). Abnormal patterns of DNA methylation are common molecular changes in human neoplasms, including colorectal cancer. *p16* methylation is closely associated with K-*ras* mutations (Guan et al, 1999). Also, aberrant methylation is associated with the microsatellite instability (MSI) phenotype in colorectal cancer. Recent studies showed that hypermethylation of the *MLH1* promoter region is common in MSI-positive sporadic colorectal cancers (Cunningham et al, 1998). Hypermethylation of *MLH1* is also associated with the absence of immunoreactive MLH1 protein (Miyakura et al, 2001).

Most sporadic cancers with an MSI phenotype are hypermethylated in the promoter region of *hMLH1*, whereas mutations and allelic loss cause the MSI phenotype in most HNPCC cancers (Wheeler et al, 2000).

GENE-GENE INTERACTIONS

Recognizing the important role that familial and genetic factors have in determining individual risk for colorectal cancer, our interdisciplinary group at M. D. Anderson has focused primarily on the elucidation of genetic factors influencing colorectal cancer susceptibility. For the study of subjects with DNA mismatch repair defects, we have used a retrospective cohort approach to study the time to onset for colorectal cancer. This type of design is powerful for identifying effects from genetic factors but does not readily yield reliable estimates of the absolute risks for cancer, because the study participants are derived from a clinic population. As population-based frequencies of cancer in families become available through the Cancer Genetics Network and the Cooperative Family Registries studies, which are collaborative studies established by the National Cancer Institute, it may be possible to embed the observed family structures that we are studying into the population-based structures. In the absence of these correction methods, we can still obtain unbiased estimates of the relative risk for cancer from genetic factors by comparing the time to onset of cancer among those with or without at-risk genotypes.

In studying individuals with DNA mismatch repair mutations, we found a strong association between time to onset of colorectal cancer and a polymorphism of cyclin D1 that inserts an adenosine (A) for a guanine (G) in codon 242, which results in alternate splicing and higher levels of this protein (Kong et al, 2000). Increased levels of cyclin D1 induce the transition from the G1 to the S phase, and higher levels of cyclin D1 may lead to decreased ability to repair DNA damage. We found that a cyclin D1 polymorphism that increased altered splicing of the cyclin D1 RNA had a major influence on the age of onset of HNPCC. The results showed that individuals with AA or AG genotypes had a 2.5-fold higher rate of cancer per year compared to individuals with the GG genotype. We also observed an association of cyclin D1 polymorphism with earlier-onset sporadic colorectal cancer in a case-control design (Kong et al, 2001).

Mutations in N-acetyltransferase 2 (NAT2), a highly polymorphic enzyme involved in the metabolism of xenobiotics and carcinogens, may affect colorectal cancer risk, especially among individuals with germline mutations in DNA mismatch repair genes. We found that individuals with the NAT2*7 variant had a significantly higher risk of colorectal cancer (hazard ratio = 2.96; $P = .012$) and all cancers (hazard ratio = 3.37, $P = .00004$) than individuals homozygous for the wild type at the NAT2*7 allele (Frazier et al, 2001). These findings suggest that the NAT2 genotype may be an important factor in the tumorigenesis of colorectal cancer and cancers related to HNPCC.

ENVIRONMENTAL FACTORS RELATED TO HEREDITARY AND FAMILIAL COLORECTAL CANCER

Familial colorectal cancer may reflect the influence of multiple genetic factors along with environmental cofactors. Fuchs et al (2002) found that women with high folate intake who had a first-degree relative with colorectal cancer were not at increased risk for colorectal cancer. However, women with low folate intake who had a relative with colorectal cancer had about a 2.5-fold increased relative risk for colorectal cancer compared with women with low folate intake and no family history of colorectal cancer. The effect of environmental exposures on risk for cancer among individuals with inherited susceptibility has not yet been studied. However, exposures, such as low folate intake, that are thought to impair DNA repair capacity would be expected to further increase the risk for colorectal cancer among individuals with mismatch repair defects.

Several studies have elucidated relationships between certain environmental exposures and genetic markers in colorectal carcinogenesis. For example, *p53* mutations can provide clues to the nature of exogenous agents and endogenous cellular events that are important to the natural history of human cancer. A recent study from Singapore showed K-*ras* mutations in 28% of 50 specimens from the period 1988–1992 versus 0% in 18 archival specimens from the period 1968–1972 (Tang et al, 1999). The study's researchers concluded that the increase seen over the 30-year period may have been due to the consumption of a western diet, along with increased intake of cooked meat and heterocyclic amines such as 2-amino-3-methylimidazo[4,5-f]quinoline and a resulting increase in aberrant crypt foci, as suggested by tests in experimental animals (Snyderwine et al, 2002).

The rate of mutation in tumors originating in the ascending colon is significantly higher than that in tumors originating in the descending colon, consistent with a decreasing gradient of a mutagen along the length of human colorectum. As such, K-*ras* activation is potentially a "fingerprint" marker of an as yet unknown exogenous mutagen.

CONCLUSIONS

The most important determinants of colorectal cancer risk are age and family history. In addition, environmental factors—such as a diet rich in saturated fats, high in red meats, and low in fiber or fruits and vegetables—appear to increase the risk for colorectal cancer. NSAID use is associated with a decreased risk for colorectal cancer in observational studies. NSAIDs decrease COX-2 levels. Clinical trials in individuals with FAP documented decreased development of adenomas from chemoprevention by COX-2 inhibitors. Therefore, chemoprevention with COX-2 inhibitors is likely to be an effective approach for decreasing risk for colorectal cancer, particularly in individuals with FAP, but possibly for the broader population as well. Interactions between genetic and environmental factors are likely to create subpopulations of individuals at much higher risk for colorectal cancer development. Further studies to identify and reliably estimate the risks for these subgroups are under way at M. D. Anderson and at other centers. To assemble sufficient numbers of individuals, collaborative efforts are required across institutions, both for observational studies and for clinical trials investigating novel chemopreventive agents and screening modalities.

KEY PRACTICE POINTS

- A family history of colorectal cancer increases the risk in first-degree relatives by about 2.3-fold.

- Rare genetic syndromes or additional family history further increases risk.

- In the collection of family histories, the number of affected relatives and their ages are important. It is useful to collect information about all cancers, but only data from first-degree relatives are reliable without additional confirmatory information.

- Other epidemiologic risk factors have a less clear impact on risk for cancer. Diets deficient in folate, calcium, and fiber and high in red meats and saturated fats increase risks for colorectal cancers. Smoking and alcohol use have only a small impact on risk for colorectal cancer.

- Cohort studies provide more readily interpretable risk information than do case-control studies but are more difficult to conduct and may not be as readily generalized in some cases.

- Use of NSAIDs is associated with a decreased risk for colorectal cancer.

- Some subsets of individuals with combinations of risk factors may be at particularly elevated risks for colorectal cancer, but further studies are required to better define these risk patterns.

SUGGESTED READINGS

Aaltonen LA, Salovaara R, Kristo P, et al. Incidence of hereditary nonpolyposis colorectal cancer and the feasibility of molecular screening for the disease. *N Engl J Med* 1998;338:1481–1487.

American Cancer Society. *Cancer Facts and Figures, 2002.* Atlanta, Ga: American Cancer Society; 2003.

Amos CI, Rubin LA. Major gene analysis for disease and disorders of complex etiology. *Exp Clin Immunogenet* 1995;12:141–155.

Antoniou AC, Pharoah PD, McMullan G, et al. A comprehensive model for familial breast cancer incorporating BRCA1, BRCA2 and other genes. *Br J Cancer* 2002;86:76–83.

Boardman LA, Thibodeau SN, Schaid DJ, et al. Increased risk for cancer in patients with the Peutz-Jeghers syndrome. *Ann Intern Med* 1998;128:896–899.

Burn J, Chapman P, Delhanty J, et al. The UK northern region genetic register for familial adenomatous polyposis coli: use of age of onset, congenital hypertrophy of the retinal pigment epithelium, and DNA markers in risk calculations. *J Med Genet* 1991;28:289–296.

Cunningham JM, Christensen ER, Tester DJ, et al. Hypermethylation of the hMLH1 promoter in colon cancer with microsatellite instability. *Cancer Res* 1998;58: 3455–3460.

Demenais FM. Regressive logistic models for familial diseases. A formulation assuming an underlying liability model. *Am J Hum Genet* 1991;49:773–785.

Dubrow R, Johansen C, Skov T, et al. Age-period-cohort modelling of large-bowel-cancer incidence by anatomic sub-site and sex in Denmark. *Int J Cancer* 1994; 58:324–329.

Ekbom A, Helmick C, Zack M, et al. Ulcerative colitis and colorectal cancer: a population-based study. *N Engl J Med* 1990;323:1228–1233.

Frazier ML, O'Donnell FT, Kong S, et al. Age associated risk of cancer among individuals with NAT2 mutations and mutations in DNA mismatch repair genes. *Cancer Res* 2001;61:1269–1271.

Fuchs CS, Willett WC, Colditz GA, et al. The influence of folate and multivitamin use on the familial risk of colon cancer in women. *Cancer Epidemiol Biomarkers Prev* 2002;11:227–234.

Giardiello FM, Brensinger JD, Tersmette AC, et al. Very high risk of cancer in familial Peutz-Jeghers syndrome. *Gastroenterology* 2000;119:1447–1453.

Gillen CD, Walmsley RS, Prior P, et al. Ulcerative colitis and Crohn's disease: a comparison of the colorectal cancer risk in extensive colitis. *Gut* 1994;35:1590–1592.

Giovannucci E. Modifiable risk factors for colon cancer. *Gastroenterol Clin North Am* 2002;31:925–943.

Giovannucci E, Rimm EB, Ascherio A, et al. Alcohol, low-methionine–low-folate diets, and risk of colon cancer in men. *J Natl Cancer Inst* 1995;87:265–273.

Giovannucci E, Stampfer MJ, Colditz GA, et al. Multivitamin use, folate, and colon cancer in women in the Nurses' Health Study. *Ann Intern Med* 1998;129: 517–524.

Gridley G, McLaughlin JK, Ekbom A, et al. Incidence of cancer among patients with rheumatoid arthritis. *J Natl Cancer Inst* 1993;85:307–311.

Grodstein F, Newcomb PA, Stampfer MJ. Post menopausal hormone therapy and the risk of colorectal cancer: a review and meta-analysis. *Am J Med* 1999;106: 574–582.

Guan RJ, Fu Y, Holt PR, et al. Association of K-ras mutations with p16 methylation in human colon cancer. *Gastroenterology* 1999;116:1063–1071.

Johns LE, Houlston RS. A systematic review and meta-analysis of familial colorectal cancer risk. *Am J Gastroenterol* 2001;96:2992–3003.

Kampman E, Potter JD, Slattery ML, et al. Hormone replacement therapy, reproductive history, and colon cancer: a multicenter, case-control study in the United States. *Cancer Causes Control* 1997;8:146–158.

Kane MF, Loda M, Gaida GM, et al. Methylation of the hMLH1 promoter correlates with lack of expression of hMLH1 in sporadic colon tumors and the mismatch repair-defective human tumor cell lines. *Cancer Res* 1997;57:808–811.

King TM, Tong L, Pack RJ, et al. Accuracy of family history of cancer as reported by men with prostate cancer. *Urology* 2002;59:546–550.

Kong S, Amos CI, Luthra R, et al. Effects of cyclin D1 polymorphism on age of onset of hereditary nonpolyposis colorectal cancer. *Cancer Res* 2000;60:249–252.

Kong SM, Wei QY, Amos CI, et al. Cyclin D1 polymorphism and increased risk of colorectal cancer at young age. *J Natl Cancer Inst* 2001;93:1106–1108.

Lalouel JM, Rao DC, Morton NE, et al. A unified model for complex segregation analysis. *Am J Hum Genet* 1983;35:816–826.

Le Marchand L, Wilkens LR, Hankin JH, et al. Independent and joint effects of family history and lifestyle on colorectal cancer risk: implications for prevention. *Cancer Epidemiol Biomarkers Prev* 1999;8:45–51.

Longnecker MP, Orza MJ, Adams ME, et al. A meta-analysis of alcoholic beverage consumption in relation to risk of colorectal cancer. *Cancer Causes Control* 1990; 1:59–68.

Mandel JS, Church TR, Bond JH, et al. The effect of fecal occult-blood screening on the incidence of colorectal cancer. *N Engl J Med* 2000;343:1603–1607.

McGarrity TJ, Peiffer LP, Amos CI, Frazier ML, Ward MG, Howett MK. Overexpression of cyclooxygenase 2 in hamartomatous polyps of Peutz-Jeghers syndrome. *Am J Gastroenterol* 2003;51:1665–1672.

Miyakura Y, Sugano K, Konishi F, et al. Extensive methylation of hMLH1 promoter region predominates in proximal colon cancer with microsatellite instability. *Gastroenterology* 2001;121:1300–1309.

Peltomaki P. Role of DNA mismatch repair defects in the pathogenesis of human cancer. *J Clin Oncol* 2003;21:1174–1179.

Potter JD. Colorectal cancer: molecules and populations. *J Natl Cancer Inst* 1999;91: 916–932.

Potter JD, Hunter D. Colorectal cancer. In: Adami H-O, Hunter D, Trichopoulos D, eds. *Textbook of Cancer Epidemiology*. New York, NY: Oxford University Press; 2002:188–211.

Rodriguez-Bigas MA, Boland CR, Hamilton SR, et al. A National Cancer Institute workshop on hereditary nonpolyposis colorectal cancer syndrome: meeting highlights and Bethesda guidelines. *J Natl Cancer Inst* 1997;89:1758–1762.

Rosenberg L, Louik C, Shapiro S. Nonsteroidal anti-inflammatory drug use and reduced risk of large bowel carcinoma. *Cancer* 1998;82:2326–2333.

Rossi DJ, Ylikorkala A, Korsisaari N, et al. Induction of cyclooxygenase-2 in a mouse model of Peutz-Jeghers polyposis. *Proc Natl Acad Sci USA* 2002;99:12327–12332.

Rossouw JE, Anderson GL, Prentice RL, et al. Risks and benefits of estrogen plus progestin in healthy postmenopausal women: principal results from the Women's Health Initiative randomized controlled trial. *JAMA* 2002;288: 321–333.

Rothman, Kenneth J. *Epidemiology: An Introduction*. New York, NY: Oxford University Press; 2002.

Rubio CA, Befrits R, Ljung T, et al. Colorectal carcinoma in ulcerative colitis is decreasing in Scandinavian countries. *Anticancer Res* 2001;21:2921–2924.

Sandhu MS, White IR, McPherson K. Systematic review of the prospective cohort studies on meat consumption and colorectal cancer risk: a meta-analytical approach. *Cancer Epidemiol Biomarkers Prev* 2001;10:439–446.

Selvin S. *Epidemiologic Analysis: A Case-Oriented Approach*. New York, NY: Oxford University Press; 2001.

Slattery ML, Edwards SL, Ma K-N, et al. Physical activity and colon cancer: a public health perspective. *Ann Epidemiol* 1997;7:137–145.

Slattery ML, Potter JD. Physical activity and colon cancer: confounding or interaction? *Med Sci Sports Exerc* 2002;34:913–919.

Slattery ML, Potter JD, Ma K-N, et al. Western diet, family history of colorectal cancer, NAT2, GSTM1 and risk of colon cancer. *Cancer Causes Control* 2000; 11:1–8.

Snyderwine EG, Yu M, Schut HA, et al. Effect of CYP1A2 deficiency on hetero-cyclic amine DNA adduct levels in mice. *Food Chem Toxicol* 2002;40:1529–1533.

Soliman AS, Bondy ML, El-Badawy SA, et al. Contrasting molecular pathology of colorectal carcinoma in Egyptian and western patients. *Br J Cancer* 2001;85:1037–1046.

Soliman AS, Smith MA, Cooper SP, et al. Serum organochlorine pesticide levels in patients with colorectal cancer in Egypt. *Arch Environ Health* 1997;52:409–415.

Steinbach G, Lynch PM, Phillips RK, et al. The effect of celecoxib, a cyclooxyge-nase-2 inhibitor, in familial adenomatous polyposis. *N Engl J Med* 2000;342:1946–1952.

Sturmer T, Glynn RJ, Lee I-M, et al. Aspirin use and colorectal cancer: post-trial follow-up data from the physicians' health study. *Ann Intern Med* 1998;128:713–720.

Su LK, Barnes CJ, Yao W, et al. Inactivation of germline mutant APC alleles by attenuated somatic mutations: a molecular genetic mechanism for attenuated familial adenomatous polyposis. *Am J Hum Genet* 2000;67:582–590.

Su LK, Kohlmann W, Ward PA, et al. Different familial adenomatous polyposis phenotypes resulting from deletions of the entire APC exon 15. *Hum Genet* 2002;111:88–95.

Tang WY, Elnatan J, Lee YS, et al. c-Ki-ras mutations in colorectal adenocarcino-mas from a country with a rapidly changing colorectal cancer incidence. *Br J Cancer* 1999;81:237–241.

Terry PD, Miller AB, Rohan TE. Obesity and colorectal cancer risk in women. *Gut* 2002;51:191–194.

Thun MJ, Henley SJ, Patrono C. Nonsteroidal anti-inflammatory drugs as anti-cancer agents: mechanistic, pharmacologic, and clinical issues. *J Natl Cancer Inst* 2002;94:252–266.

Vasen HF, Stormorken A, Menko FH, et al. MSH2 mutation carriers are at higher risk of cancer than MLH1 mutation carriers: a study of hereditary nonpolypo-sis colorectal cancer families. *J Clin Oncol* 2001;19:4074–4080.

Wacholder S, Hartge P, Struewing JP, et al. The kin-cohort study for estimating penetrance. *Am J Epidemiol* 1998;148:623–630.

Wacholder S, Silverman DT, McLaughlin JK, et al. Selection of controls in case-control studies. II. Types of controls. *Am J Epidemiol* 1992;135:1029–1041.

Wheeler JM, Loukola A, Aaltonen LA, et al. The role of hypermethylation of the hMLH1 promoter region in HNPCC versus MSI+ sporadic colorectal cancers. *J Med Genet* 2000;37:588–592.

Winawer SJ, Zauber AG, Ho MN, et al. Prevention of colorectal cancer by colono-scopic polypectomy. *N Engl J Med* 1993;329:1977–1981.

Woodage T, King SM, Wacholder S, et al. The APCI1307K allele and cancer risk in a community-based study of Ashkenazi Jews. *Nat Genet* 1998;20:62–65.

Wu K, Willett WC, Fuchs CS, et al. Calcium intake and risk of colon cancer in women and men. *J Natl Cancer Inst* 2002;94:437–446.

7   COLORECTAL CANCER: SCREENING AND PRIMARY PREVENTION

Patrick M. Lynch

CHAPTER OVERVIEW

Colorectal cancer is one of the most common and serious cancers. The predictable adenoma-to-carcinoma sequence and the relative accessibility of the colon to available screening measures allow many opportunities for early detection and prevention. Accepted screening measures include testing for fecal occult blood, barium enema, flexible sigmoidoscopy, and more recently, colonoscopy. Newer screening techniques include computed tomography colonography and stool-based DNA testing. All of the above have to do with early detection and, in the case of colonoscopy, treatment of early colorectal neoplasia. Because these are still secondary prevention measures, primary prevention through "chemoprevention" is a focal point at M. D. Anderson Cancer Center and elsewhere. Epidemiologic and experimental background have provided a basis for recent clinical trials demonstrating a role for nonselective and selective cyclo-oxygenase-2 inhibition of adenoma progression in an important human condition, familial adenomatous polyposis. One ongoing trial involves use of a combination of agents (celecoxib and difluoromethylornithine) with different proposed mechanisms of action: COX-2 inhibition and ornithine decarboxylase inhibition. Another trial is investigating the role of COX-2 inhibition in potentially delaying onset of first adenomas in young carriers of *APC* gene mutations responsible for familial adenomatous polyposis.

Introduction

Over the past 50 years, there has been a shift in emphasis from tertiary to secondary to primary prevention of colorectal cancer. In this volume, other chapters will concentrate on surgical, chemotherapeutic, and radiotherapeutic measures to minimize the morbidity and mortality associated with the treatment of established malignancy, all of which can be thought of as tertiary prevention. In this chapter, initial attention will be devoted to a brief review of secondary prevention, which we can think of as screening to achieve the earliest possible detection of colorectal neoplasia. Ideally, this detection is at the adenoma stage, at which removal of the precancerous lesion is associated, in principle at least, with the literal prevention of invasive colorectal cancer. Most of this chapter will then discuss primary prevention, the prevention of colorectal cancer by manipulating the underlying risk factors in such a way as to reduce the rate of formation of neoplasia.

Why should investigators be concerned with the primary prevention of colorectal cancer? First, colorectal cancer is among the top 4 cancers (along with lung, breast, and prostate cancer) in terms of overall incidence and mortality. It is therefore a serious problem warranting serious attention on a broad front. Second, there is reason to believe that elimination of environmental (dietary) risk factors could make a difference in the occurrence of colorectal cancer, not unlike the rationale for reducing lung cancer risk by not smoking or by stopping smoking. Third, demonstration of an adenoma-to-carcinoma sequence provides an excellent model for monitoring the effect of drugs or dietary manipulation on a key cancer precursor. Fourth, because of advances in the technology of adenoma and cancer detection (colonoscopy today, perhaps "virtual colonoscopy" with computed tomography tomorrow), monitoring for early lesions is quite feasible.

In this chapter, I will briefly review the development of the several converging areas of investigation that have led to the current generation of clinical colorectal chemoprevention trials. Epidemiologic clues and experimental bases for undertaking specific trials will be recalled. Discussion of the rationale for trial design will be followed by a presentation of our own completed and ongoing trials at M. D. Anderson Cancer Center.

PRINCIPLES OF SCREENING

A successful screening test should be inexpensive, safe, easy to perform, well accepted by consumers and providers, sensitive (identify persons with the disease in question), and specific (exclude persons lacking disease).

Screening for colorectal cancer and precancerous polyps must be carried out with knowledge of the costs, benefits, risks, and limitations. For those who would actually order or perform any of the available tests, a basic understanding of technique is helpful as well.

Several epidemiologic principles should be borne in mind in considering the performance characteristics of commonly employed screening tests. Fecal occult blood testing (FOBT), the test most commonly used, provides a good framework for a brief discussion of factors that affect such important variables as sensitivity, specificity, and positive and negative predictive value.

Sensitivity is the ratio of persons with the disease having positive test results to all subjects with disease. The category of "all with disease" includes both those with positive test results and those with negative test results. The formula for sensitivity then is $TP/(TP + FN)$, where TP = true positive and FN = false negative. From this it can be seen that the most critical factor in determining sensitivity is the rate of false negatives—that is, those persons with the disease in question whose disease is missed by the test. Conversely, *specificity* is the ratio of healthy (disease-free) subjects with a negative test result to the total persons without disease [$TN/(TN + FP)$], where TN = true negative and FP = false positive. Here, the factor adversely affecting specificity is the proportion of false positives. Other important performance characteristics of a test are *positive predictive value* [$TP/(TP + FP)$] and *negative predictive value* [$TN/(TN + FN)$]. Using FOBT to illustrate these, consider the effect of rehydrating FOBT slides. It has been shown that by increasing the positivity rate for FOBT from a range of 2% to 4% up to 6% to 10%, rehydration increases the rate of detection of colorectal cancers. Hence, rehydration improves the sensitivity of the test. However, because colonoscopy performed to follow up such positive test results often yields negative findings, a substantial rate of false positivity is shown to exist for rehydrated slides, representing a compromise in positive predictive value. A trade-off thus exists, and the practitioner or policy-maker must decide, on the basis of other considerations, whether the rate of negative follow-up colonoscopies is an acceptable trade-off in relation to the improved test sensitivity. In fact, those who take into account all the costs and benefits generally conclude that rehydration is not worthwhile.

CURRENT SCREENING RECOMMENDATIONS AND LIMITATIONS

Several measures are currently recommended for colorectal cancer screening, and no single test can be considered ideal (Rex et al, 2000; Smith et al, 2001; Winawer et al, 2003). The options include FOBT (Mandel et al, 1993); flexible sigmoidoscopy (Selby et al, 1992), used alone or in combination with other tests (Lieberman et al, 2001); double-contrast barium enema, often used in combination with flexible sigmoidoscopy; and a more recently discussed approach, "primary" colonoscopy. Firm randomized-trial data support a mortality reduction through the use of FOBT, though significant limitations are conceded, including relatively high false-positive and false-negative rates (Mandel et al, 1993). Nearly as compelling are case-control data showing a mortality advantage of sigmoidoscopy for lesions within reach of the scope (Selby et al, 1992). No data from well-designed trials have been presented to make a case for double-contrast barium enema in achieving a mortality reduction or definite stage-shift in subjects undergoing the test; long history of use and indirect data combine to support recommendations for its use (Rex et al, 1997; Winawer et al, 2000).

Colonoscopy, while a gold standard for finding colorectal neoplasia and removing precancerous adenomas (Lieberman et al, 2000), has been criticized as excessively expensive and risky for use in routine average-risk screening. It has been shown to carry a mortality advantage when used in high-risk groups, such as subjects at risk for hereditary nonpolyposis colorectal cancer (HNPCC). Figure 7–1 shows illustrative portions of 1 representative set of screening guidelines, that of the National Comprehensive Cancer Network. These guidelines differ in only minor respects from those adopted by the American Cancer Society and the American Gastroenterology Association. Similarly detailed National Comprehensive Cancer Network guidelines exist for familial and genetic high-risk screening (see www.nccn.org for a detailed online presentation).

FECAL OCCULT BLOOD TESTING

Randomized trials have shown a consistent 15% to 33% reduction in colorectal cancer mortality through the implementation of annual FOBT (Mandel et al, 1993). In addition, FOBT is certainly the cheapest form of screening available. Although these investigations provide the most concrete evidence favoring screening, the effect of this particular intervention must be considered modest, leading to an examination of its limitations. The low cost of FOBT screening must be weighed against the cost of performing examinations, typically colonoscopy, to follow up positive test results. As noted above, the use of slide rehydration, while improving sensitivity, comes at the cost of a much higher rate of colonoscopy to work

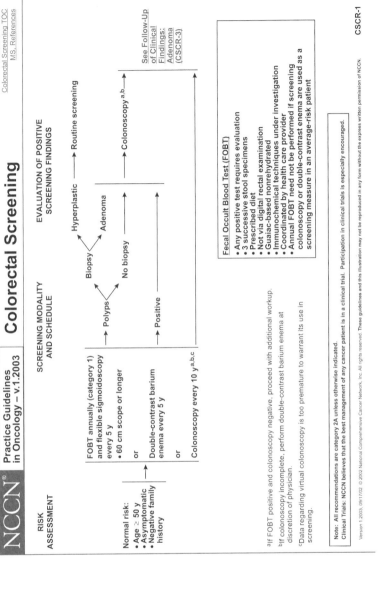

Figure 7-1. National Comprehensive Cancer Network practice guidelines for colorectal screening. These guidelines are a work in progress that will be refined as often as new significant data become available. Reprinted with permission from NCCN 2003 Colorectal Screening Guideline (version 1.2003), "The Complete Library of NCCN Oncology Practice Guidelines" [CD-ROM], (May 2003), Jenkintown, Pennsylvania. To view the most recent and complete version of the guideline, go online to www.nccn.org.

Continued

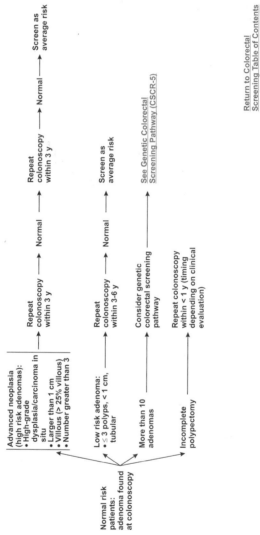

Figure 7-1. *Continued*

up positive screens. In fact, it has been argued that the FOBT trials actually demonstrated the salutary effect of colonoscopy. The additional cost of treating cancers *not* detected by FOBT must be factored into any critical assessment of FOBT performance.

FLEXIBLE SIGMOIDOSCOPY

Flexible sigmoidoscopy is reasonably inexpensive, safe, relatively easy to perform, and accurate in identifying and excluding lesions within its reach. Though the best mortality-improvement data actually come from the era of rigid proctoscopy, investigators have uniformly concluded that flexible sigmoidoscopy is associated with better patient acceptance. In principle, the greater depth of insertion should also achieve the identification of an even higher proportion of lesions. In reality, this last advantage points up the main limitation of flexible sigmoidoscopy, namely its complete lack of sensitivity for lesions beyond its reach. In the most widely cited trial (Selby et al, 1992), no improvement in mortality was observed in subjects ultimately diagnosed with lesions beyond the reach of the (in that study, rigid) scope. This has led to recommendations for *combined* use of FOBT and flexible sigmoidoscopy, thought to perhaps achieve a mortality reduction of as much as 80%. A tremendous amount of study has attempted to determine whether a flexible sigmoidoscopy finding positive for adenomas is predictive of proximal neoplasia. Controversy has existed over whether distal hyperplastic polyps predict proximal neoplasia. The National Polyp Study rather convincingly indicated no increased risk of proximal neoplasia if the only flexible sigmoidoscopy finding is 1 or more hyperplastic polyps (Winawer et al, 1993). The risk of proximal neoplasia is increased if distal adenomas are large (>1 cm) or multiple or show villous architecture. Some controversy persists over whether small (<1 cm) adenomas represent a risk of proximal neoplasia high enough to warrant colonoscopy. In the United States, the standard of care has been to evaluate the entire colon if any adenoma is identified by flexible sigmoidoscopy. Because doubt has been expressed about the magnitude of this risk (Atkin et al, 1992), the issue remains unresolved.

BARIUM ENEMA

No prospective randomized trial of air contrast barium enema (ACBE) has been conducted in average-risk populations. ACBE has been shown to be at least 70% sensitive for identifying large polyps and cancer. Despite the absence of definitive, prospective data, the long history of clinical application of ACBE has earned this modality a place in the recommendations of authoritative groups (American Cancer Society, American Gastroenterology Association, American College of Gastroenterology, and others).

As an adjunct to the National Polyp Study (colonoscopy follow-up of patients after adenoma polypectomy), paired ACBE and colonoscopy was performed in nearly 600 subjects as follow-up after endoscopic polypectomy (Winawer et al, 2000). If colonoscopy is taken as a "gold standard," ACBE was 32% sensitive for the detection of polyps up to 5 mm, 53% sensitive for the detection of 6- to 10-mm polyps, and 48% sensitive for the detection of polyps larger than 10 mm. In fact, colonoscopy did miss a small number of adenomas. Overall, colonoscopy was considered superior. It should be emphasized that the population was by no means average risk. Although by definition all subjects were regarded as at high risk by virtue of their adenoma history, all had already undergone removal of these adenomas at least once, perhaps rendering these patients at low risk.

Colonoscopy

In recent years, the possibility of primary colonoscopy has been entertained. Primary colonoscopy can be considered the use of colonoscopy as the initial or only screening test for persons at average risk of colorectal cancer. While no prospective trial has been able to demonstrate a reduction in mortality, a reduction in invasive cancer has been suggested.

For a number of years, colonoscopy has been considered the appropriate screening test for high-risk subjects, such as persons with inflammatory bowel disease, a personal history of adenomas or invasive adenocarcinoma, or a family history of colorectal cancer. The current guidelines of the American Cancer Society and the National Comprehensive Cancer Network suggest that colonoscopy is the preferred tool for such persons. Subjects with a positive family history have a high prevalence of lesions beyond the reach of the flexible sigmoidoscope. As noted above, in a head-to-head prospective comparison of colonoscopy and barium enema in subjects with previous adenomas, colonoscopy was more sensitive for the detection of adenomas larger than 1 cm (Winawer et al, 2000).

Colonoscopy has been accepted as an appropriate tool for surveillance of persons with a significant family history of colorectal cancer (Jarvinen et al, 2000). But is everyone with, for example, 1 or 2 colorectal cancer–affected first-degree relatives at about the same risk, or is some stratification possible? If there are differences in risk, are they important enough to investigate? Or is colonoscopy so universally attractive that even crude estimates of increased risk are sufficient to warrant the test? Many studies have shown that there is an increased relative risk of colorectal cancer and of adenomas in first-degree relatives of colorectal cancer patients. This risk increases as age at onset of cancer in the relative in question decreases. This is the basis for the common recommendation that screening should begin at age 40 in such families or at 10 years younger than the youngest affected individual in the family. However, it is also recognized that there is tremendous heterogeneity within the group of subjects with a positive family history. At one extreme are cases in which only 1 first-degree relative has colorectal cancer, typically but not always at an early age, and HNPCC is demonstrated by mutation analysis. Indeed, population studies have shown this to be so. Aaltonen et al (1998) performed microsatellite instability testing on a large series of unselected Finnish patients. Microsatellite instability, a marker of HNPCC risk, was found in 12%. Of these, few were found to have pathologic mismatch-repair gene mutations for HNPCC. Close relatives of such individuals are at 50% risk of being mismatch-repair gene mutation carriers themselves, with an attendant 80% lifetime risk of colorectal cancer. Any large series of "family history positive, not otherwise specified" subjects will include a small proportion, perhaps 2% to 3%, who actually have HNPCC. Another small group will have attenuated familial adenomatous polyposis (FAP), with a sufficiently late onset, often after age 50, and modest enough adenoma burden as to escape being labeled as FAP. At the other extreme will be a much larger group of patients, typically with later-onset disease, the main cause of which will have been environmental (dietary). In this last group, the dietary risk will be modulated by a more modest genetic modifier of risk.

Considerable effort is being devoted to the study of genetic polymorphisms that account for variability in hepatic xenobiotic metabolizing activity. At present, such genetic modifiers of essentially ubiquitous dietary carcinogens probably constitute too weak an influence to be of immediate clinical utility in risk stratification.

Assuming colonoscopy is to be performed, should follow-up of those with adenomas and a positive family history be more aggressive than follow-up of those at average risk who for one reason or another are found to have an adenoma? Likewise, if results of a baseline examination are negative, should a repeat examination be performed at a shorter interval than for those undergoing average-risk screening?

Keeping in mind that subjects with a positive family history represent a truly heterogeneous group, one must consider the range of follow-up strategies. If a person at average risk is found to have an adenoma, he or she is, from that point on, considered at increased risk of developing recurrent adenomas. The National Polyp Study concluded that for subjects with small, solitary adenomas without severe dysplasia, repeat colonoscopy can safely be put off for 3 years. If results of such a follow-up examination are normal, repeat examinations at intervals of 3 to 5 years are acceptable. Conversely, subjects with HNPCC who are found to have adenomas are followed up very aggressively, at intervals of 1 to 2 years and with no lengthening of the interval as negative results ensue. This is because adenomas in persons with HNPCC are often flat, subtle, and dysplastic out of proportion to their size, indicating an accelerated adenoma-to-carcinoma sequence. For persons at moderately increased adenoma risk because of their family history, there are no good data regarding the long-term yield of more aggressive as opposed to less aggressive follow-up.

Investigational Measures for Colorectal Cancer Screening

Two new methodologies, virtual colonoscopy (also known as computed tomography colonography) and stool-based testing for mutated DNA, are exciting and of considerable interest. Virtual colonoscopy entails the use of spiral computed tomography with very thin cuts (otherwise, small lesions would be missed) and new computer techniques for 3-dimensional reconstruction. Currently, standard bowel preparations are required and elimination of all effluent is important. Efforts are under way to develop oral contrast agents that mix with enteral contents so that they may be subtracted from images, eliminating the bowel preparation, which many patients find more noxious than the colonoscopy itself. Several single-institution trials have yielded virtual colonoscopy sensitivities of greater than 90% for the detection of adenomas larger than 1 cm. In one study (Pickhardt et al, 2003) of CT with 3-dimensional endoluminal display vs conventional colonoscopy in 1233 asymptomatic adults, CT colonography yielded a 94% sensitivity for adenomas 10 mm or larger, with 96% specificity. This was actually a better sensitivity than was provided by conventional or "optical" colonoscopy. In a smaller study (Cotton et al, 2004; 615 subjects) using several different CT software platforms, the sensitivity for adenomas 10 mm or larger was only 55% with CT colonography. The difference may be attributed to better CT technique and oral contrast in the Pickhardt study. Notably, experience on the part of the CT radiologists did not seem to be an important determinant of test sensitivity. For now, the role of CT colonography in clinical screening for colorectal cancer in average-risk populations remains uncertain. Additional data with optimal CT techniques appear to be warranted.

It is known that in the course of the adenoma-to-carcinoma sequence in the colon, a variety of genetic mutations are acquired in key regulatory genes and their targets. Exfoliated colonic epithelium can be retrieved, and its DNA can be extracted and amplified and subjected to mutation analysis. Ahlquist et al (2000) have reported encouraging data on the use of a panel of markers, including *APC*, *p53*, *Ras*, and *Bat 26*. So far, most data pertain to established malignancies rather than adenomas.

So which test is appropriate for persons at increased risk? FOBT and flexible sigmoidoscopy are not, and barium enema is appropriate only if colonoscopy cannot be performed for some reason. Virtual colonoscopy and mutational analysis, if better validated, may someday be appropriate. For now, colonoscopy is the only appropriate choice.

COLON CANCER CHEMOPREVENTION

Chemoprevention of colorectal cancer has come to imply the use of orally administered agents, whether dietary or strictly pharmacologic, to reduce the risk of developing adenocarcinoma.

Epidemiologic data strongly point to geographic differences in colorectal cancer incidence. Rates have been highest in northwestern Europe, North America, Oceania, and Argentina and lowest in sub-Sahara Africa. As such differences were explored in greater detail, specific factors in the diet came to be implicated. Several studies have led to the conclusion that diets high in animal fat and total energy intake increased risk, while diets high in total fiber, whether fruit, vegetable, or bran, were associated with lower risk.

Although well accepted as a key paradigm in carcinogenesis and taken for granted in many ways, the adenoma-to-carcinoma sequence is very important to our understanding of chemoprevention. Even though most adenomas do not progress to invasive adenocarcinoma, essentially all adenocarcinomas arise from adenoma precursors. Most would agree that elimination of adenomas, such as by colonoscopic polypectomy, dramatically reduces colon cancer risk, and several key trials have so demonstrated. Primary prevention of adenomas should accomplish the same goal. Thus, because adenomas are more common than cancers (30% to 70% lifetime risk for adenomas vs 3% to 7% lifetime risk of colon cancer), they are a more attractive target for clinical trials. Adenoma occurrence and recurrence can be monitored with relative ease by means of colonoscopy. Importantly, the U.S. Food and Drug Administration has accepted adenoma prevention as a clinically relevant surrogate endpoint, as opposed to invasive cancer and mortality. The latter endpoints require far longer study durations and larger sample sizes in order to demonstrate efficacy.

Human chemoprevention clinical trials have several elements in common. There should be a rationale for the selection of agent or agents. Ideally, this selection should be based on sound epidemiologic grounds, with experimental evidence of minimal toxicity as well as efficacy in laboratory animals, including an attempt to understand the mechanism of drug action in anticarcinogenesis. The endpoint of the trial should have biological relevance. Fortunately, in the case of colorectal neoplasia, the endpoint of adenoma incidence (and in some instances, regression) is a reasonable alternative to an endpoint of cancer itself.

GROUPS AT HIGH RISK FOR COLORECTAL CANCER AS TARGETS FOR CHEMOPREVENTION TRIALS

The vast majority of colorectal cancers must be considered sporadic. Most persons in the United States are at average risk of colorectal cancer, though this risk is actually high when considered in the context of worldwide patterns of occurrence. Subjects who have already developed adenomas are at increased risk of recurrent polyps and have been the target population in several sporadic adenoma trials. However, these trials are very expensive and require huge numbers of subjects. Typically, more than 1,000 subjects are required in the current generation of placebo-controlled trials of such agents as supplemental fiber, calcium, and nonsteroidal anti-inflammatory drugs (NSAIDs).

Our group has taken a different approach, targeting individuals at the highest risk of adenomas and cancer, namely members of families with conditions such as FAP and HNPCC.

FAP has for a century been one of the most commonly recognized inherited cancer-predisposing disorders. Its inheritance is autosomal dominant, with high penetrance. Adenomas typically occur by age 10 to 15 years, gradually increasing in number and distribution over the next decade. Molecular diagnosis through testing for germline mutations in the adenomatous polyposis coli (*APC*) gene is now possible and should become routine. However, for genetic testing to be utilized effectively, the critical role of genetic counseling must be recognized, as discussed in chapter 8.

The medical oncologist as chemotherapist will have few encounters with the FAP patient. A typical scenario includes the patient who presents with advanced colorectal cancer in the presence of a de novo mutation. Such patients will develop cancer at an early age and often present with a history of minimal symptoms. This might include rectal bleeding that is attributed to hemorrhoids and not worked up because of the young age of the patient. Presentation with advanced malignancy is uncommon in patients with a known family history of FAP but does still occasionally occur.

The nearly universal occurrence of multiple adenomas in patients with FAP makes for a readily evaluable population for studies of adenoma regression and adenoma prevention. The NSAID sulindac showed some promise in an early uncontrolled study. This led to a series of randomized prospective placebo-controlled clinical trials. In one European trial (Labayle et al, 1991) employing a crossover design, use of sulindac at standard anti-inflammatory doses dramatically reduced residual rectal adenomas in FAP subjects after colectomy. This effect was seen in just a few months but was short-lived, with recurrence of adenomas following crossover to the placebo arm of the trial. In the key United States trial, Giardiello et al (1993) demonstrated a 56% reduction in adenoma count and a 65% reduction in adenoma size, though no subjects achieved complete regression of adenomas. Maximum effect was seen at 6 months, and both number and size of adenomas increased during the 3 months following cessation of sulindac, paralleling the findings in the Labayle trial.

Sulindac was reported to be well tolerated in Giardiello's small trial. Nevertheless, the toxic effects of NSAIDs, including sulindac, can be life-threatening in a small proportion of subjects. The most common serious adverse effect of NSAIDs is gastrointestinal toxicity, mainly gastroduodenal ulcers and bleeding in the upper gastrointestinal tract. Because of this and other toxic effects, considerable effort has been devoted to the development of safer NSAIDs. A key breakthrough in this area was the development of selective cyclooxygenase (COX) inhibitors. COX is a key enzyme in the pathway of arachidonic acid metabolism to various prostaglandins. There are 2 isoforms, COX-1 and COX-2. COX-1 is constitutively expressed and is involved in mediation of mucosal integrity and platelet function. COX-2 is inducible and mediates inflammation and, apparently, neoplasia. When a selective inhibitor of COX-2 was developed, there was an opportunity to inhibit the "bad" COX (COX-2) while leaving the "good" COX (COX-1) alone. In large-scale clinical trials involving osteoarthritis and rheumatoid arthritis, such selective COX-2 inhibitors as celecoxib and rofecoxib yielded the desired anti-inflammatory effects with fewer gastrointestinal and other side effects compared with more traditional NSAIDS.

The first concrete evidence of a favorable COX-2 effect on human colorectal neoplasia came in our FAP adenoma regression trial (Steinbach et al, 2000). Initially, 75 patients were randomly assigned to receive celecoxib (Celebrex, Pfizer Inc., New York, NY), either 100 or 400 mg orally twice daily, or a look-alike placebo for 6 months, with the study duration and adenoma regression endpoint based on previous trials of sulindac that had shown efficacy. Comprehensive compliance and patient safety monitoring were performed throughout the trial, with adverse events graded in accordance with National Cancer Institute Common Toxicity Criteria.

Colonoscopy or sigmoidoscopy (if colectomy was previously done) and duodenoscopy were performed at baseline and off study at month 6. The examinations were documented by videotape and a series of photographs.

After 6 months of therapy at the highest dose of celecoxib (400 mg twice a day, twice the usual antiarthritic dose), as measured by still photographs in designated regions of interest, there was a statistically significant ($P =$ .003) reduction in adenoma burden, compared with baseline. Specifically, the high-dose group experienced a mean 28% reduction in adenoma count, compared with a 4.5% reduction in the placebo group, and an intermediate reduction of 12% in the 100-mg-twice-a-day group. This effect persisted after adjustment for age, sex, previous surgery (colectomy vs intact colon), baseline polyp burden, and investigating institution. The celecoxib was well tolerated, with 68%, 56%, and 57% of subjects in the placebo, low-dose, and high-dose groups, respectively, reporting a grade 2 or worse adverse event, including diarrhea and abdominal pain. Adverse events requiring subject withdrawal from the trial included suicide (celecoxib 100-mg arm, in a patient with a prior suicide attempt), acute allergic reaction (celecoxib 400-mg arm), and dyspepsia (celecoxib 400-mg arm, although no ulcer was observed on upper gastrointestinal endoscopy). No significant changes occurred in hematologic or chemical profiles.

In the aggregate, these data indicate that COX-2 is an important factor in colorectal carcinogenesis and that its selective inhibition may retard the formation or progression of adenomas, at least in patients with FAP. It remains to be seen whether intervention with COX-2 inhibitors will be able to prevent or at least delay the initial occurrence of adenomas in young FAP carriers with FAP. If so, there may be settings in which colectomy or proctocolectomy could be postponed for years, enabling such young subjects to be more active participants in their own disease management. Meanwhile, celecoxib may be used to treat patients who have already undergone colectomy and who develop recurrent rectal polyps. Most such patients and their surgeons are eager to avoid a second operation. If the use of celecoxib is to be considered an adjunct to endoscopic polypectomy in such patients, it is important that careful attention be paid to appropriate follow-up. Anecdotal cases of progression to overt malignancy have been documented in subjects treated with sulindac, even as regression of adenomas was documented. Clearly, individualized management of patients is imperative.

At the time celecoxib was being approved for use in FAP, the U.S. Food and Drug Administration requested that several additional, postmarketing studies be performed. One such investigation was to be the use of celecoxib in clinical trials to prevent the onset of first adenomas in young genotype-positive and phenotype-negative children carrying APC gene mutations. The phase I, dose-finding phase is nearing completion.

Yet another FAP trial is accruing here at M. D. Anderson, St. Mark's in London, and the Cleveland Clinic. This is a 2-arm, randomized, prospective, double-blind trial involving FAP subjects with residual colorectal (no previous colectomy) or rectal (postcolectomy) polyps. The trial employs celecoxib 400 mg orally twice a day vs celecoxib 400 mg orally twice a day plus difluoromethylornithine (DFMO) at a dose of 0.5 mg/m^2 (rounded to the nearest 250 mg). Target accrual is 152 subjects. Endoscopic evaluation is at 0 and 6 months. The primary endpoint is adenoma regression, as in the original celecoxib trial. DFMO is an irreversible enzyme-activated inhibitor of ornithine decarboxylase, which in turn is rate limiting in the polyamine pathway (Pegg, 1988). Although its pathway differs from that of COX-2 inhibitors, DFMO has been shown to decrease carcinogen-induced tumors in rodents (Kingsnorth et al, 1983). That it employs a different pathway will be capitalized upon in achieving hoped-for synergy in reducing and preventing adenomas in FAP.

Until recently, HNPCC was a clinical diagnosis involving the familial pattern of early-onset or multiple primary colorectal cancer, with or without the presence of certain extracolonic tumors. In many families, colonic tumors occur most frequently in the right colon. Adenomas may be completely absent and rarely number more than a few.

As with FAP, management of HNPCC involves recognition of risk, followed by appropriate surveillance and surgical intervention. These must be enhanced, compared with interventions in the patient at average risk. In sufficiently striking families, colorectal cancer risk to offspring of affected parents approaches 50%. Molecular genetic testing will detect mutations in 1 of the HNPCC-related genes in up to 85% of families. Assuming such a mutation is identified, offspring of affected parents can be segregated into 2 groups, those at population risk (noncarriers) and those whose risk approaches 100% (carriers). In carriers, colonoscopy is recommended, beginning at age 20 to 30 years and repeated at intervals of 1 to 5 years (the broad range reflects a lack of definitive data and lack of consensus). Noncarriers require no further enhanced evaluation, assuming accuracy of the genetic testing. When adenocarcinomas are detected, subtotal colectomy with ileorectal anastomosis is urged. Residual risk to the rectum exists after colectomy, but its magnitude is uncertain and probably not great enough to warrant proctectomy. The approach to the patient with an adenoma is uncertain. Most surgeons would perform simple endoscopic polypectomy, but the possibility of prophylactic colectomy may be increasingly considered in known mutation carriers, especially when difficult-to-remove right-sided sessile lesions are involved. Surveillance for extracolonic tumors has received little attention.

With recognition of HNPCC as a distinct entity with predictable colorectal cancer risk, efforts in chemoprevention began. Cats et al (1995) employed oral calcium in a small series of subjects at risk of HNPCC tumors. The trial endpoint was epithelial proliferation or labeling index, as measured by bromodeoxyuridine incorporation. No significant difference in posttreatment labeling index was observed between the study group receiving 1.5 g of $CaCO_3$ and the control group. The design of our ongoing study utilizing celecoxib is outlined below. Another multicenter trial, centered in Europe but intercontinental in scope, employs aspirin and resistant (high amylase, fermentable) starch (novelose) in a factorial design. Its accrual goals are very ambitious, approximately 1,200 subjects from 55 institutions, and accrual is under way at this time. It is intended to have sufficient power to identify a treatment effect, namely reduction in adenoma incidence among HNPCC subjects, during a follow-up period of at least 2 years for each enrolled subject. Eligibility criteria are very similar to those employed in our HNPCC celecoxib trial.

Studies have shown that although COX-2 expression occurs in colorectal adenomas and cancers, it may not be as great in colorectal adenomas and cancers in HNPCC as it is in FAP or sporadic colorectal cancer. In our series (Sinicrope et al, 1999) 16 (67%) of 24 HNPCC tumors and 24 (92%) of 26 sporadic tumors showed evidence of COX-2 immunoreactivity. If confirmed in additional investigations, this would constitute another manner in which the "HNPCC pathway," characterized by instability in microsatellite markers and a relative paucity of tumor-suppressor gene mutations and allelic losses, differs from both FAP and sporadic colorectal cancer. Further, to the extent that COX-2 is relatively underexpressed, inhibitors of COX-2 ought to be less effective in HNPCC.

Because of the relatively low incidence of adenomas in HNPCC, it would be very difficult to conduct clinical trials having statistical power sufficient to demonstrate a reduction in adenoma incidence. Nevertheless, we undertook an evaluation of the effect of celecoxib on various intermediate markers in HNPCC. Accrual was recently completed, and our study included 77 subjects with either a mismatch-repair gene mutation or previous microsatellite instability–positive colorectal cancer in the appropriate family history setting. It followed a design somewhat akin to that employed in the first FAP trial. The 3 arms were placebo, celecoxib 200 mg twice daily, and celecoxib 400 mg twice daily. Subjects underwent colonoscopy at baseline, and the off-study examination was performed at month 12. In this HNPCC cohort, pretreatment mucosal biomarker data showed significant differences in microarray gene expression between the right and left colon (Glebov et al, 2003). That these may be physiologic and not necessarily intrinsic features of HNPCC is supported by the demonstration of a very similar pattern of microarray expression in a control, average-risk screening population. It remains to be seen whether there may be more specific patterns of expression that distinguish mucosa in HNPCC patients from that in normal patients.

COX-2 Inhibition in Patients with Sporadic Colorectal Adenoma

Epidemiologic and case-control series have for years supported the notion that NSAIDs reduce the risk of colorectal neoplasia. One randomized, prospective, placebo-controlled trial has now shown that low-dose aspirin (81 mg/day) reduces the risk of recurrent adenomas in patients with endoscopically removed adenomas (Baron et al, 2003).

The first large-scale COX-2 inhibitor trial involving subjects with a history of sporadic colorectal adenoma has recently begun (Bertagnolli, personal communication). This is a phase III, prospective, randomized, double-blind, 3-arm, multicenter trial in which celecoxib at multiple doses (200 mg twice daily and 400 mg twice daily) is compared with placebo. Subjects will have undergone endoscopic polypectomy of adenoma (1 adenoma ≥ 1 cm, or 2 or more adenomas of any size) within 3 months of study entry. The primary endpoint will be recurrence of adenomas at 12 and 36 months after study entry. As in our FAP and HNPCC trials, this trial of sporadic adenoma will include measures of surrogate endpoints in a nested subgroup of subjects. Anticipated enrollment is 650 subjects per arm, or 1,950 subjects in total.

An international trial of sporadic adenoma, sponsored by Pfizer and very similar in design to the Bertagnolli study, is being conducted in parallel. This study would, if adenoma prevention efficacy were demonstrated, provide a basis for approval of celecoxib in other countries. The principal investigators are Bernard Levin of M. D. Anderson and Nadil Arber of Tel Aviv, Israel. Accrual is progressing well at this time.

THE FUTURE

It is an exciting time to be involved in colorectal cancer chemoprevention clinical trials. If ongoing trials of aspirin and selective COX-2 inhibitors demonstrate effectiveness in reducing risk of sporadic and familial adenomas, widespread use of these agents for this purpose can be anticipated. It will then be necessary to monitor a number of outcomes. What really will be the extent of use of these agents in the population? Will they be used appropriately or abused in ways difficult to predict? At what age will their use be initiated? At what dose and frequency? Will subjects simply take an occasional low dose of cheap aspirin and hope for the best, opting out of the expense and discomfort of clinical tests? Will their health care

---

KEY PRACTICE POINTS

- FOBT has been shown to reduce colorectal cancer mortality and is widely recommended for screening. However, it suffers from limited sensitivity because polyps and even some cancers may not bleed enough to yield a positive test result. FOBT also had limited specificity owing to high false-positive rates resulting in nondiagnostic colonoscopy follow-up.

- Sigmoidoscopy has been shown to reduce colorectal cancer mortality through detection of early lesions in the distal colorectum and is widely recommended for screening. However, it is limited by the anatomic incompleteness of the examination and suboptimal patient acceptance.

- Colonoscopy is the gold standard for evaluation of the colon because of high sensitivity, specificity, and therapeutic potential, even though mortality reduction has not been conclusively established. Colonoscopy is limited by its higher cost, lesser availability, greater risk, and suboptimal patient acceptance.

- Newer screening methods, computed tomography colonography and testing for mutated DNA in the stool, offer some real promise but have yet to be adequately validated.

- Chemoprevention by means of NSAIDs seems well validated in FAP.

- In patients with a history of nonfamilial adenomas, low-dose (81 mg/day) aspirin reduces the risk of polyp recurrence. Trials of COX-2 inhibitors are under way in similar populations.

- There is insufficient evidence to support relaxation of colorectal neoplasia screening/surveillance measures in patients engaged in chemoprevention measures.

providers go along with such an approach and become less vigorous in urging colorectal cancer screening? Will consumers conclude that NSAIDs are so effective in reducing cancer risk that they veer away from a more healthful diet and lifestyle? If NSAID use becomes widespread, will we see a significant downturn in colorectal cancer incidence? If so, will it be possible to sort out the NSAID effect from such confounders as screening behavior and diet?

The above questions perhaps naively assume that colorectal cancer prevention by means of NSAIDs, selective or not, *will* become a significant fact of life for Americans. Whether or not this comes to pass, scientific activity will continue on other fronts. Combinations of agents will be evaluated, capitalizing on advances in our knowledge of the mechanisms of adenoma-to-carcinoma formation and their pharmacologic manipulation. By the targeting of complementary pathways, synergy will continue to be sought in chemoprevention, just as it is in cancer therapy. Novel agents will of course continue to be developed and brought along more quickly through in vitro and animal models. Those of us interested in high-risk groups will need to closely monitor such developments, as these populations will most likely continue to be in the forefront of clinical trial testing of new drugs and combinations.

Suggested Readings

Aaltonen LA, Salovaara R, Kristo P, et al. Incidence of hereditary nonpolyposis colorectal cancer and the feasibility of molecular screening for the disease. *N Engl J Med* 1998;338:1481–1487.

Ahlquist DA, Skoletsky JE, Boynton KA, et al. Colorectal cancer screening by detection of altered human DNA in stool: feasibility of a multitarget assay panel. *Gastroenterology* 2000;119:1219–1227.

Atkin WS, Morson BC, Cuzick J. Long-term risk of colorectal cancer after excision of rectosigmoid adenomas. *N Engl J Med* 1992;326:658–662.

Baron JA, Cole BF, Sandler RS, et al. A randomized trial of aspirin to prevent colorectal adenomas. *N Engl J Med* 2003;348:891–899.

Cats A, Kleibeuker JH, van der Meer R, et al. Randomized, double-blinded, placebo-controlled intervention study with supplemental calcium in families with hereditary nonpolyposis colorectal cancer. *J Natl Cancer Inst* 1995;87:598–603.

Cotton PB, Durkalski VL, Pineau BC, et al. Computed tomographic colonography (virtual colonoscopy): a multicenter comparison with standard colonoscopy for detection of colorectal neoplasia. *JAMA* 2004;291:1713–1719.

Giardiello FM, Hamilton SR, Krush AJ, et al. Treatment of colonic and rectal adenomas with sulindac in familial adenomatous polyposis. *N Engl J Med* 1993;328:1313–1316.

Glebov OK, Rodriguez LM, Nakahara K, et al. Distinguishing right from left colon by the pattern of gene expression. *Cancer Epidemiol Biomarkers Prev* 2003;12:755–762.

Jarvinen HJ, Aarnio M, Mustonen H, et al. Controlled 15-year trial on screening for colorectal cancer in families with hereditary nonpolyposis colorectal cancer. *Gastroenterology* 2000;118:829–834.

Kingsnorth AN, King WWK, Diekema KA, et al. Inhibition of ornithine decarboxylase with 2-difluoro-methylornithine: reduced incidence of dimethylhydrazine-induced colon tumors in mice. *Cancer Res* 1983;43:2545–2549.

Labayle D, Fischer D, Vielh P, et al. Sulindac causes regression of rectal polyps in familial adenomatous polyposis. *Gastroenterology* 1991;101:635–639.

Lieberman DA, Weiss DG, Bond JH, et al. Use of colonoscopy to screen asymptomatic adults for colorectal cancer. *N Engl J Med* 2000;343:162–168.

Lieberman DA, Weiss DG. Veterans Affairs Cooperative Study Group 380. One-time screening for colorectal cancers with combined fecal occult-blood testing and examination of the distal colon. *N Engl J Med* 2001;345:555–560.

Mandel JS, Bond JH, Church TR, et al. Reducing mortality from colorectal cancer by screening for fecal occult blood. *N Engl J Med* 1993;328:1365–1371.

Pegg AE. Polyamine metabolism and its importance in neoplastic growth and as a target for chemotherapy. *Cancer Res* 1988;48:759–774.

Pickhardt PJ, Choi R, Hwang I, et al. Computed tomography virtual colonoscopy to screen for colorectal neoplasia in asymptomatic adults. *N Engl J Med* 2003;349:2191–2200.

Rex DK, Johnson DA, Lieberman DA, et al. Colorectal cancer prevention 2000: screening recommendations of the American College of Gastroenterology. *Am J Gastroenterol* 2000;95:868–877.

Rex DK, Rahmani EY, Haseman JH, et al. Relative sensitivity of colonoscopy and barium enema for detection of colorectal cancer in clinical practice. *Gastroenterology* 1997;112:17–23.

Selby JV, Friedman GD, Quesenberry CP, et al. A case control study of screening sigmoidoscopy and mortality from colorectal cancer. *N Engl J Med* 1992;26: 653–657.

Sinicrope FA, Lemoine M, Xi L, et al. Reduced expression of cyclooxygenase-2 proteins in hereditary nonpolyposis colorectal cancers relative to sporadic cancers. *Gastroenterology* 1999;117:1–10.

Smith RA, von Eschenbach AC, Wender R, et al. American Cancer Society guidelines for the early detection of cancer: update on early detection guidelines for prostate, colorectal, and endometrial cancers. *CA Cancer J Clin* 2001;51:38–75.

Steinbach G, Lynch PM, Phillips RKS, et al. The effect of celecoxib, a cyclooxygenase-2 inhibitor, in familial adenomatous polyposis. *N Engl J Med* 2000;342: 1946–1952.

Winawer S, Fletcher R, Rex D, et al. Colorectal cancer screening and surveillance: clinical guidelines and rationale-update based on new evidence. *Gastroenterology* 2003;124:544–560.

Winawer SJ, Stewart ET, Zauber AG, et al. A comparison of colonoscopy and double-contrast barium enema for surveillance after polypectomy. National Polyp Study Work Group. *N Engl J Med* 2000;342:1766–1772.

Winawer SJ, Zauber AG, Ho MN, et al. Prevention of colorectal cancer by colonoscopic polypectomy. The National Polyp Study Workgroup. *N Engl J Med* 1993; 329:1977–1981.

8 HEREDITARY NONPOLYPOSIS COLORECTAL CANCER AND GENETIC COUNSELING

Miguel A. Rodriguez-Bigas and Patrick M. Lynch

CHAPTER OVERVIEW

Patients who present with suspected hereditary nonpolyposis colorectal cancer (HNPCC) require specialized counseling and treatment. The characteristics of HNPCC, the availability of genetic testing for HNPCC, and the potential implications of positive and negative test results must be discussed with patients and family members in detail. In patients who decide to proceed with genetic testing, results must be communicated in an appropriate manner, and follow-up is essential. Treatment for patients with colon cancer who are members of an HNPCC kindred must be individualized, but the treatment of choice is total abdominal colectomy with an ileorectal anastomosis.

HEREDITARY NONPOLYPOSIS COLORECTAL CANCER

Hereditary nonpolyposis colorectal cancer (HNPCC) is the most common of the inherited gastrointestinal syndromes predisposing to colorectal cancer. The syndrome accounts for approximately 2% to 3% of all colorectal cancers (Westlake et al, 1991; Salovaara et al, 2000). HNPCC is an autosomal dominant heritable syndrome. Therefore, 50% of the children of an affected individual will develop the syndrome. The penetrance of HNPCC has been estimated to be between 80% and 85% (Lynch et al, 1983; Vasen et al, 1996); thus, not all affected individuals will develop cancer in their lifetime.

HNPCC is characterized by early age at onset, excess synchronous and metachronous lesions, right-sided predominance, and extracolonic manifestations. The median age of diagnosis of colorectal cancer in persons with HNPCC is approximately 45 years. Although most patients present with right-sided colon malignancies, up to 40% of patients present with left-sided colorectal tumors. In patients with HNPCC, the risk of developing synchronous colorectal neoplasms has been reported to be as high as 18%, and the risk of developing metachronous lesions has been reported to be 25% to 30% (Aarnio et al, 1995; Box et al, 1999; Lynch and de la Chapelle, 1999). The most common extracolonic tumor in HNPCC is endometrial cancer, which is present in 30% to 40% of affected women (Aarnio et al, 1995; Lynch and de la Chapelle, 1999). Other extracolonic cancers common in the syndrome are transitional cell carcinoma of the renal pelvis and ureter, small bowel adenocarcinoma, and sebaceous skin tumors (Muir-Torre syndrome). Less commonly reported in HNPCC are hepatobiliary, gastric, ovarian, renal cell, bladder, and brain tumors.

At the molecular level, HNPCC is characterized by germline mutations in the mismatch repair genes. These genes include *hMLH1*, *hMSH2*, *hMSH6*, *hPMS1*, and *hPMS2*. Mutations in these genes lead to microsatellite instability (MSI), which is found in more than 85% of colorectal tumors from patients with HNPCC (Lynch and de la Chapelle, 1999). A germline mutation in transforming growth factor beta type II has been described in an atypical family (Lu et al, 1998). *hMSH6* mutations tend to occur in families with endometrial cancer and in older patients with colorectal cancer.

Pathologically, colorectal cancers from HNPCC patients are characterized by poor differentiation, mucin production, Crohn's-like reaction, and an intense lymphocytic infiltrate (Jass et al, 1994). Even though some of these characteristics (mucin and poor differentiation) indicate a worse prognosis, HNPCC patients with colorectal cancer have been reported to have a better prognosis stage for stage than patients with sporadic colorectal cancer (Watson et al, 1998; Lynch and de la Chapelle, 1999). It is important to note that adenomas do occur in patients with HNPCC. Currently it is believed that adenomas in patients with HNPCC progress to carcinoma more quickly than do adenomas in patients with sporadic colorectal cancer.

Approach to Patients with Suspected HNPCC

The most important component of the management of HNPCC is identifying the affected individuals and their families. HNPCC has been defined by the Amsterdam Criteria: 3 affected individuals on the same side of the family; 2 successive generations; 1 affected individual who is a first-degree relative of the other 2; and colorectal cancer diagnosed before age 50 years (Vasen et al, 1991). These criteria were established to identify high-risk families for genetic studies in an attempt to identify the genes causing the syndrome. Some HNPCC families do not meet the Amsterdam Criteria. Because the original Amsterdam Criteria did not include extracolonic malignancies, the criteria were modified to include endometrial cancer, renal pelvis and ureter transitional cell carcinoma, and small bowel adenocarcinoma. The Amsterdam II Criteria (Vasen et al, 1999) include any combination of the latter 3 extracolonic malignances as well as colorectal cancer that affects 3 individuals in a family and 2 successive generations, with 1 of the individuals diagnosed before the age of 50 years and with the affected individual a first-degree relative of the other 2. Other criteria have been reported in an attempt to identify at-risk and affected individuals, but the most important aspect in identifying a potential HNPCC patient is the suspicion that the individual could be affected, with suspicion based on the clinical history, family history, age at diagnosis, or histopathologic characteristics of the tumor.

Discussion of Therapeutic Options

Once a patient is identified as a potential HNPCC patient, the most important aspect of care is the multidisciplinary approach. This is emphasized in our Gastrointestinal Center at M. D. Anderson Cancer Center. During the first visit of a patient to our Gastrointestinal Center, a complete history and physical examination are performed, including a detailed family history. During this visit, the therapeutic options for the specific condition are discussed with the patient. In addition, the clinician gives a general overview of HNPCC and answers any questions that the patient has.

Genetic Counseling, Genetic Testing, and Communication of Results

Once the therapeutic decisions have been made, a genetic counseling session is arranged. This session is usually scheduled for after the patient has recovered from surgery; however, for patients who have already had surgery, the meeting is arranged at the patient's convenience. The genetic counseling session is a multidisciplinary session and generally is led by one of our genetic counselors. However, a clinician with special interest in HNPCC is always available to answer any questions regarding treatment. For some individuals, the first genetic-counseling session is relatively straightforward because they already have an idea that there is a problem within the family. For others, 1 session may not suffice for the patient to understand the implications of potentially being a member of a kindred with HNPCC. During this visit, the patient is given a more extensive overview of the syndrome, including genetics, inheritance patterns, manifestations, and genetic testing. Ample time is allowed for the patient to ask questions.

Next comes the question of how to confirm a suspected diagnosis. One of the crucial aspects of genetic testing is deciding what is to be done with the information obtained. Are there benefits for those affected individuals and their families? What are the downsides to knowing the mutation status? What if a mutation is not identified? Our genetic counselors discuss all these aspects with the patient in subsequent counseling sessions. Most patients require more than 1 visit to have their questions addressed. It is important to emphasize to patients that genetic testing is not simple and can have major implications throughout the patient's lifetime.

Once all questions are answered, patients are asked whether they want to proceed with genetic testing. If the answer is affirmative, written informed consent is obtained and then a blood sample is collected. Genetic testing is performed in a Clinical Laboratory Improvement Amendment–certified laboratory. Results are given to patients in person, although some individuals are not immediately ready to get the results and choose to delay their appointment. Again, the genetic counselor and physician are available for any questions after the results are given. In case the need for psychological support arises, our team includes a qualified psychologist who is available for intervention. The clinical implications of the results are discussed with the patient.

It cannot be overemphasized that ample time should be given to genetic counseling prior to genetic testing. A detailed discussion of the potential implications of both a positive and a negative test result should be undertaken. If a number of family members are to be tested, the discussions can be held both privately and for the family as a group. However, we give the results of the testing in private. The patients are contacted 1 and 6 months after the test so that we can answer any questions they may have as well as to give follow-up.

An important aspect of genetic counseling is choosing whom to test. As discussed earlier, several criteria help both the clinicians and the genetic counselors in selecting the individuals who most likely will be members of HNPCC kindreds. Nevertheless, any individual who undergoes genetic testing with negative findings for a mutation must understand that if he or she is the first individual to be tested in the family, a negative test result is not informative. If HNPCC is strongly suspected, surveillance for that individual and at-risk family members should be consistent with the surveillance criteria of the International Collaborative Group on HNPCC (Table 8–1). A negative mutation result will be informative for individuals who are at risk and have a mutation identified in their families. Such

Table 8–1.   International Collaborative Group on HNPCC Guidelines for
Screening of Genetic Carriers or At-Risk Individuals

Site at Risk	Procedure	Age to Start, years	Frequency
Colon	Colonoscopy	20–25	Every 2 years
Endometrium and ovaries	Pelvic examination, transvaginal sonography, measurement of CA-125	30–35	Every 1–2 years
Stomach*	Upper endoscopy	30–35	Every 1–2 years
Urinary tract*	Sonography, urinalysis	30–35	Every 1–2 years

* Individuals with a family history of these neoplasms.
Modified from International Collaborative Group on Hereditary Non-Polyposis Colorectal
Cancer (2003). Used with permission.

patients still have the same risk of developing cancer as the general
population.

At M. D. Anderson, colorectal cancers from individuals suspected of
having HNPCC are tested for hMLH1, hMSH2, and hMSH6 protein
expression by immunohistochemical analysis. We used to test these
tumors for MSI since MSI is present in more than 85% of colorectal cancers
from HNPCC patients. However, a recently published study evaluating
hMLH1 and hMSH2 protein expression reported a 92% sensitivity and a
100% positive predictive value for MSI with absence of hMLH1 and
hMSH2 protein expression (Lindor et al, 2002). Therefore, immunohistochemical analysis appears to be a reliable method to screen for MSI, and
in fact, the absence of protein expression serves as a guide as to which
gene to test for mutation. Nevertheless, we still use MSI testing in selected
situations.

TREATMENT FOR PATIENTS WITH HNPCC

Because of the increased incidence of synchronous and metachronous
colorectal neoplasms in patients with HNPCC, the treatment of choice for
patients with HNPCC is a total abdominal colectomy with ileorectal anastomosis. However, no prospective studies show a survival advantage
for this treatment over segmental resection. Therefore, even though the
treatment of choice is a total abdominal colectomy with ileorectal anastomosis, the procedure should be individualized. In women who are postmenopausal or who have completed their family, consideration should be
given to prophylactic hysterectomy and bilateral salpingo-oophorectomy.
However, there are no data to suggest a survival benefit from the latter
procedure. In HNPCC patients treated with less than an abdominal colectomy, surveillance should be the mainstay of treatment, and inclusion in

KEY PRACTICE POINTS

- The most important component of the management of HNPCC is identifying the affected individuals and their families.

- Patients identified as being at high risk for HNPCC should be treated with a multidisciplinary approach.

- Ample time must be allowed for genetic counseling prior to genetic testing.

- During genetic counseling, the potential implications of positive and negative test results must be discussed in detail.

- During genetic counseling, it must be emphasized to patients that genetic testing is not simple and can have major implications throughout a patient's lifetime.

- A negative mutation-testing result does not mean that the individual tested does not carry a mutation unless an affected individual in the kindred carries a mutation.

- The treatment of choice for patients with HNPCC is total abdominal colectomy with an ileorectal anastomosis, but management should be individualized.

chemoprevention studies should be considered. These patients and patients who are at risk but are members of families in which no mutation has been found after genetic testing should be monitored as if they were affected. Prophylactic colectomy has been proposed as an option in certain cases in gene carriers (Burke et al, 1997).

Summary

In summary, at M. D. Anderson, genetic counseling is an integral part of the management of patients suspected of having a hereditary cancer syndrome. A multidisciplinary approach to genetic counseling is utilized at our center.

Suggested Readings

Aarnio M, Mecklin JP, Aaltonen L, et al. Life-time risk of different cancers in hereditary nonpolyposis colorectal cancer (HNPCC) syndrome. *Int J Cancer* 1995;64:430–433.

Box JC, Rodriguez-Bigas MA, Weber TK, et al. The incidence and clinical implications of multiple colorectal carcinomas in hereditary nonpolyposis colorectal cancer. *Dis Colon Rectum* 1999;42:717–721.

Burke W, Petersen GM, Lynch P, et al. Recommendations for follow-up care of individuals with an inherited predisposition to cancer: hereditary nonpolyposis colorectal cancer. *JAMA* 1997;277:915–919.

International Collaborative Group on Hereditary Non-Polyposis Colorectal Cancer. Guidelines for management recommended by ICG-HNPCC. Available at http://www.nfdht.nl/. Accessed October 29, 2003.

Jass JR, Smyrk TC, Stewart SM, et al. Pathology of hereditary nonpolyposis colorectal cancer. *Anticancer Res* 1994;14:1631–1635.

Lindor N, Burgart LJ, Leontovich O, et al. Immunohistochemistry versus microsatellite instability testing in phenotyping colorectal tumors. *J Clin Oncol* 2002; 20:1043–1048.

Lu SL, Kawabata M, Imamura T, et al. HNPCC associated with germline mutation in the TGF-β type II receptor gene. *Nat Genet* 1998;19:17–18.

Lynch HT, Albano WA, Ruma TA, et al. Surveillance/management of an obligate gene carrier: the cancer family syndrome. *Gastroenterology* 1983;84:404–408.

Lynch HT, de la Chapelle A. Genetic susceptibility to non-polyposis colorectal cancer. *J Med Genet* 1999;36:801–818.

Miyaki M, Konishi M, Tanaka K, et al. Germline mutation of MSH6 as the cause of hereditary nonpolyposis colorectal cancer. *Nat Genet* 1997;17:271–272.

Salovaara R, Loukola A, Kristo P, et al. Population-based molecular detection of hereditary nonpolyposis colorectal cancer. *J Clin Oncol* 2000;18:2193–2200.

Vasen HFA, Mecklin JP, Meera Khan P, et al. The International Collaborative Group on Hereditary Non-Polyposis Colorectal Cancer (ICG-HNPCC). *Dis Colon Rectum* 1991;34:424–425.

Vasen HFA, Watson P, Mecklin JP, et al. New criteria for hereditary nonpolyposis colorectal cancer (HNPCC, Lynch Syndrome) proposed by the International Collaborative Group on HNPCC (ICG-HNPCC). *Gastroenterology* 1999;116: 1453–1456.

Vasen HFA, Wijnen JTH, Menko FH, et al. Cancer risk in families with hereditary nonpolyposis colorectal cancer diagnosed by mutation analysis. *Gastroenterology* 1996;110:1020–1027.

Watson P, Lin K, Rodriguez-Bigas MA, et al. Colorectal cancer survival in hereditary nonpolyposis colorectal cancer. *Cancer* 1998;83:259–266.

Westlake PJ, Bryant HE, Huchcroft SA, et al. Frequency of hereditary nonpolyposis colorectal cancer in southern Alberta. *Dig Dis Sci* 1991;36:1441–1447.

Wijnen J, de Leeuw W, Vasen H, et al. Familial endometrial cancer in female carriers of MSH6 germline mutations. *Nat Genet* 1999;23:142–144.

9 COLON CANCER

Edward H. Lin and Henry Q. Xiong

CHAPTER OVERVIEW

For decades, 5-fluorouracil was the only chemotherapy agent known to be active against colorectal cancer. In recent years, many new cytotoxic agents have been introduced, including targeted therapies, and therapeutic options have been greatly expanded. The main focus of treatment for patients with stage I colon cancer is secondary prevention of new adenomatous polyps. The goal of treatment of patients with stage II and III colon cancer is cure; therefore, patients should undergo adequate surgical staging and optimal adjuvant therapy. In the majority of patients with metastatic (stage IV) disease, the therapeutic goal is palliation; potentially curative treatment is possible only in selected cases. Therefore, treatment should aim to maximize survival with the least negative impact on quality of life.

INTRODUCTION

Colon cancer is a very common malignancy yet is also preventable if appropriate screening and preventative measures are undertaken. Surgery is the curative modality for patients with stage I, II, and III colon cancer and for selected patients with advanced disease. The use of adjuvant chemotherapy for patients with stage II colon cancer is controversial and should be individualized. Adjuvant chemotherapy for patients with stage III colon cancer improves both disease-free and overall survival. Newer cytotoxic and targeted therapies and molecular markers and genomics will be integrated into the increasingly individualized, multidisciplinary treatment paradigm for colon cancer, with the goals of maximizing tumor control, enhancing survival, and improving patients' overall quality of life.

In this chapter, we will emphasize the experience in colon cancer management at M. D. Anderson Cancer Center while providing readers with perspective on a number of pivotal trials of 5-fluorouracil (5-FU), irinotecan, capecitabine, and oxaliplatin in patients with colon cancer. The integration of molecular prognostic markers and targeted therapy in the treatment of colon cancer will be discussed, as will the management of treatment-related side effects.

EPIDEMIOLOGY

Of the 130,000 cases of colorectal cancer expected in 2000, it was estimated that 93,800 would be classified as colon cancer. Colon cancer ranks fourth in overall cancer incidence and is the third leading cause of cancer-specific mortality in both men and women. Colon cancer has no sex predilection. About 56,000 patients with colon and rectal cancer die of metastatic disease each year (Jemal et al, 2002).

The risk of colon cancer rises with age. The overall risk of colon cancer increases from 1 in 1,600 to 1,900 among individuals aged 39 years or less, to 1 in 120 to 150 among individuals aged 40 to 59 years, to 1 in 30 among individuals aged 60 to 79 years. More than 90% of cases occur in people who are 50 years of age or older.

One of the recognized risk factors for colon cancer is the Western diet high in saturated fat but low in fiber and antioxidants. The protective effects of fiber and calcium have turned out to be not as important as the protective effects of antioxidants. Physical inactivity is a stronger risk factor than obesity in colon cancer. Alcohol use increases colon cancer risk by about twofold, but smoking does not seem to be linked to colon cancer. Patients with a long-standing history of inflammatory bowel disease have an incremental risk of developing colon cancer of 9% at 10 years, 20% at 20 years, and more than 35% at 30 years. Patients with pancolitis are at higher risk than those with segmental colitis. Patients with a history of ulcerative colitis of more than 8 years' duration should undergo surveillance colonoscopy every 6 to 12 months for the detection of dysplastic changes or cancerous polyps, which may be technically challenging owing to the infiltrative nature of the cancer. Detection of precancerous or cancerous lesions should prompt counseling regarding prophylactic total colectomy.

About 15% to 18% of colon cancer patients have an underlying genetic condition that predisposes to colon cancer, such as familial adenomatous polyposis (FAP) (1%) or hereditary nonpolyposis colorectal cancer (15%). FAP is an autosomal-dominant syndrome that occurs in approximately 1 in every 7,500 live births. It is caused by a mutation of the adenomatous polyposis coli (*APC*) gene, which is located on the long arm of chromosome 5 (region 5q21–q22). Individuals with FAP develop hundreds to thousands of colonic and rectal adenomatous polyps by the third decade of life. Left untreated, virtually every FAP patient will develop invasive adenocarcinoma by age 50 years.

Stage for stage, colorectal cancer patients with FAP have the same prognosis as those with sporadic colorectal cancer except for patients with delayed diagnosis or detection or late secondary complications from desmoid tumors and other secondary malignancies. In contrast, colon cancer patients with microsatellite-unstable tumors (hereditary nonpolyposis colorectal cancer) have a better prognosis than do patients with microsatellite-stable cancer. The observed better survival is not due to the effects of adjuvant chemotherapy (Ribic et al, 2003).

Regular use of aspirin has been associated with a significant reduction in the risk of colorectal cancer (hazard ratio, 0.56 to 0.75) in a number of large retrospective analyses. Two large prospective randomized placebo-controlled studies confirmed that daily aspirin use—particularly at a dose of 81 mg daily rather than 325 mg daily—was effective in preventing villous or tubulo-villous polyp formation in patients with a history of adenomatous polyps or colorectal cancer (Baron et al, 2003; Sandler et al, 2003). Specific cyclooxygenase-2 (COX-2) inhibitors, such as celecoxib, which have been shown to cause regression of polyps in patients with FAP, are being studied in patients with sporadic colorectal polyps (Steinbach et al, 2000). The role of estrogen replacement therapy for colon cancer prevention is not well defined.

Colonoscopy is the single most effective measure for colon cancer screening, detection, and prevention. At M. D. Anderson, colonoscopy is routinely performed as the primary mode of screening and follow-up in patients with a history of colorectal cancer. Other potentially cost-effective screening measures include fecal occult blood testing, barium enema, sigmoidoscopy, and computerized tomography colonography ("virtual colonoscopy").

CLINICAL PRESENTATIONS

The most common clinical presentations of colon cancer include occult to frank gastrointestinal bleeding with or without evidence of iron-deficiency anemia. Altered bowel habits, fatigue, and unexplained weight loss are uncommon; the presence of unexplained fatigue or gastrointestinal symptoms should prompt clinical evaluation. Right-sided colon cancer tends to be associated with more profound anemia than left-sided colon cancer, as left-sided tumors often present with early warning signs of altered bowel habits and early gastrointestinal bleeding. Patients—even those with advanced colon cancer—may have no clinical symptoms. Jaundice is uncommon unless there is biliary duct obstruction.

DIAGNOSIS AND STAGING

Most colon cancer cases are clinically silent; therefore, colon cancer is often detected on either routine laboratory testing or colonoscopy screening. Once the pathology findings are confirmed, all patients in whom invasive colon cancer is suspected should undergo a thorough history and physical examination as well as laboratory testing including complete blood cell counts; measurement of electrolytes; liver function panels; measurement of prothrombin time, partial thromboplastin time, and carcinoembryonic antigen (CEA); electrocardiography; chest radiography; and a baseline computed tomography scan of the abdomen and pelvis.

More than 95% of colon cancers are adenocarcinoma; rare pathologic subtypes include adenocarcinoma with carcinoid or neuroendocrine features and small cell carcinoma of the large bowel. Pathologic features associated with a poor prognosis include the presence of nodal metastasis (the strongest prognostic factor); poor histologic grade, as determined by the degree of glandular differentiation; the presence of either intracellular mucin (also known as signet ring) or extracellular mucin; and perineural, lymphovascular, or vascular invasion. Adenocarcinoma with mucinous differentiation and lymphocyte infiltration in the tumor is highly suggestive of a microsatellite-unstable tumor. Occasionally, ovarian cancer masquerades as colon cancer or vice versa. The distinction can often be made clinically through histologic examination (orientation of tumor invasion within the colon wall or outside the colon wall). In addition, ovarian cancer is often positive for cytokeratin-7, whereas colon cancers are often positive for cytokeratin-20 but always negative for cytokeratin-7. Mucinous ovarian tumors may also be positive for cytokeratin-20.

Colon cancers are staged surgically. Colon cancer is staged according to the TNM (tumor, nodes, metastasis) staging classification in the 6th edition of the American Joint Commission on Cancer's *AJCC Cancer Staging Manual* (Greene et al, 2002). The TNM system (see chapter 1, Table 1–6) has replaced the previously used Duke's colon cancer staging system and modified Astler-Coller system and is further simplified by the M. D. Anderson color-matrix cancer staging system.

Half of patients with colon cancer develop distant metastases, and about 25% of patients present with metastases at the time of colon cancer diagnosis. Five-year survival rates in patients with colon cancer correlate with tumor stage. The overall 5-year survival rates for patients with stage I, II, III, and IV colon cancers are 90%, 70% to 80%, 40% to 65%, and less than 10%, respectively.

TENETS OF MANAGEMENT

Surgery achieves tumor control through zero-order kinetics; therefore, adequate resection margins and higher number of lymph nodes sampled are associated with improved disease-free and overall survival. Patients with 10 or fewer lymph nodes removed have significantly lower 5-year survival rates than patients with 20 to 40 lymph nodes removed. Hemicolectomy with regional lymph node dissection is indicated for patients with stage I, II, or III colon cancer; for patients who present with resectable or low-volume synchronous metastatic colon cancer; and for patients with perforation or obstruction.

Resection of liver or lung metastases, anastomotic recurrence, or recurrence in draining lymph nodes is associated with 5-year survival rates of 20% to 40%. Only rarely do patients benefit from resection of peritoneal metastases or retroperitoneal lymph nodes. It is important to note that the surgical series are highly selected retrospective review series in which survival was calculated without inclusion of all stage IV patients in the denominator. Nonetheless, 7 factors are significant and independent predictors of poor long-term outcome after metastasectomy: positive surgical margins, extrahepatic disease, node-positive primary tumor, disease-free interval between diagnosis of primary tumor and diagnosis of metastases of less than 12 months, number of hepatic tumors greater than 1, largest hepatic tumor larger than 5 cm, and CEA level greater than 200 ng/ml. Patients with 3, 4, or 5 of these predictors should be considered for experimental trials of adjuvant chemotherapy (Fong et al, 1999). Newer ablative techniques, such as radiofrequency ablation, are increasingly used alone or in conjunction with surgery. In general, 75% of patients with successful metastasectomy have a recurrence within the first 2–3 years.

Twenty percent to 50% of patients with stage II or III disease eventually develop metastatic disease or locally recurrent disease because of occult micrometastases or inadequate resection of tumor. Cytotoxic chemotherapy achieves tumor control through first-order kinetics. Cytotoxic chemotherapy has 3 major roles: (1) To provide effective adjuvant treatment to eliminate or reduce the overall tumor micrometastasis burden. (2) To convert patients with unresectable disease into candidates for surgical resection. The newer combination-chemotherapy regimens are particularly effective in producing tumor response and are therefore more effective in reduction of tumor burden. (3) To palliate tumor-related symptoms or prolong time to tumor progression and overall survival and improve quality of life in patients with metastatic colon cancer.

In line with the above-mentioned therapeutic goals are the 5 following treatment principles: (1) familiarity with agent-specific and regimen-specific toxicity; (2) timely adjustments of dose and schedule as well as institution of treatment breaks or preventative measures to minimize treatment-related side effects; (3) selection of patients for 5-FU monotherapy versus combination chemotherapy or alternating therapy to maximize the duration of tumor control with minimal induction of chemoresistance; (4) appropriate utilization of chemoradiation for palliation and neoadjuvant treatment of metastatic disease; and (5) early identification and timely referral of patients with potentially resectable disease.

CHEMOTHERAPY

For decades, 5-FU was the only chemotherapy agent known to be active against colorectal cancer. In recent years, many new chemotherapeutic agents have been introduced, and therapeutic options have been greatly expanded.

Fluorouracil

As an antimetabolite, 5-FU inhibits both the DNA and RNA synthesis pathways in cancer. 5-FU is converted to 5-FUdR by thymidine phosphorylase and then to FdUMP through thymidine kinase. FdUMP inhibits DNA synthesis by binding to thymidylate synthase (the process is facilitated by leucovorin) to form a stable ternary complex.

Because for 4 decades 5-FU was the only active agent for the treatment of colon cancer, numerous clinical trials have been conducted of strategies designed to modulate 5-FU activity, either through manipulation of its infusion schedule (continuous infusion, bolus administration, or circadian) or through addition of response modifiers such as levamisole, leucovorin, interferon, and N-(phosphonacetyl)-L-aspartic acid (PALA). The highlights of the study findings are as follows: (1) 5-FU alone produced responses in 15% of patients with metastatic colon cancer, and the addition of levamisole, interferon, or PALA to 5-FU provided no benefits but increased treatment toxicity. (2) Compared with bolus administration of 5-FU, continuous infusion of 5-FU was associated with a modest improvement in the tumor response rate (from 15% to 20%), improvement in tumor control by about 4 weeks, and reduction in the rate of systemic grade 3 and 4 hematologic and nonhematologic side effects (12% vs 35%) except for hand-foot syndrome (34% vs 12%). (3) The addition of leucovorin enhanced 5-FU activity in vitro and in vivo, but the absolute survival benefit of leucovorin was 2% to 4%. (4) A 6-month course of adjuvant 5-FU produced an effect equivalent to that of a 12-month course of 5-FU and leucovorin (O'Dwyer et al, 2001; Rodriguez et al, 2003).

Irinotecan

Irinotecan is a camptothecin derivative that acts as a topoisomerase I inhibitor. Irinotecan was first shown to be active as a single agent in patients in whom treatment with 5-FU failed. Irinotecan in these patients produced a 41% longer median overall survival (9.2 months vs 6.5 months) than best supportive care and was associated with better quality-of-life scores (Cunningham et al, 1998). Compared with infusional 5-FU in patients in whom prior 5-FU failed, irinotecan again produced longer median overall survival (10.8 months vs 8.5 months; P = .02) (Rougier et al, 1998).

Various combinations of irinotecan, 5-FU, and leucovorin were then compared with 5-FU and leucovorin as front-line treatment for metastatic colorectal cancer. The regimens used are described in Table 9–1, and the studies are summarized in Table 9–2. The one U.S. study (Saltz et al, 2000) explored weekly bolus 5-FU and leucovorin plus weekly irinotecan (the so-called IFL regimen), whereas 2 European studies (Douillard et al, 2000; Kohne et al, 2003) explored infusional 5-FU and leucovorin plus irinotecan administered either weekly or biweekly (the so-called FOLFIRI and AIO + irinotecan regimens).

The major findings of these studies were as follows: (1) The combination of irinotecan, 5-FU, and leucovorin consistently produced higher overall tumor response rates (35% to 54.2% vs 18% to 31.5%), longer time to tumor progression (6.7 to 8.5 months vs 4.2 to 6.3 months), and better overall survival (14.8 to 20.1 months vs 12.6 to 16.9 months). (2) The AIO + irinotecan (infusional-5-FU) regimen appeared to be associated with the least treatment-related toxicity and better treatment outcomes (response rate, time to progression, and overall survival) than the respective 5-FU/leucovorin control arms. Interestingly, the AIO 5-FU/leucovorin regimen was associated with a response rate of 31.5%, time to progression of 6.3 months, and median overall survival of 16.9 months, similar to the outcomes seen with the IFL regimen.

Table 9–1. Commonly Used Chemotherapy Regimens for First- and Second-Line Treatment of Metastatic Colorectal Cancer*

Regimen Name	Drug Doses and Schedules	Incidence of Grade 3 or More Severe Toxic Effects	Reference
Regimens with Leucovorin, 5-FU, and Irinotecan			
AIO + Irinotecan	Leucovorin 500 mg/m² IV over 2 hours weeks 1, 2, 3, 4, 5, and 6 5-FU 2000 mg/m² CI IV over 24 hours weeks 1, 2, 3, 4, 5, and 6 Irinotecan 80 mg/m² IV over 30 minutes weeks 1, 2, 3, 4, 5, and 6	Diarrhea, 20% Stomatitis, 5% Neutropenia, 8% Cardiovascular, 1%	Kohne et al, 2003
FOLFIRI	Leucovorin 200 mg IV over 2 hours days 1 and 2 5-FU 400 mg/m² IV bolus days 1 and 2 5-FU 600 mg/m² CI IV over 22 hours days 1 and 2 Irinotecan 180 mg/m² day 1 only Repeat cycle every 2 weeks	Diarrhea, 44% Stomatitis, 5% Neutropenia, 29% Vomiting, 11%	Douillard et al, 2000
IFL	Leucovorin 20 mg/m² IV over 2 hours weeks 1, 2, 3, and 4, then 2 weeks off 5-FU 425–500 mg/m² IV over 15 minutes weeks 1, 2, 3, and 4 Irinotecan 100–125 mg/m² IV over 90 minutes weeks 1, 2, 3, and 4 Repeat cycle every 6 weeks or 2 weeks on 1 week off	Neutropenia, 54% Diarrhea, 23% Nausea, 10% Cardiovascular, 2% 60-day mortality, 3.4%	Saltz et al, 2000
Regimens with Leucovorin, 5-FU, and Oxaliplatin			
FOLFOX4	Leucovorin 200 mg IV over 2 hours days 1 and 2 5-FU 400 mg/m² IV bolus days 1 and 2 5-FU 600 mg/m² CI IV over 22 hours days 1 and 2 Oxaliplatin 85 mg/m² day 1 only Repeat cycle every 2 weeks	Neutropenia, 50% Diarrhea, 12% Neuropathy, 18%	de Gramont et al, 2000, and Pitot et al, 2003

Regimen	Dosing	Toxicity	Reference
FOLFOX6	Leucovorin 400 mg IV over 2 hours day 1 5-FU 400 mg/m² IV bolus day 1 5-FU 2400–3000 mg/m² CI IV over 46 hours Oxaliplatin 100 mg/m² day 1 only Repeat cycle every 2 weeks	Neutropenia, 26% Diarrhea, 11% Paresthesia, 34%	Tournigand et al, 2001
FOLFOX7-5FU/ LV-FOLFOX7 (OPTIMOX)	Leucovorin 400 mg IV over 2 hours day 1 5-FU 2400 mg/m² CI IV over 46 hours Oxaliplatin 130 mg/m² day 1 only Repeat cycle every 2 weeks	Neuropathy, 10.8% Neutropenia, 21.2%	Andre et al, 2003

Regimen with Irinotecan and Oxaliplatin

Regimen	Dosing	Toxicity	Reference
IROX	Irinotecan 80–100 mg IV over 90 minutes Oxaliplatin 85–125 mg IV over 30 minutes Repeat cycle every 21 days	Neutropenia, 36% Diarrhea, 24% Vomiting, 22% Paresthesia, 7%	Pitot et al, 2003

Regimens with Capecitabine and Irinotecan

Regimen	Dosing	Toxicity	Reference
XELIRI (CAPIRI)	Capecitabine (X) 1000 mg/m²/day by mouth days 1–14 (total dose = 2000 mg/m²/day) Irinotecan 200–250 mg IV day 1[1,2] Or Irinotecan 80 mg IV on day 1 and day 8[2] Repeat cycle every 21 days	Neutropenia, 10% Hand-foot syndrome, 6% Diarrhea, 5% Anorexia, 2%	Patt et al, 2003, and Grothey et al, 2003
XELOX (CAPOX)	Capecitabine (X) 1000 mg/m²/day by mouth days 1–14 (total dose = 2000 mg/m²/day) Oxaliplatin 130 mg IV day 1 Repeat cycle every 21 days	Neutropenia, 10% Neuropathy, 6% Diarrhea	Diaz-Rubio et al, 2002

Abbreviations: CI, continuous infusion; IV, intravenously.

* Both irinotecan- and oxaliplatin-based regimens were active in second-line therapy, producing tumor response rates of about 10% to 15%. The expected approval of cetuximab will lead to use of this drug in third-line treatment of colorectal cancer. The expected approval of bevacizumab will add another front-line treatment for metastatic colorectal cancer.

Table 9–2. Pivotal Phase III Trials in the First-Line Treatment of Metastatic Colorectal Cancer

First Author and Year	No. of Patients	Regimens*	Response Rate (%)	Progression-Free Survival Rate (%)	Median Overall Survival (months)
Saltz, 2000	231	IFL	39†	7.0†	14.8†
	226	Irinotecan	21	4.3	12.6
	220	Bolus 5-FU and leucovorin	18	4.2	12
Douillard, 2000	187	de Gramont or AIO	22	4.4	14.1
	198	FOLFIRI	35†	6.7†	17.4†
Kohne, 2003	214	AIO	31.5	6.4	16.9
	216	AIO + irinotecan	54.2†	8.5†	20.1
Giacchetti, 2000	100	Infusional 5-FU and leucovorin	16	6.1	19.9
	100	Infusional 5-FU and leucovorin + oxaliplatin	53	8.7†	19.4
de Gramont, 2000	210	de Gramont	22.3	6.2	14.7
	210	FOLFOX4	50.7†	9.0†	16.2
Pitot, 2003	267	IFL	31	6.9	14.8
	264	IROX	34	6.5	17.4
	267	FOLFOX4	45	8.7†	19.5†

* Regimens are described in Table 9–1.
† Statistically significant.

The hallmark side effects of irinotecan are watery diarrhea and a small increase in the risk of thrombotic complications (Cunningham et al, 1998; Rougier et al, 1998; Douillard et al, 2000; Saltz et al, 2000).

Oxaliplatin

Oxaliplatin is a water-soluble platinum derivative and is an inactive prodrug that requires in vivo biotransformation. There is no evidence of cytochrome P_{450} metabolism of the DACH ring in vitro. The route of elimination is predominantly (54%) urinary; fecal excretion accounts for 2% of elimination.

Oxaliplatin has synergistic antitumor activity with 5-FU against a broad spectrum of different cisplatin-resistant cell lines. Oxaliplatin's major mechanism of action is DNA adduct formation through platinum interstrand and intrastrand DNA cross-links, leading to inhibition of DNA replication, interference with transcriptional activation, and induction of tumor cell apoptosis.

Three pivotal phase III trials of oxaliplatin in the frontline treatment of metastatic colorectal cancer are summarized in Table 9–2. In 2 trials (de Gramont et al, 2000; Giacchetti et al, 2000), the combination of oxaliplatin with infusional 5-FU and leucovorin was compared with infusional 5-FU and leucovorin. The 3-drug combinations were associated with improved tumor response rates and improved time to progression but had no impact on overall survival (Table 9–2). The lack of survival benefit was thought to be due in large part to crossover or sample size.

The North Central Cancer Treatment Group (Pitot et al, 2003) then compared the IFL regimen, the regimen of irinotecan and oxaliplatin (IROX), and FOLFOX4 in patients with metastatic colorectal cancer. Compared with IFL, FOLFOX4 demonstrated a superior response rate (45% vs 31%), time to progression (8.7 months vs 6.9 months), and median overall survival (19.5 months vs 14.8 months) and an improved side effect profile. IROX also appeared to be superior to IFL. Three caveats need to be emphasized: (1) Sixty percent of patients in the FOLFOX4 arm received irinotecan for salvage therapy, while only 25% of patients in the IFL arm received oxaliplatin as second-line therapy; (2) FOLFOX4 employed infusional 5-FU, which is superior to the bolus 5-FU used in the IFL arm; and (3) exposure to all 3 active agents is associated with longer median survival.

FOLFOX4 was also studied as second-line therapy in patients in whom IFL failed. Compared with 5-FU and leucovorin, FOLFOX4 was associated with an improved response rate (9.8% vs 0.7%) and time to tumor progression (5.6 months vs 2.6 months). There was also a trend toward a survival benefit (9.8 months vs 8.7 months; $P = .07$) (Rothenberg et al, 2001).

The side effects of oxaliplatin include acute dysthesia during oxaliplatin infusion, cumulative sensory neuropathy, and thrombocytopenia.

Capecitabine

If 5-FU is administered orally, 90% of the 5-FU is metabolized by dipyrimidine dehydrogenase in the gut or peripheral blood monocytes.
Administration of oral fluoropyrimidines combined with either a reversible dipyrimidine dehydrogenase inhibitor (e.g., tegafur) or an irreversible
dipyrimidine dehydrogenase inhibitor (e.g., eniluracil) did not result in
significant therapeutic advantages over intravenous infusion of 5-FU and
leucovorin.

Capecitabine, a 5-FU prodrug, is more active than bolus 5-FU and leucovorin and has a side effect profile similar to that of infusional 5-FU.
Capecitabine is converted to 5-FU by a 3-step enzymatic reaction—by car-
boxylesterase in the gut, cytidine deaminase in the liver and tumor, and
finally, thymidine phosphorylase, the level of which is 3- to 15-fold higher
in tumor tissue than in adjacent normal tissue. Because of the enzymatic
conversion and preferential conversion to 5-FU by high levels of thymidine phosphorylase in tumor tissue, the mean concentration of 5-FU ratios
was more than 3 times as high in primary tumor tissue as in adjacent
healthy tissue and more than 21 times as high in primary tumor tissue as
in plasma. In contrast, administration ratios of tumor to healthy tissue or
plasma were all close to 1, indicating no tumor selectivity.

Despite these pharmacologic advantages of capecitabine, 2 large randomized phase III trials conducted in the United States and Europe (Hoff
et al, 2001; Van Cutsem et al, 2001) showed that although capecitabine
produced a higher tumor response rate (25% vs 14%) than bolus 5-FU and
leucovorin, capecitabine was not associated with benefits in terms of time
to tumor progression or overall survival. However, the toxicity profile of
capecitabine was better than that of 5-FU and leucovorin and similar to
that of continuous-infusion 5-FU.

Capecitabine may be administered alone or in combination with either
irinotecan (regimen known as XELIRI) or oxaliplatin (regimen known as
XELOX) in the frontline treatment of metastatic colorectal cancer. The
phase II data showed that XELIRI or XELOX may replace the inconvenient
infusional 5-FU without compromising the response rate and safety
profiles. In a phase II study conduced at M. D. Anderson (Patt et al, 2003),
XELIRI was associated with a response rate of 42%, an overall tumor
control rate of 74%, and median time to progression of 7.1 months. Randomized phase III trials comparing capecitabine-based combination
regimens to the standard FOLFIRI or FOLFOX regimens are ongoing.

Two common side effects of capecitabine are hand-foot syndrome and
diarrhea (Patt et al, 2003; Van Cutsem et al, 2003).

TARGETED THERAPY

In recent years, there has been exponential growth in our knowledge of
cancer cell growth and survival. Cancer cells have 6 essential hallmarks:

self-sufficiency in growth signals, insensitivity to antigrowth signals, tissue invasion and metastasis, limitless replicative potential, sustained angiogenesis, and evasion of apoptosis. In turn, understanding of the mechanisms underlying cancer growth, invasion, and survival advantage has led to the identification of molecular targets and the development of molecular therapies for all malignancies, including colon cancer.

Bevacizumab

Vascular endothelial growth factor (VEGF) is a very potent angiogenic factor. It is overexpressed in 70% to 80% of colorectal cancers and is associated with poor prognosis. Bevacizumab (Avastin) is a recombinant humanized (93%) chimeric immunoglobulin-G monoclonal antibody with a serum half-life in humans of 17 to 21 days. Bevacizumab blocks all VEGF isoforms with high affinity and high specificity and prevents VEGF binding to all VEGF receptors. Bevacizumab also blocks angiogenesis, preventing activation through VEGF and activation of downstream signaling pathways and endothelial cell proliferation and migration. A phase II study showed that addition of bevacizumab (5 mg/kg intravenously every 2 weeks) to 5-FU and leucovorin improved tumor response rate, enhanced median time to tumor progression to 9 months, and enhanced median overall survival to 21.5 months (Kabbinavar et al, 2003). In a randomized phase III study comparing bevacizumab (5 mg/kg intravenously every 2 weeks) plus the IFL regimen versus IFL alone in front-line treatment of stage IV colorectal cancer, the regimen with bevacizumab was associated with an enhanced response rate (44.9% vs 34.7%) and improved median time to tumor progression (10.4 months vs 7.1 months, $P = .0014$) and median overall survival (20.3 months vs 15.6 months; $P = .00003$). The unique side effects of bevacizumab included manageable hypertension (10% of patients), proteinuria, and rare abdominal perforations (Hurwitz et al, 2003). It is interesting that a randomized phase III study failed to show that adding the tyrosine kinase inhibitor SU5416 (a VEGF inhibitor) to the IFL regimen failed to produce a survival advantage over IFL alone. It is important to note that bevacizumab plus 5-FU and leucovorin without irinotecan produced median survival close to 20 months. Bevacizumab is now approved for firstline treatment of metastatic colorectal cancer. Other VEGF tyrosine kinase inhibitors—for example, PTK-787—are currently in phase III clinical development.

Cetuximab

In colorectal cancer, epidermal growth factor receptor (EGFR) has been associated with all 6 of the hallmarks of cancer mentioned at the beginning of the Targeted Therapy section. Overexpression of EGFR is noted in 70% to 80% of colorectal cancers. In vitro and in vivo models support EGFR as a valid molecular target for many solid tumors, including colorectal cancer.

Cetuximab (Erbitux) is a human-murine chimeric anti-EGFR immunoglobulin G monoclonal antibody. Cetuximab binds to EGFR with a binding affinity approximately one log higher than that of the natural ligand, transforming growth factor beta, preventing EGFR receptor dimerization and blocking EGFR signaling pathways. A phase II study in 121 patients previously treated with the IFL regimen showed that cetuximab plus IFL produced a response in 22.5% of patients and stable disease in 26.7% (Saltz et al, 2002). Cetuximab alone is associated with a response rate of 10% and with a median response duration of 6 months. In a randomized study, cetuximab (loading dose of 400 mg/m^2 intravenously, then 250 mg/m^2 intravenously weekly) plus irinotecan (100 to 125 mg/m^2 intravenously weekly for 4 weeks or 200 to 250 mg/m^2 intravenously every 3 weeks) also produced a response rate of 22% with a median response duration of 4 months in heavily pretreated patients previously treated with irinotecan or oxaliplatin. All clinical parameters except the development of an acneiform rash, including EGFR expression, were predictors of response. Anaphylactic reaction occurs in less than 5% and acneiform skin rash occurs in about 50% of patients treated with cetuximab (Saltz et al, 2000; Cunningham et al, 2003).

Other EGFR antagonists, including small-molecule tyrosine kinase inhibitors (e.g., gefitinib [Iressa]) and monoclonal antibodies (e.g., EMD 2000), have also been developed.

Celecoxib

Overexpression of COX-2 is seen in 70% to 80% of colorectal cancers and is also a strong prognostic factor. Celecoxib is a specific COX-2 inhibitor that is already approved for treatment of osteoarthritis and rheumatoid arthritis and prevention of colon polyps in patients with FAP. COX-2 inhibitors avoid the side effects of COX-1 inhibition, which include increased risk of gastritis, peptic ulcers, and gastrointestinal bleeding. The preliminary M. D. Anderson experience suggests that concurrent use of celecoxib and capecitabine with or without radiotherapy reduces the incidence of capecitabine-induced hand-foot syndrome while significantly enhancing the overall tumor response rate, time to tumor progression, and overall survival (Lin et al, 2002). A number of prospective randomized phase III studies involving celecoxib are currently in progress.

MANAGEMENT OF COLON CANCER BY STAGE

Carcinoma In Situ

Carcinoma in situ can almost always be cured by polypectomy alone or repeated polypectomy if complete endoscopic removal of the carcinoma in situ cannot be documented. Polypectomy may also be adequate for small T1 tumors that are margin-negative (i.e., no adenocarcinoma within 3 mm of the cauterized margin), well or moderately differentiated, and without lymphovascular or vascular invasion.

Stage I Colon Cancer

Polypectomy with negative margins is usually adequate for treatment of carcinoma in situ or small, well-differentiated T1 tumors with greater-than-3 mm cauterized margins and absence of lymphovascular invasion. Hemicolectomy with local-regional lymph node dissection is required for T1 tumors that are poorly differentiated, were previously treated with piecemeal polypectomy without clearly defined margins, or have evidence of lymphovascular invasion and for T2 or more advanced tumors.

The 10-year survival rate for patients with stage I colon cancer exceeds 90%. The primary goal of management of stage I disease is secondary prevention of new adenomatous polyps. Follow-up clinical examinations (measurement of CEA) should be conducted every 6 months for 2 years, then yearly for 5 years. Surveillance colonoscopy should be done within the first year after diagnosis and every 3 to 5 years thereafter. Low-dose aspirin therapy (81 mg by mouth daily) may be appropriate.

Stage II Colon Cancer

The 5-year survival rate for patients with stage II colon cancer treated with surgery alone is about 80%. The role of adjuvant 5-FU and leucovorin in patients with stage II colon cancer is controversial. Dozens of individual studies failed to demonstrate a statistically significant benefit of 5-FU-based adjuvant treatment over observation alone; however, 3 meta-analyses suggested that adjuvant 5-FU and leucovorin produced an overall survival benefit of 2%, raising the overall survival rate from 81% to 83% (Erlichman, 1997; IMPACT, 1999; Mamounas et al, 1999). Therefore, it is imperative to discuss the pros and cons of 5-FU adjuvant treatment with patients, taking into account factors such as the patient's age, life expectancy, and general health.

The subset of patients with perforated T4 tumors have a much higher risk of locoregional recurrence—up to 50%—after treatment with surgery alone. Therefore, these patients should be offered not only systemic adjuvant chemotherapy but also chemoradiation with an optimal fluoropyrimidine plus radiotherapy at 45 Gy for 5 weeks (Willett et al, 1993, 1999). In patients with stage II colon cancer in the MOSAIC study (discussed in detail in the next section), the FOLFOX4 regimen achieved a relative risk reduction of 18%, or a gain in disease-free survival from 83.9% to 86.6% (de Gramont et al, 2003).

Other poor prognostic markers (high tumor grade and perineural, lymphatic, or vascular invasion) are useful in estimating the risk of recurrence but have not been prospectively validated as a guide for adjuvant treatment (Erlichman, 1997).

Stage III Colon Cancer

The 5-year survival rate for patients with stage III colon cancer treated with surgery alone is 40% to 60%. Lymph node metastasis is the strongest predictor of survival. Results of the many pivotal studies of adjuvant therapy for patients with stage III disease are as follows: (1) Adjuvant 5-FU and levamisole for 1 year improved the disease-free survival and overall survival rates by 30% and 20%, respectively, over observation. (2) Adjuvant 5-FU and leucovorin for 6 months produced survival rates equivalent to those seen with 5-FU and levamisole for 1 year, and the addition of levamisole to 5-FU and leucovorin did not increase the effect of 5-FU and leucovorin alone but did increase toxicity.

The Mayo Clinic and Roswell Park regimens (Table 9–3) are the 2 most commonly used regimens for adjuvant treatment of colon cancer. It is important to bear in mind that the Mayo Clinic regimen was associated with a far higher incidence of neutropenia than was the Roswell Park regimen, and that the Roswell Park regimen was associated with a higher incidence of diarrhea (Moertel et al, 1995; O'Connell et al, 1998; O'Dwyer et al, 2001). It is also important to point out that elderly patients (those older than 70 years) benefit from adjuvant 5-FU and leucovorin to the same degree as do younger patients (Sargent et al, 2001). A large randomized phase III study that compared capecitabine versus the Mayo Clinic regimen demonstrated improved safety in favor of capecitabine (Twelves et al, 2003).

In a large randomized phase III study (the MOSAIC study) in patients with stage II and III colon cancer, the FOLFOX4 regimen resulted in superior 3-year disease-free survival (78% vs 73%; $P < .01$) compared with

Table 9–3. Commonly Used Adjuvant Chemotherapy Regimens for Patients with Stage III Colon Cancer*

Mayo Clinic Regimen	More likely to cause
5-FU 425 mg/m² IV bolus daily × 5	myelosuppression
Leucovorin 20 mg/m² IV daily × 5	
Repeat every 4–5 weeks for 6 cycles	
Roswell Park Regimen	More likely to cause diarrhea
Leucovorin 500 mg/m² over 2 hours	
5-FU 500 mg/m² bolus mid of leucovorin	
Weekly × 6 followed by a 2-week rest for 4 cycles	

* The pros and cons of adding oxaliplatin to 5-FU in the adjuvant treatment of colon cancer should be discussed with patients prior to initiation of treatment.

5-FU and leucovorin, achieving a relative risk reduction of 23% in both stage II and stage III patients. In subset analyses, FOLFOX4 improved disease-free survival from 65% to 71% in patients with stage III disease, with a relative risk reduction of 24% (hazard ratio, 0.76). FOLFOX4 was very safe—it was associated with an all-cause mortality rate of 0.5% in both arms, and the incidence of febrile neutropenia was less than 2%. Of concern was the development of grade 2 and grade 3 sensory neuropathy in 31.5% and 12.4%, respectively, of patients. Fortunately, the grade 3 sensory neuropathy was reversible: the percentage of patients with this side effect after 1 year of follow-up had declined to 1%. Although the median follow-up time is short at 3 years, this is the first clinical trial to show that addition of a new class of cytotoxic agent, oxaliplatin, to 5-FU and leucovorin produced improved disease-free survival at 3 years (de Gramont et al, 2003). In contrast, the Cancer and Leukemia Group B 89803 trial, which compared the IFL regimen versus 5-FU and leucovorin (Roswell Park regimen) in patients with stage III colon cancer, reported unexpected 60-day mortality rates of 2.2% in the experimental IFL arm. The final analysis demonstrated neither a disease-free nor an overall survival difference between the 2 regimens.

Stage IV Colon Cancer

About half of all patients with colon cancer die of metastatic or recurrent disease, and one quarter of patients present with synchronous stage IV disease. Sites of metastasis often include lymph nodes in the primary tumor drainage basin or in the para-aortic retroperitoneal chain. The liver is the most common visceral-organ site of colon cancer metastasis, followed by the lungs, peritoneum, and bone. Rare metastases to the adrenal gland, brain, and thyroid gland have also been reported. Mucinous tumors, especially of signet-ring-cell type, have a predilection for causing abdominal carcinomatosis, similar to presentations of ovarian cancer. The differential diagnosis is often straightforward; however, immunohistochemical studies with cytokeratin markers may be required. Second colon cancer primary tumors are more commonly encountered in younger patients and patients with an underlying genetic predisposition, such as patients with hereditary nonpolyposis colorectal cancer.

Even though an increasing number of therapeutic regimens are available for the first-line and second-line treatment of metastatic colorectal cancer, all eligible patients should be strongly encouraged to participate in well-designed clinical trials. Moreover, treatment of patients should be individualized on the basis of many clinical variables that affect the clinical outcome. Some of these variables are performance status, synchronous or metachronous metastasis, pattern and sites of metastasis, disease-free interval from primary tumor diagnosis or treatment, surgical resectability, feasibility of palliative or definitive chemoradiation, comorbid conditions, patient age, and patient preference and lifestyle.

Patients with synchronous resectable or borderline resectable metastases should undergo surgical removal of the primary tumor first and then combination chemotherapy before metastasectomy is explored. Patients with high-volume systemic metastases, unless there are emergent surgical indications (e.g., bleeding, perforation, or obstruction), should preferably proceed to chemotherapy before surgery for the primary tumor. Hemicolectomy with or without colostomy is indicated if there is evidence of bowel perforation, obstruction, or bleeding. Occasionally, bowel obstruction can be successfully managed with the deployment of colonic stents or argon laser ablation.

For patients with high-volume unresectable metastases involving multiple visceral sites, the goal of therapy is to prolong survival and maintain or improve the patient's overall quality of life. The median survival for patients with metastatic colorectal cancer has increased from 9 months with best supportive care to 12 months with 5-FU and leucovorin to 14 to 17 months with combination chemotherapy to 20 months with an optimal fluoropyrimidine plus either irinotecan or oxaliplatin or combination treatment with bevacizumab and IFL.

The pros and cons of irinotecan versus oxaliplatin are as follows: (1) Infusional 5-FU is the optimal way of administering 5-FU. The de Gramont and AIO infusional-5-FU-plus-leucovorin regimens are the most commonly used in combination with irinotecan (e.g., FOLFIRI) and oxaliplatin (e.g., FOLFOX4). (2) FOLFOX4 is superior to IFL in terms of clinical outcomes but is equivalent to FOLFIRI. Furthermore, the optimal sequential monotherapy has not been carefully studied. Exposure to all active agents is associated with optimal survival benefits (3). The combination of 5-FU and leucovorin is synergistic with oxaliplatin but likely additive with irinotecan. Single-agent oxaliplatin produces weak antitumor activity, whereas irinotecan is an effective antitumor agent, producing a response rate of 25% when given as monotherapy in the first-line and second-line settings. (4) Cumulative sensory neuropathy secondary to oxaliplatin does not occur after 4 to 6 cycles of treatment, and efficacy is evident within the first 2 cycles of treatment. However, the tradeoff is cumulative neuropathy, hypersensitivity reactions, and thrombocytopenia. In contrast, with irinotecan, diarrhea is not a cumulative toxicity, but fatigue occurs in some patients (Kohne et al, 2003; Pitot et al, 2003).

Resectable recurrences include anastomotic recurrence, isolated liver or lung metastasis, recurrence in regional draining lymph nodes, and isolated peritoneal metastasis on a case-by-case basis. The liver is the most common site of visceral metastases, and isolated liver metastases can be treated with segmentectomy or extended left or right trisegmentectomy with or without radiofrequency ablation (Goldberg et al, 1998). Similarly, pulmonary metastases can be resected through lobectomy, partial lobectomy, or wedge resection depending on the size and number of lesions. The role of adjuvant chemotherapy after metastasectomy is controversial.

Because the risk of recurrence after metastasectomy is approximately 70% to 80%, it would be prudent to recommend adjuvant treatment with infusional 5-FU with either oxaliplatin or irinotecan in certain patients; other patients could be offered observation. The selection of patients for adjuvant treatment should be largely based on whether patients previously received 5-FU and leucovorin or duration of response to neoadjuvant chemotherapy and, importantly, the disease-free interval prior to tumor resection.

Treatment with adjuvant 5-FU and leucovorin plus hepatic arterial infusion of FUdR improves the hepatic disease-free survival rate at 2 years but not the median overall survival over treatment with 5-FU and leucovorin alone. Even though hepatic arterial infusion with FUdR for liver metastasis from colorectal cancer improved the tumor response rates (range, 35% to 80%), the improved response rates did not translate into meaningful survival benefits (Kemeny et al, 1999). With the advent of newer targeted and cytotoxic chemotherapy for colorectal cancer, use of hepatic arterial infusion has largely fallen out of favor at M. D. Anderson because of the lack of systemic effect and the serious short-term and long-term complications.

For symptomatic or life-threatening metastases that can be encompassed by the radiation portal, chemoradiation is a highly effective but underutilized therapeutic tool. With 3-dimensional conformal planning techniques, metastases that can be safely irradiated include regional nodal metastases, unilateral liver or lung metastases, limited bone metastases, and metastases associated with impending cord compression. Either infusional 5-FU (250 to $300\,mg/m^2/day$ continuous infusion) or capecitabine is used as the radiation sensitizer. Radiation activates already upregulated thymidine phosphorylase in the tumor tissue, and thymidine phosphorylase converts capecitabine to 5-FU preferentially in the tumor tissue. The dose of capecitabine is either 900 to $1,000\,mg/m^2$ twice daily Monday through Friday or $825\,mg/m^2$ twice daily Monday through Sunday during radiotherapy. Long-term survival has been observed in patients who received radiotherapy with or without surgery.

MANAGEMENT OF SIDE EFFECTS

Diarrhea

Diarrhea is a common side effect of all colorectal cancer chemotherapy regimens, especially those that include irinotecan administered weekly rather than on an every-3-week schedule. Irinotecan produces both acute and delayed diarrhea. The acute phase occurs with 12 hours of irinotecan infusion and manifests as acute salivation, nausea, abdominal cramping, and diarrhea due to an exaggerated vagal response. Acute diarrhea responds well to atropine. The delayed phase occurs within 4 to 6 weeks of irinotecan exposure and manifests as onset of acute abdominal cramping, followed by progressive cholera-like watery diarrhea that can lead to vascular collapse in the absence of prompt intervention. Patients should receive loperamide or diphenoxylate at the first sign of loose stool or abdominal cramping and then every 2 to 4 hours until the diarrhea resolves. Laxatives, stool softeners, and bowel motility agents, as well as dairy products, fruit juice, alcohol, and coffee, need to be discontinued. For patients who cannot maintain adequate oral hydration, parenteral fluid may be needed. The so-called BRAT diet (bananas, rice, applesauce, and toast) or a low-fiber diet (crackers, soft noodles, and chicken) is recommended. Fever greater than 101°F (38.3°C), diarrhea persisting more than 24 hours, and bloody stools are indications for hospitalization. Patients should receive parenteral fluid or nutrition, antibiotics, antidiarrheal medications, opium tincture, and octreotide. The dose and schedule of octreotide (subcutaneous, intravenous, and depot) should be based on the severity of diarrhea.

Severe diarrhea secondary to 5-FU is less common and may be due to underlying dipyrimidine dehydrogenase (DPD) deficiency. With only 1 dose of 5-FU, patients with DPD deficiency can develop severe diarrhea, mucositis, neutropenia, cerebellar side effects, and skin rash. Both capecitabine and 5-FU are contraindicated in patients in whom DPD deficiency is suspected.

Hand-Foot Syndrome

The mechanism of hand-foot syndrome is unknown. It appears to be dose related and may be the result of inflammation. The role of high-dose pyridoxine (vitamin B6) in the treatment of hand-foot syndrome is not clear. The M. D. Anderson experience suggests that concurrent use of celecoxib significantly reduces the overall incidence and severity of capecitabine-induced hand-foot syndrome, by about 30% to 50% (Lin et al, 2002).

Neuropathy

Sensory neuropathy induced by oxaliplatin can be reduced with concurrent infusion of calcium gluconate at 1 gram and $MgSO_4$ at 1 gram. A stop-and-go strategy (termed OPTIMOX) has also been suggested: (1) Stop when there is evidence of grade 2 or greater neuropathy or the cumulative dose level is reached. (2) Go when the sensory neuropathy has regressed to grade 1 or less or when disease progresses with 5-FU and leucovorin alone.

SURVEILLANCE AFTER TREATMENT

The risk of colon cancer recurrence is highest during the first 2 to 3 years after diagnosis; more than 90% of recurrences occur within the first 5 years.

CEA is a nonspecific tumor-associated antigen, the level of which may be elevated 3 to 6 months before radiographic evidence of disease becomes apparent. CEA levels can be quite elevated in other malignancies (e.g., lung cancer, breast cancer, and thyroid cancer) and as a result of smoking, alcohol use, hepatitis, and inflammatory bowel disease (but the level is usually less than 6 ng/ml). CEA level remains normal in approximately 20% of patients with colorectal cancer, so CEA is not a useful marker for screening (Benson et al, 2000; Bast et al, 2001). Either CA19.9 or CA125 is also elevated in some colon cancer cases.

General guidelines for surveillance for patients with stage II or III colon cancer at M. D. Anderson are as follows: (1) Clinical examination and CEA testing every 3 months for the first year, every 4 months for the second year, every 6 months for the next 3 years, and then annually. Complete blood cell count and measurement of liver enzymes are optional. (2) Chest radiography and computed tomography every 6 months for the first 2 years, then annually. These tests are especially important for patients with a higher risk of recurrence (N2 disease) or with negative CEA findings.

Because of the high risk of recurrence, surveillance for patients who have undergone metastasectomy is more intense: (1) Clinical examination, measurement of CEA level, chest radiography (or computed tomography of the chest in patients with lung metastases), and CT scan of the abdomen and pelvis every 3 to 4 months for the first 2 years and every 6 months thereafter.

Surveillance colonoscopy should be performed in all patients with a history of colorectal cancer within 1 year after the initial diagnosis and then every 3 to 5 years.

FUTURE DIRECTIONS

Molecular and genetic studies of colon cancer have delineated molecular pathways of carcinogenesis and identified a plethora of molecular prognostic markers, including DNA proliferative index, p53, pRb, bcl-2, DCC (18q) deletion, microsatellite instability, transforming growth factor receptor-II, and overexpression of DPD, thymidine phosphorylase, thymidylate synthase, COX-2, EGFR, and VEGF. Microsatellite instability and transforming growth factor receptor-II appear to be favorable prognostic factors (Takahashi et al, 1998; Ioachim et al, 1999; van Triest et al, 1999; Watanabe et al, 2001). Integration and validation of these molecular markers in prospective clinical trials would be an important first step toward individualizing therapy in patients with colon cancer. Markers might be useful in identifying high-risk stage II and III patients for adjuvant treatment. Or they might be used to determine sensitivity or resistance to chemotherapy—e.g., low-level expression of DPD, thymidine phosphorylase, and thymidylate synthase predicts 5-FU sensitivity, while high levels of DPD,

KEY PRACTICE POINTS

- Colon cancer is highly preventable if appropriate screening with colonoscopy is performed.

- Patients with carcinoma in situ or small T1 tumors can be cured with simple polypectomy. However, all T2 or more extensive tumors require treatment with hemicolectomy and lymph node dissection.

- After surgical resection, the standard treatment for patients with stage II disease remains observation, but it is important to discuss with patients the potential benefits of adjuvant treatment.

- All patients with stage IIB colon cancer (i.e., perforation [T4] or obstruction) benefit from chemoradiation plus adjuvant chemotherapy.

- Patients with stage III colon cancer should receive 6 months of treatment with 5-FU and leucovorin with or without oxaliplatin.

- Adjuvant capecitabine has a better safety profile than the Mayo Clinic 5-FU-plus-leucovorin schedule except for hand-foot syndrome. Survival data are currently not available.

- Frontline treatment for metastatic colorectal cancer involves the use of infusional 5-FU administered according to either the de Gramont schedule or the AIO schedule with or without irinotecan or oxaliplatin ± bevacizumab.

- The IFL regimen plus bevacizumab produced a median overall survival of 20 months, similar to that seen with infusional 5-FU plus either irinotecan or oxaliplatin. Use of IFL is not recommended. Currently there are no survival data on adding bevacizumab to FOLFOX or FOLFIRI.

- Substitution of infusional 5-FU with oral capecitabine in combination treatment produced similar antitumor efficacies and favorable side effect profiles. There are no data on use of capecitabine with bevacizumab.

- Irinotecan plus cetuximab or FOLFOX4 produced response rates of 20% and 10%, respectively, in second-line treatment of patients in whom IFL had failed. The median duration of tumor control after second-line therapy is about 6 months.

- Metastasectomy results in 5-year survival in selected subsets of patients with stage IV colon cancer that involves only liver or lung, the site of the anastomosis, or regional draining lymph nodes.

- Patients who undergo metastasectomy can be observed or can be treated with either preoperative or postoperative combination chemotherapy or monotherapy with or without chemoradiation, depending on the sites of metastasis, disease-free interval, prior chemotherapy, disease burden, probability of margin-free resection, and medical comorbid conditions.

thymidine phosphorylase, or thymidylate synthase predicts 5-FU resistance (Salonga et al, 2000). Other molecular markers are being developed to predict tumor response to oxaliplatin (ERCC1) or susceptibility to irinotecan side effects (UGT1A1 gene polymorphism) (Iqbal and Lenz, 2001). Integration of molecular markers plus genomics and proteomics will one day be used to refine and enhance clinicians' ability to gauge patients' prognosis and make better treatment decisions.

SUGGESTED READINGS

Andre T, Figer A, Cervantes A, et al. FOLFOX7 compared to FOLFOX4: preliminary results of the randomized optimox study. *Proc Am Soc Clin Oncol* 2003; 22:253. Abstract 1016.

Baron JA, Cole BF, Sandler RS. A randomized trial of aspirin to prevent colorectal adenomas. *N Engl J Med* 2003;348:891–899.

Bast RC Jr, Ravdin P, Hayes DF, et al. 2000 update of recommendations for the use of tumor markers in breast and colorectal cancer: clinical practice guidelines of the American Society of Clinical Oncology. *J Clin Oncol* 2001;19:1865–1878.

Benson AB III, Desch CE, Flynn PJ. 2000 update of American Society of Clinical Oncology colorectal cancer surveillance guidelines. *J Clin Oncol* 2000;18:3586–3588.

Cunningham D, Humblet Y, Siena S, et al. Cetuximab (C225) alone or in combination with irinotecan (CPT-11) in patients with epidermal growth factor receptor (EGFR)-positive, irinotecan-refractory metastatic colorectal cancer (MCRC). *Proc Am Soc Clin Oncol* 2003;22:252. Abstract 1012.

Cunningham D, Pyrhonen S, James RD, et al. Randomised trial of irinotecan plus supportive care versus supportive care alone after fluorouracil failure for patients with metastatic colorectal cancer. *Lancet* 1998;352:1413–1418.

de Gramont A, Figer A, Seymour M, et al. Leucovorin and fluorouracil with or without oxaliplatin as first-line treatment in advanced colorectal cancer. *J Clin Oncol* 2000;18:2938–2947.

de Gramont A, Banzi M, Navarro M, et al. Oxaliplatin/5-FU/LV in adjuvant colon cancer: results of the international randomized MOSAIC trial. *Proc Am Soc Clin Oncol* 2003;22:253. Abstract 1015.

Diaz-Rubio E, Evans TR, Tabemero J, et al. Capecitabine (Xeloda) in combination with oxaliplatin: a phase I, dose-escalation study in patients with advanced or metastatic solid tumors. *Ann Oncol* 2002;13:558–565.

Douillard JY, Cunningham D, Roth AD, et al. Irinotecan combined with fluorouracil compared with fluorouracil alone as first-line treatment for metastatic colorectal cancer: a multicentre randomised trial. *Lancet* 2000;355:1041–1047.

Erlichman C. Metaanalysis of adjuvant therapy for stage II colon cancer. *J Clin Oncol* 1997;16:280a.

Fong Y, Fortner J, Sun RL, et al. Clinical score for predicting recurrence after hepatic resection for metastatic colorectal cancer: analysis of 1001 consecutive cases. *Ann Surg* 1999;230:309–318.

Giacchetti S, Perpoint B, Zidani R, et al. Phase III multicenter randomized trial of oxaliplatin added to chronomodulated fluorouracil-leucovorin as first-line treatment of metastatic colorectal cancer. *J Clin Oncol* 2000;18:136–147.

Goldberg RM, Fleming TR, Tangen CM, et al. Surgery for recurrent colon cancer: strategies for identifying resectable recurrence and success rates after resection. Eastern Cooperative Oncology Group, the North Central Cancer Treatment Group, and the Southwest Oncology Group. *Ann Intern Med* 1998;129:27–35.

Greene FL, Page DL, Fleming ED, Fritz AG, Balch CM, Haller DG, Morrow M, eds. *AJCC Cancer Staging Manual*. 6th ed. New York, NY: Springer-Verlag New York, Inc.; 2002:131–132.

Grothey A, Jordan K, Kellner O, et al. Randomized phase II trial of capecitabine plus irinotecan (CapIri) vs capecitabine plus oxaliplatin (CapOx) as first-line therapy of advanced colorectal cancer (ACRC). *Proc Am Soc Clin Oncol* 2003; 22:255. Abstract 1022.

Hoff PM, Ansari R, Batist G, et al. Comparison of oral capecitabine versus intravenous fluorouracil plus leucovorin as first-line treatment in 605 patients with metastatic colorectal cancer: results of a randomized phase III study. *J Clin Oncol* 2001;19:2282–2292.

Hurwitz H, Fehrenbacher L, Cartwright T, et al. Bevacizumab (a monoclonal antibody to vascular endothelial growth factor) prolongs survival in first-line colorectal cancer (CRC): results of a phase III trial of bevacizumab in combination with bolus IFL (irinotecan, 5-fluorouracil, leucovorin) as first-line therapy in subjects with metastatic CRC. *Proc Am Soc Clin Oncol* 2003. Abstract 3646.

IMPACT. Efficacy of adjuvant fluorouracil and folinic acid in B2 colon cancer. International Multicenter Pooled Analysis of B2 Colon Cancer Trials (IMPACT B2) Investigators. *J Clin Oncol* 1999;17:1356–1363.

Ioachim EE, Goussia AC, Machera M, et al. Immunohistochemical evaluation of cathepsin D expression in colorectal tumours: a correlation with extracellular matrix components, p53, pRb, bcl-2, c-erbB-2, EGFR and proliferation indices. *Anticancer Res* 1999;19:2147–2155.

Iqbal S, Lenz HJ. Determinants of prognosis and response to therapy in colorectal cancer. *Curr Oncol Rep* 2001;2:102–108.

Jemal A, Thomas A, Murray T, Thun M. Cancer statistics 2002. *CA Cancer J Clin* 2002;52:23–47.

Kabbinivar F, Hurwitz HI, Fehrenbacher L, et al. Phase II, randomized trial comparing bevacizumab plus fluorouracil (FU)/leucovorin (LV) with FU/LV alone in patients with metastatic colorectal cancer. *J Clin Oncol* 2003;21:60–65.

Kohne CH, Van Cutsem E, Wils JA, et al. Irinotecan improves the activity of the AIO regimen in metastatic colorectal cancer: results of EORTC GI Group study 40986. *Proc Am Soc Clin Oncol* 2003;22:254. Abstract 1018.

Kemeny N, Huang Y, Cohen AM, et al. Hepatic arterial infusion of chemotherapy after resection of hepatic metastases from colorectal cancer. *N Engl J Med* 1999; 341:2039–2048.

Lin E, Morris J, Ayer G. Effect of celecoxib on capecitabine-induced hand-foot syndrome and antitumor activity. *Oncology (Huntingt)* 2002;16(12 suppl 14): 31–37.

Mamounas E, Wieand S, Wolmark N, et al. Comparative efficacy of adjuvant chemotherapy in patients with Dukes' B versus Dukes' C colon cancer: results from four National Surgical Adjuvant Breast and Bowel Project adjuvant studies (C-01, C-02, C-03, and C-04). *J Clin Oncol* 1999;17:1349–1355.

Masunaga R, Kohno H, Dhar DK, et al. Cyclooxygenase-2 expression correlates with tumor neovascularization and prognosis in human colorectal carcinoma patients. *Clin Cancer Res* 2000;6:4064–4068.

Moertel CG, Fleming TR, Macdonald JS, et al. Fluorouracil plus levamisole as effective adjuvant therapy after resection of stage III colon carcinoma: a final report. *Ann Intern Med* 1995;122:321–326.

O'Connell MJ, Laurie JA, Kahn M, et al. Prospectively randomized trial of postoperative adjuvant chemotherapy in patients with high-risk colon cancer. *J Clin Oncol* 1998;16:295–300.

O'Dwyer PJ, Manola J, Valone FH, et al. Fluorouracil modulation in colorectal cancer: lack of improvement with N-phosphonoacetyl-l-aspartic acid or oral leucovorin or interferon, but enhanced therapeutic index with weekly 24-hour infusion schedule—an Eastern Cooperative Oncology Group/Cancer and Leukemia Group B Study. *J Clin Oncol* 2001;19:2413–2421.

Patt YZ, Lin E, Leibmann J, et al. Capecitabine plus irinotecan for chemotherapy-naïve patients with metastatic colorectal cancer (MCRC): US multicenter phase II trial. *Proc Am Soc Clin Oncol* 2003;22:281. Abstract 1130.

Pitot HC, Wiesenfeld M, Mahoney MR, et al. A phase II trial of oxaliplatin (Oxal), 5-fluorouracil (5Fu), and leucovorin (LV) in patients (pts) with metastatic colon cancer (M-CRC) refractory to irinotecan (CPT11) based therapy: a North Central Cancer Treatment Group (NCCTG) study. *Proc Am Soc Clin Oncol* 2003;22:261. Abstract 1048.

Ribic CM, Sargent DJ, Moore MJ. Tumor microsatellite instability status as a predictor of benefit from fluorouracil based adjuvant chemotherapy for colon cancer. *N Engl J Med* 2003;349:247–257.

Rodriguez M, Lin E, Crane C. Colorectal cancer. In: Kufe DW, Holland JF, Frie E, Bast RC, Pollock RE, eds. *Cancer Medicine*. 6th ed. Hamilton, Ontario: BC Decker; 2003:1635–1666.

Rothenberg ML, Meropol NJ, Poplin EA, et al. Mortality associated with irinotecan plus bolus fluorouracil/leucovorin: summary findings of an independent panel. *J Clin Oncol* 2001;19:3801–3807.

Rougier P, Van Cutsem E, Bajetta E, et al. Randomised trial of irinotecan versus fluorouracil by continuous infusion after fluorouracil failure in patients with metastatic colorectal cancer. *Lancet* 1998;352(9138):1407–1412.

Salonga D, Danenberg KD, Johnson M, et al. Colorectal tumors responding to 5-fluorouracil have low gene expression levels of dihydropyrimidine dehydrogenase, thymidylate synthase, and thymidine phosphorylase. *Clin Cancer Res* 2000;6:1322–1327.

Saltz LB, Cox JV, Blanke C, et al. Irinotecan plus fluorouracil and leucovorin for metastatic colorectal cancer. Irinotecan Study Group. *N Engl J Med* 2000;343: 905–914.

Saltz LB, Meropol NJ, Loehrer PJ, et al. Single agent IMC-C225 (Erbitux™) has activity in CPT-11-refractory colorectal cancer (CRC) that expresses the epidermal growth factor receptor (EGFR). *Proc Am Soc Clin Oncol* 2002. Abstract 504.

Sandler RS, Halabi S, Baron JA. A randomized trial of aspirin to prevent colorectal adenomas in patients with previous colorectal cancer. *N Engl J Med* 2003; 348:883–890.

Sargent DJ, Goldberg RM, Jacobson SD, et al. A pooled analysis of adjuvant chemotherapy for resected colon cancer in elderly patients. *N Engl J Med* 2001; 345:1091–1097.

Steinbach G, Lynch PM, Phillips RKS, et al. The effect of celecoxib, a cyclooxygenase inhibitor, on familial adenomatous polyposis. *N Engl J Med* 2000;342: 1946–1952.

Takahashi Y, Bucana CD, Cleary KR, et al. p53, vessel count, and vascular endothelial growth factor expression in human colon cancer. *Int J Cancer* 1998;79:34–38.

Tournigand C. FOLFIRI followed by FOLFOX versus FOLFOX followed by FOLFIRI in metastatic colorectal cancer (MCRC): final results of a phase III study. *Proc Am Soc Clin Oncol* 2001;20. Abstract 494.

Twelves C, Wong A, Nowacki MP, et al. Improved safety results of a phase III trial of capecitabine vs bolus 5-FU/leucovorin (LV) as adjuvant therapy for colon cancer (the X-ACT Study). *Proc Am Soc Clin Oncol* 2003;22:294. Abstract 1182.

Van Cutsem E, Twelves C, Cassidy J, et al. Xeloda Colorectal Cancer Study Group. Oral capecitabine compared with intravenous fluorouracil plus leucovorin in patients with metastatic colorectal cancer: results of a large phase III study. *J Clin Oncol* 2001;19:4097–4106.

Van Cutsem E, Twelves C, Tabernero J, et al. XELOX: mature results of a multinational, phase II trial of capecitabine plus oxaliplatin, an effective 1st line option for patients (pts) with metastatic colorectal cancer (MCRC). *Proc Am Soc Clin Oncol* 2003;22:255. Abstract 1023.

van Triest B, Pinedo HM, van Hensbergen Y, et al. Thymidylate synthase level as the main predictive parameter for sensitivity to 5-fluorouracil, but not for folate-based thymidylate synthase inhibitors, in 13 nonselected colon cancer cell lines. *Clin Cancer Res* 1999;5:643–654.

Watanabe T, Wu TT, Catalano PJ, et al. Molecular predictors of survival after adjuvant chemotherapy for colon cancer. *N Engl J Med* 2001;344:1196–1206.

Willett CG, Fung CY, Kaufman DS, et al. Postoperative radiation therapy for high-risk colon carcinoma. *J Clin Oncol* 1993;11:1112–1117.

Willett CG, Goldberg S, Shellito PC, et al. Does postoperative irradiation play a role in the adjuvant therapy of stage T4 colon cancer? *Cancer J Sci Am* 1999; 5:242–247.

10 RECTAL CANCER

Nora A. Janjan, Edward H. Lin,
Marc E. Delclos, Christopher Crane,
Miguel A. Rodriguez-Bigas, and John M. Skibber

CHAPTER OVERVIEW

A multimodality approach is required for the treatment of rectal cancer.
All disciplines must understand and exploit the biological basis of the
components of therapy. Adjuvant chemotherapy has allowed significant
advances in disease-free and overall survival. Adjuvant radiation therapy
has provided tremendous benefit by improving local control rates and
sparing patients the morbidity of recurrent disease. Tumor regression with
preoperative chemoradiation has allowed sphincter-preserving surgical
procedures with excellent functional outcome, even among patients with

locally advanced distal rectal tumors. Even higher rates of sphincter preservation may be possible with further surgical advances and newer chemotherapeutic agents that have improved synergy with radiation and increased systemic activity.

INTRODUCTION

Colorectal cancer is among the 4 most commonly diagnosed cancers. More than 90,000 new cases of colon cancer and more than 35,000 new cases of rectal cancer are diagnosed each year. Colorectal cancer is linked to specific genetic syndromes, breast and ovarian cancers, and nutritional factors.

Colorectal cancer generally arises from an adenomatous polyp that forms in a field of epithelial cell hyperproliferation and crypt dysplasia. The National Polyp Study (Winawer, 1999) demonstrated that two thirds of all polyps removed were adenomatous polyps, which have a potential for malignant transformation. The transformation of a polyp into a cancer took about 5.5 years for polyps larger than 1 cm and about 10 years for smaller polyps. This study also showed that removing polyps sharply decreased the expected incidence of colorectal cancer.

Data from the Surveillance, Epidemiology, and End Results program and the National Cancer Database (Mettlin et al, 1997) have shown that most colorectal cancers arise in the proximal colon. Fifteen percent of colorectal cancers and adenomatous polyps occur in the cecum or appendix, 14% occur in the ascending colon or hepatic flexure, 14% occur in the transverse colon or splenic flexure and descending colon, 24% occur in the sigmoid colon, and 28% occur in the rectosigmoid and rectum. Although 30% to 50% of individuals have adenomatous polyps, only 6% develop clinically diagnosed colorectal cancer.

HEREDITARY COLORECTAL CANCER

The difficulties of dealing with hereditary colorectal cancers can be divided into 3 categories: confidentiality, coordination, and communication. It is often difficult for physicians to differentiate between sporadic, familial (at least 1 relative affected but no clear Mendelian pattern of inheritance or known mutation), and inherited (a single gene mutation playing a causative role) colorectal cancer cases. If familial or inherited disease is suspected, referral should be made to a center for genetic assessment. Another resource is the Online Mendelian Inheritance in Man database, which can be accessed at www3.ncbi.nlm.nih.gov/Omim/searchomim.html. For detailed information about genetic counseling for patients with hereditary disease, see chapter 8.

Hereditary nonpolyposis colorectal cancer (HNPCC) accounts for only about 5% of all cases of colorectal cancer, and there are no specific histopathologic characteristics that differentiate HNPCC from sporadic colorectal cancers. The Amsterdam Criteria for HNPCC are the following: (a) 3 relatives with colon cancer, of whom 2 must be first-degree relatives of the third, (b) colon cancer that spans 2 generations, and (c) 1 case of colon cancer diagnosed before 50 years of age (Rex et al, 2000). Several molecular pathways exist for the development of colorectal cancer. Among these are the adenomatous polyposis coli–β-catenin pathway and the pathways that involve abnormalities of DNA mismatch repair. Both of these pathways are involved in both sporadic colorectal cancer and inherited colorectal-cancer syndromes, including familial adenomatous polyposis and HNPCC.

Microsatellite instability, indicative of frequent genetic mutations throughout the genome, is found in virtually all colon cancers from patients with HNPCC but in only 15% of sporadic cancers. Overexpression of the *cyclooxygenase-2* gene has also been identified in sporadic and HNPCC colonic adenomas. Administration of cyclooxygenase-2 inhibitors resulted in regression of adenomas, and no malignancies were detected during prolonged follow-up. To identify patients with HNPCC, the Bethesda Guidelines for testing of colorectal tumors for microsatellite instability (Table 10–1) should be applied.

Table 10–1. Bethesda Guidelines for Testing of Colorectal Tumors for Microsatellite Instability

1. Individuals with cancer in families that meet the Amsterdam criteria
2. Individuals with 2 HNPCC-related cancers, including synchronous and metachronous colorectal cancers or associated extracolonic cancers*
3. Individuals with colorectal cancer and a first-degree relative with colorectal cancer and/or HNPCC-related extracolonic cancer and/or a colorectal adenoma; one of the cancers diagnosed at age <45 y, and the adenoma diagnosed at age <40 y
4. Individuals with colorectal cancer or endometrial cancer diagnosed at age <45 y
5. Individuals with right-sided colorectal cancer with an undifferentiated pattern (solid/cribriform) on histopathology diagnosed at age <45 y†
6. Individuals with a signet-ring-cell-type colorectal cancer diagnosed at age <45 y‡
7. Individuals with adenomas diagnosed at age <40 y

Abbreviation: HNPCC, hereditary nonpolyposis colorectal cancer.
* Endometrial, ovarian, gastric, hepatobiliary, or small-bowel cancer or transitional cell carcinoma of the renal pelvis or ureter.
† Solid/cribriform defined as poorly differentiated or undifferentiated carcinoma composed of irregular, solid sheets of large eosinophilic cells and containing small gland-like spaces.
‡ Composed of >50% signet ring cells.
Reprinted with permission from Rodriguez-Bigas MA, Boland CR, Hamilton SR, et al. Journal of the National Cancer Institute, vol. 89:1758–1762,1997.

Screening

Screening for colorectal cancer is recommended because of the defined risk of transformation of benign lesions into cancer.

In the Minnesota Colon Cancer Control Study (Church et al, 1997), annual fecal occult blood studies were performed over a 13-year period. If 1 sample was positive, a diagnostic work-up, including a colonoscopy, was performed. The sensitivity of fecal occult blood studies in the detection of colorectal cancer was about 90%, the cure rate for early colorectal cancer was about 90%, and the screening strategy reduced the mortality from colorectal cancer by one third among patients over the age of 50 years.

Colonoscopy reveals twice as many polyps as are detected with flexible sigmoidoscopy. In a study by Blumberg et al (2000), a screening and 2 follow-up colonoscopy procedures were performed among 204 patients with a history of adenomatous polyps. The results are summarized in Figure 10–1. By 4 years, the risk of adenoma formation was the same whether or not the findings on interim colonoscopy were negative. On the basis of this finding, surveillance colonoscopy was recommended at 4- to 5-year intervals.

Screening for colorectal cancer is often not done because of the nature of the procedures. Virtual colonoscopy is a possible alternative to endoscopic colonoscopy; however, patients require the same preparative regimen as with endoscopic colonoscopy, some discomfort is experienced with the insufflation of air during the procedure, and more technical

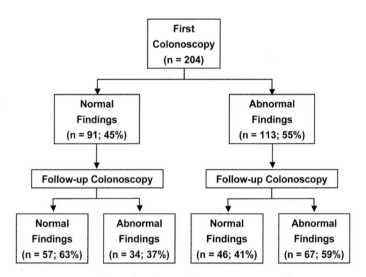

Figure 10–1. Results of colonoscopy screening.

expertise is needed than is needed for endoscopic colonoscopy to ensure the accuracy of the procedure.

For the average-risk individual, defined as someone 50 years of age or older who has no risk factors for colorectal cancer except older age, the preferred screening strategy is a colonoscopy every 5 years because it permits evaluation of the entire colon and clears adenomas by polypectomy, reducing the incidence of and deaths from colorectal cancer.

SURVEILLANCE AFTER TREATMENT

The majority of recurrences of colorectal cancer occur within 5 years and most recurrences occur within 3 years after surgery. The American Society of Clinical Oncology has created guidelines for colorectal cancer surveillance using evidence-based criteria (Desch et al, 1999). Standard follow-up includes regular history, physical examination, and diagnostic studies (complete blood cell count, liver function studies, carcinoembryonic antigen [CEA] testing, and fecal occult blood testing). Other evaluations include yearly chest radiography, computed tomography (CT) of the liver, and colonoscopy. Routine CEA testing detects metastatic disease 5 months before routine clinical evaluations, but 30% of recurrent tumors do not produce CEA, and a false-negative CEA finding is more common in poorly differentiated tumors.

In a study by Giess et al (1998), metastatic disease was found in 34% of CT studies performed in 1,119 patients with colorectal cancer. Thirty-three percent of the studies (1,007/3,073) showed metastases in the abdomen, 7% (227/3,073) showed metastases in the pelvis, and 6% (194/3,073) showed metastases in both the abdomen and pelvis. Whole-body positron emission tomography (PET) has been used to identify recurrent disease before it is evident on other imaging studies; with resectable colorectal cancer, there was a 20% diagnostic value with fluorodeoxyglucose-PET in detecting disease. Sensitivity and specificity in the detection of recurrent colorectal cancer were about 95% for fluorodeoxyglucose-PET, compared to 69% and 98%, respectively, for CT (Flanagan et al, 1998).

STAGING

The TNM staging system used for rectal cancer is outlined in chapter 1 (Table 1–6). The T classification is determined by a combination of physical examination, including proctoscopy, and imaging (transrectal sonography, CT, or magnetic resonance imaging [MRI] with an intrarectal coil). To detect liver metastases, specialized techniques should be used for the administration of contrast agents and the CT scan time.

While CT and MRI are more than 90% accurate in determining metastatic spread, these techniques have limitations in the evaluation of local disease extension of rectal cancer. The ability to detect the primary tumor depends on its size and location. In a study of 158 patients, CT identified the primary tumor in only 75% of cases (Horton et al, 2000). CT identifies perirectal fat involvement in 50% to 75% of cases. The accuracy of transrectal MRI in the detection of tumor involvement of the perirectal fat is 85% in a number of series. Accuracy in the evaluation of perirectal lymph node involvement is about 60% for both CT and MRI.

Primary rectal cancers should be staged before surgery or preoperative chemoradiation. The overall accuracy of preoperative endorectal sonography (Figure 10–2) in determining the depth of wall penetration ranges from 72% to 97%, with up to 12% of tumors overstaged and 9% understaged. Potential sources of errors on endorectal sonography include certain tumor locations, stenosis, peritumoral inflammation, postbiopsy and postsurgical changes, hemorrhage, and pedunculated or villous tumors. Tumors at or near the anal verge can easily be missed with endorectal sonography. Normal perirectal lymph nodes are less than 3 mm in diameter and are not usually visualized by endorectal sonography. When lymph nodes are seen, they may contain metastatic disease, or they may be inflamed. A node is generally considered to contain metastatic disease if it has discrete margins and is uniformly hypoechoic or has

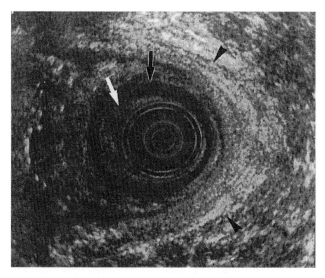

Figure 10–2. Endorectal ultrasound appearance of the normal rectal wall and a tumor. Perirectal lymph node involvement can be detected with a hypoechoic lesion outside the rectal wall.

the same echotexture as the primary tumor. The accuracy of endorectal sonography in predicting perirectal lymph node invasion ranges from 60% to 85%.

Brief Overview of Treatment by Disease Stage

The M. D. Anderson Cancer Center approach to the treatment of rectal cancer strategically combines key therapeutic factors.

Early-Stage Disease

Patients with early-stage rectal cancer (T1 or T2 tumor without clinical lymph node involvement) are usually treated with surgery alone. Surgical approaches include local excision and resection with total mesorectal excision. After total mesorectal excision, radiation therapy is not usually required for pathologic T1 or T2 N0 tumors. After local excision, radiation therapy is unnecessary for T1 tumors with favorable characteristics because the risk of local failure in such cases is less than 10%. Radiation therapy after local excision is recommended for T1 tumors with unfavorable characteristics and for all T2 tumors because the risk of local failure in such cases is about 20%. Unfavorable characteristics include tumor ulceration, histologic evidence of lymphatic, vascular, or perineural invasion, and poor differentiation.

Locally Advanced Disease

Locally advanced rectal cancer is defined as a T3 or T4 tumor or any tumor associated with positive regional lymph nodes. Complete surgical resection with mesorectal excision is recommended for patients with T3 and T4 tumors because of the risk of tumor cut-through and inadequate lymph node resection with local excision. Combined-modality therapy has significantly improved local and distant disease control and is now the standard of care for locally advanced rectal cancer.

Combined-Modality Therapy

Several prospective randomized trials have shown the benefit of adjuvant radiation therapy and chemotherapy for locally advanced rectal cancer, defined as a T3 or T4 primary tumor or any tumor with positive regional lymph nodes.

Studies Demonstrating Benefit

The 3 major trials that demonstrated the need for all treatment modalities in locally advanced rectal cancer are the National Surgical Adjuvant Breast and Bowel Project R-01 trial (Fisher et al, 1988), the Gastrointestinal Tumor

Table 10–2. Results of the National Surgical Adjuvant Breast and Bowel Project R-01 Trial*

| | Treatment | | |
Outcome	S	S + CTX	S + XRT
Overall survival rate, %	38	46	39
Disease-free survival rate, %	30	37	34
Local failure rate, %	16	12	10

Abbreviations: S, surgery; CTX, chemotherapy; XRT, radiation therapy.
* A total of 528 patients were randomly assigned to surgery only; surgery and
  postoperative chemotherapy (fluorouracil, semustine, and vincristine); or surgery and
  postoperative radiation therapy (40 to 47 Gy).
Data from Fisher et al (1988).

Study Group trial (GTSG, 1985, 1986), and the Mayo Clinic/North Central Cancer Treatment Group trial (Krook et al, 1991).

The results of the National Surgical Adjuvant Breast and Bowel Project R-01 trial are listed in Table 10–2. This trial showed that compared with surgery alone, surgery plus postoperative radiation therapy decreased the local recurrence rate but did not affect survival. Surgery plus postoperative chemotherapy significantly improved disease-free survival and overall survival but did not reduce the risk of local failure compared with surgery alone.

The Gastrointestinal Tumor Study Group and the Mayo Clinic/North Central Cancer Treatment Group trials showed reductions in local recurrence rates and improvements in disease-free and overall survival when postoperative radiation therapy and chemotherapy were administered to patients with Duke's stages B2 and C rectal cancer. In the Gastrointestinal Tumor Study Group trial, there was a statistically significant recurrence-free survival and overall survival advantage for combined-modality therapy including surgery, radiation therapy, and chemotherapy over surgery alone or surgery in combination with any other component of therapy (Table 10–3). The Mayo Clinic/North Central Cancer Treatment Group trial compared outcomes for postoperative radiation therapy alone to those with postoperative radiation therapy and chemotherapy. This trial also showed that treatment with all 3 modalities provided the best local and distant disease control (Table 10–4).

The next question involved how to optimize the administration of chemotherapy. The intergroup trial was performed among 660 patients with stage II and III rectal cancer to determine if there was a difference between bolus and infusional 5-fluorouracil (5-FU) (Table 10–4). During pelvic irradiation, either a 500-mg/m^2 bolus of 5-FU was given daily for 3 consecutive days during weeks 1 and 5, or 5-FU was infused at a rate of 225 mg/m^2 seven days per week. Local control rates were similar in the 2 treatment groups, but there were significant improvements in time to

Table 10–3. Results from the Gastrointestinal Tumor Study Group 7175 Trial*

Outcome	Treatment			
	S	S + CTX	S + XRT	S + CTX + XRT
10-y overall survival rate, %	26	41	33	45
10-y disease-free survival rate, %	44	51	50	65
Recurrence rate, %	55	46	46	35
Local failure rate, %	25	27	20	10

Abbreviations: S, surgery; CTX, chemotherapy; XRT, radiation therapy.
* A total of 202 patients were randomly assigned to surgery only, surgery and postoperative chemotherapy (fluorouracil and semustine); surgery and postoperative radiation therapy (40 to 48 Gy); or surgery, chemotherapy, and radiation therapy.
Data from Gastrointestinal Tumor Study Group (1986).

relapse and overall survival with infusional 5-FU. It was thought that these results related to the higher total doses of 5-FU and the more prolonged exposure to 5-FU during treatment. The average doses of 5-FU during radiation therapy were 6,546 mg/m^2 in the infusion group and 2,499 mg/m^2 in the bolus group. The toxicity profiles were also different; bolus 5-FU was

Table 10–4. Outcomes of the Major Trials of Combined-Modality Therapy for Rectal Cancer

Trial and Regimen*	Local Relapse Rate, %	Distant Relapse Rate, %	Disease-Free Survival Rate, %	Overall Survival Rate, %	P
GITSG (202 patients)					.005
S	24	34	45	32	
S + 5-FU and Me	27	27	54	48	
S + XRT	20	30	52	45	
S + XRT + 5-FU and Me	11	26	67	57	
NCCTG (204 patients)					.025
S + XRT	25	46	38	38	
S + XRT + 5-FU and Me	14	29	58	53	
INT (660 patients)					.01
S + XRT + bolus 5-FU	NS	NS	53	60	
S + XRT + PVI 5-FU	NS	NS	63	70	

Abbreviations: GITSG, Gastrointestinal Tumor Study Group; S, surgery; 5-FU, fluorouracil; Me, semustine; XRT, radiation therapy; NCCTG, North Central Cancer Treatment Group; INT, intergroup; NS, not significant; PVI, protracted venous infusion.
* Median follow-up time was 7 years in the GITSG and NCCTG trials and 4 years in the INT trial.
Reprinted with permission from Vaughn DJ, Haller DG. Adjuvant therapy for colorectal cancer: past accomplishments, future directions. *Cancer Invest* 1997;15:435–447.

associated with more hematologic and infusional 5-FU was associated with more gastrointestinal toxicity.

Surgery

The anatomic location of the tumor and the structures involved by the tumor in the rectum often determine recommendations regarding surgery. The rectum is classically divided into 3 levels: the low rectum, midrectum, and proximal rectum (Figure 10–3). Because of variations in anatomy and body habitus, it is difficult to assign precise measurements to delineate each of these rectal segments. The American College of Surgeons has classified cancers extending from the anal verge to 15 cm as rectal cancers. Others have reported that tumors located 12 to 15 cm from the anal verge act biologically more like colon cancers than rectal cancers. Because of this, a more stringent definition of rectal tumors has been adopted: tumors located within 12 cm of the anal verge on rigid proctoscopy with the patient in the left lateral Sims position.

Important to achieving local control of rectal cancer is complete resection of the mesorectum. Incomplete resection of the mesorectal fat reproducibly results in local failure rates as high as 90% within 18 months of resection alone because of residual tumor left behind within lymph

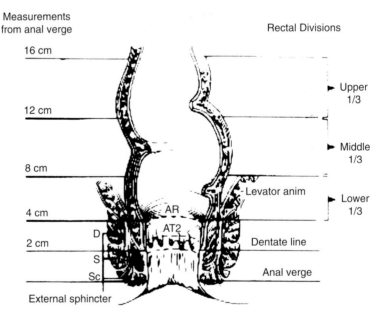

Figure 10–3. Anatomy of the rectum. D, deep; S, superficial; Sc, subcutaneous. Reprinted with permission from Janjan NA, Delclos ME, Ballo MT, Crane CH. The colon and rectum. In: Cox JD, Ang KK, eds. *Radiation Oncology: Rationale, Technique, Results.* 8th ed. St. Louis, MO: Mosby; 2003:497–536.

nodes attached to the pelvic sidewall. The visceral fascia covers the rectum and the mesorectum. The parietal fascia covers the musculoskeletal and vascular structures of the pelvic sidewalls, including the pelvic autonomic plexus. One third of patients with mesorectal lymph node involvement also have lateral pelvic lymph node involvement. Lateral lymph node involvement is also associated with transmural and extraperitoneal disease. Therefore, lateral lymph node dissection is performed when there is perirectal penetration (stage T3) or mesorectal lymph node involvement.

With surgery alone, overall recurrence rates are 65% when lateral lymph nodes are positive and 38% when lateral lymph nodes are negative; local recurrence rates are 26% and 10%, respectively, and 5-year overall survival rates are 49% and 74%, respectively. Combined-modality therapy that includes surgical resection with total mesorectal excision results in local control rates of more than 90% in locally advanced rectal cancer.

In a detailed evaluation of the lymph nodes from the surgical specimens of 164 colorectal cancer patients, a total of 12,496 lymph nodes, about 76 nodes per patient, were evaluated for metastases (DeCosse, 1997). Metastases were found in 59% of cases, and 33% of the lymph nodes with metastases had tumor deposits that were less than 4 mm in diameter. The locations of the lymph nodes indicated that 7-cm proximal and distal margins and excision of the regional mesentery are needed to encompass both the intermediate and the central lymph nodes. In a study of 1,664 patients with T3 or T4 or node-positive rectal cancer who were treated with radiation and chemotherapy, the number of nodes examined pathologically was significantly associated with the time to relapse among patients with node-negative disease (Tepper et al, 2001). Among node-negative patients who had 0 to 4, 5 to 8, 9 to 13, and 14 or more nodes examined, the 5-year relapse rates were 37%, 34%, 26%, and 19%, respectively; the corresponding 5-year survival rates were 68%, 73%, 72%, and 82%, respectively. The number of nodes evaluated pathologically made no difference in node-positive patients.

Sphincter-Preserving Surgery

Because of combined-modality therapy, sphincter preservation is now possible in the treatment of distal rectal cancer. When rectal cancer is resected with sparing of the pelvic autonomic nerves and lateral lymph node dissection, local control rates are 100% in patients with Duke's stage A and B disease, and 5-year survival rates in patients with Duke's stage A, B, and C disease are 96%, 84%, and 67%, respectively. Urinary function is preserved in 94% of patients with dissection of the unilateral pelvic plexus. When the complete pelvic plexus is preserved, 70% of males retain sexual function; if the hypogastric nerves have to be removed but the pelvic plexus is preserved, 67% of males maintain the ability to have an erection and intercourse without normal ejaculation.

Limited resection and organ preservation is also possible when the disease invades adjacent organs. Ninety percent of cases of bladder involvement can be detected with CT and cystoscopy. Pathologic involvement of the bladder occurs in 58% of patients. With partial resection of the bladder, negative pathologic margins can be obtained in 94% of cases, and rates of local control and survival are not compromised.

There are 3 types of sphincter-preserving operations. These include a standard low anterior resection, a low anterior resection with coloanal anastomosis, and a low anterior resection or coloanal anastomosis with a J-pouch colonic reservoir. All low anterior resections involve a resection and an anastomosis between a serosalized colon and the extraperitoneal nonserosalized rectum. The standard low anterior resection involves an intrapelvic anastomosis within the sacral hollow; the remaining distal segment of rectum is variable. By comparison, a coloanal anastomosis is an extrapelvic anastomosis at the apex of the anal canal or at the dentate line, and there is no remaining distal rectum. A J-pouch reconstruction can be combined with either a low anterior resection or a coloanal resection; this reconstruction recreates the reservoir function of the rectum and improves long-term bowel function. Creation of a temporary ileostomy allows healing and reduces postoperative morbidity. Extensive experience with this technique has confirmed excellent rates of tumor control and functional outcome, including fecal continence. Treatment must be indexed to the level of experience among the treating physicians and to patient factors. Perioperative complication rates decreased dramatically when more experience was gained with resection after preoperative chemoradiation. Considerable variability has been shown in the rates of local-regional recurrence and survival between surgeons and institutions; advanced stage of disease, vascular invasion, and absence of a specialty in colorectal surgery proved to be independent predictors of local and overall recurrence (Dorrance et al, 2000).

Local Excision

Although a local excision is a sphincter-preserving surgery, it is distinct from a low anterior resection or other sphincter-preserving surgery. Local excision can only cure tumors confined to the bowel wall. The most important distinction is that a mesorectal resection, which removes involved perirectal nodes, is not performed with a local excision.

The risk of lymph node involvement is 0% to 12% for T1 tumors, 12% to 28% for T2 tumors, and 36% to 79% for T3 and T4 tumors (Mellgren et al, 2000). Because of this, local failure rates with local excision alone are higher than with more comprehensive surgical approaches. There is a parallel relationship between T classification, the risk of lymph node failure, and the risk of local failure. Local failure rates with local excision were as follows: T1, 4%; T2, 16%; and T3, 23%. The depth of tumor penetration and the tumor grade are directly related to the risk of perirectal nodal involvement. Studies have also shown that tumor ulceration and histologic evidence of lymphatic, vascular, or perineural invasion are associated with an increased risk of nodal metastases. To be considered for local excision, patients should have tumors 3 cm or smaller and involving less than half of the rectal circumference. Fewer complications are associated with a transanal rather than a Kraske approach to local excision and postoperative radiation therapy.

In the study by Mellgren et al (2000), transanal excision was performed in 108 patients with T1 and T2 tumors, and the results were compared to those achieved with standard surgical approaches in 153 patients with similar characteristics. The local recurrence rate was higher after transanal excision (28% vs 4%). Outcomes were stage dependent: 18% of T1 and 47% of T2 tumors treated with transanal excision recurred, compared with 0% and 6%, respectively, of T1 and T2 tumors treated with mesorectal resection. Improvements in local control were achieved with postoperative radiation therapy even though the postoperative-radiation group had more adverse features, including higher T classification (15% T2 for local excision vs 70% T2 for local excision plus radiation). The 5-year actuarial results for 52 patients treated with local excision alone and 47 patients treated with local excision plus radiation therapy showed improved rates of local control (72% vs 90%) and relapse-free survival (66% vs 74%) in the group treated with radiation.

Despite the improvement in outcomes among patients with high-risk features treated with radiation, the use of preoperative chemoradiation followed by local excision is controversial because of the lack of pathologic data. At this time, the role of local excision in the treatment of rectal cancer is dependent on stage and other tumor characteristics and is still largely undefined. Patient selection is extremely important in performing a local excision. Attempts to maximize sphincter preservation must not result in inferior rates of tumor control or functional outcome.

Radiation Therapy

Radiation therapy has 3 general roles in rectal cancer management. First, radiation therapy is used to enhance local-regional control by eliminating microscopic residual disease around the primary tumor and in the draining lymphatics. Second, radiation therapy is administered preoperatively to locally advanced primary tumors to cause significant tumor regression and make inoperable lesions resectable or amenable to a more conservative surgical approach with sphincter preservation. Third, radiation therapy is used to palliate symptoms due to infiltration of pelvic structures or metastatic disease.

Factors associated with increased risk of local and distant recurrence include higher stage; certain tumor locations; serosal, lymphatic, and neurovascular invasion; tumor location near the anus; and posterior extension of disease (because of the limited radial [presacral] surgical margin). Adjuvant irradiation eradicates microscopic residual tumor and eliminates local recurrence in approximately 90% of patients.

Careful attention to technique is important with both preoperative and postoperative radiation therapy. Whenever possible, the small bowel should be displaced from the treatment portal. The volume of small bowel in the radiation portal has been shown to directly correlate with radiation toxicity. Radiation techniques that displace the small bowel from the radiation portal, such as the use of a belly board, also help to reduce gastrointestinal side effects. In a study that used CT treatment planning with patients in the supine position and in the prone position with the belly board (Figure 10–4), the median volume of small bowel irradiated was reduced by 54% (Koelbl et al, 1999). The median dose to the small bowel was 15 Gy with the belly board technique and 24 Gy with patients in the supine position. The median volume of the bladder irradiated was reduced 62% with the belly board technique. Exclusion of the small bowel is particularly important because patients treated with combined-modality therapy are at risk for both radiation-related and chemotherapy-related diarrhea.

In most cases, the entire pelvis is encompassed using a posterior and right and left lateral radiation treatment portals. High-energy photons, like 18-MV photons, should be used to effectively treat the pelvic structures at depth and limit the dose to the skin. Studies of patterns of spread indicate that the external iliac lymph node chain does not routinely need to be included in the treatment portals. Anterior fields should be considered only when there is anterior extension of disease to the urogenital regions. In some cases, anterior-posterior fields or a 4-field arrangement may prove necessary because of tumor extension or anatomical constraints. Adequate coverage of the tumor volume should be confirmed with treatment-planning imaging. If an anterior portal is used, there also needs to be careful estimation of the dose administered to the small bowel. The volume of small bowel in the field can be determined either with use of a contrast agent at the time of treatment simulation or with CT-based treatment planning.

Even with distal rectal involvement, including infiltration of the anal canal, the risk of inguinal node involvement is limited, and radiation treatment portals do not need to include the inguinal region. The risk of recurrence in the inguinal region in patients with distal rectal tumors is less than 5%. However, radiation techniques should be modified if inguinal lymph nodes are clinically evident and pathologically confirmed to be involved with metastatic disease. Metastatic involvement of the inguinal nodes portends an especially poor prognosis in terms of dissemination of disease.

The superior border of the radiation field, in general, should be placed at the L5–S1 interspace (Figure 10–5). However, if the rectosigmoid is involved, individual anatomy may dictate that the superior border be

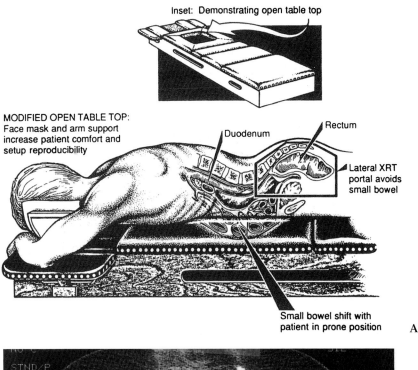

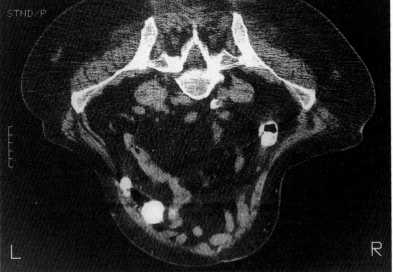

Figure 10–4. Use of a belly board in the treatment of colorectal cancer. (*A*) The patient lies prone on a modified table top. (*B*) CT scan obtained at simulation shows how the small bowel falls outside the radiation field with the belly board technique. Panel A reprinted with permission from Rich T, Ajani JA, Morrison WH, et al. Chemoradiation therapy for anal cancer: radiation plus continuous infusion of 5-fluorouracil with or without cisplatin. *Radiother Oncol* 1993;27:209–215.

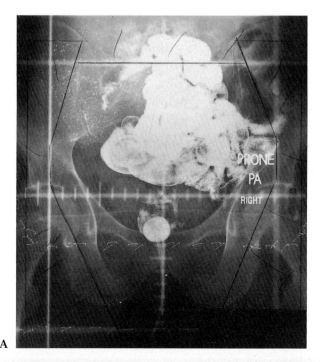

A

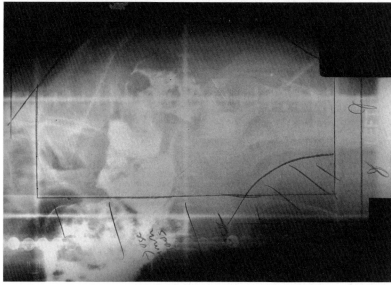

B

Figure 10–5. Routine radiation portals for rectal cancer. (*A*) Posterior field. (*B*) Lateral fields showing displacement of the bowel. Reprinted with permission from Janjan NA, Delclos ME, Ballo MT, Crane CH. The colon and rectum. In: Cox JD, Ang KK, eds. *Radiation Oncology: Rationale, Technique, Results.* 8th ed. St. Louis, MO: Mosby; 2003:497–536.

placed at the L4–L5 interspace. The inferior border of the field is dictated by the inferior extent of the tumor; generally, the inferior aspect of the field should be placed 2 cm inferior to the lowest aspect of the tumor. The anus may need to be included in the treatment field in some cases when the tumor is located in the distal rectum. Whenever possible, however, the anus should be blocked from the radiation portal to reduce treatment-related side effects like moist desquamation. For tumors located in the midrectum and proximal rectum, the inferior border of the radiation field is placed at the bottom of the obturator foramen. The lateral border should include the sacroiliac joints, and a 2-cm margin should be placed around the pelvic brim to include the internal iliac lymph node chains in the posterior treatment portal.

For the lateral treatment fields, the superior and inferior borders should be consistent with the posterior portal. With routine treatment simulation, a contrast should be placed in the rectum to ensure an adequate margin around the primary tumor. The anterior aspect of the field should be placed 2 cm in front of the most anterior aspect of the sacral promontory and anterior to the femoral heads to include the obturator nodes. Every effort should be made to exclude the small bowel. To reduce damage to the genitalia, a block should be placed anterior to the femur. Posteriorly, the entire sacrum should be included to ensure an adequate radiation dose to the radial margin of resection in the presacral region.

Using the 3-field belly board technique, the pelvis receives 45 Gy in 25 fractions (1.8 Gy per fraction) prescribed to the 95% isodose line using 18-MV photons. A concomitant boost is delivered during the last week of pelvic irradiation. With a 6-hour interfraction interval, the boost field (tumor volume plus a 2-cm margin administered with the patient in the belly board position) receives 7.5 Gy in 5 fractions (1.5 Gy per fraction) prescribed to the 95% isodose line using conformal radiation planning techniques.

Chemotherapy

Chemotherapy Administered During Radiation Therapy

In combined-modality therapy for rectal cancer, continuous-infusion 5-FU given at a dose of 300 mg/m^2 per week concurrently with 5 days per week of radiation therapy is the standard; however, the experience with oral 5-FU analogs is expanding. An oral route of administration for chemotherapy has several advantages. Among these are the ease of administration and avoidance of the inconvenience, discomfort, and cost associated with intravenous administration of either bolus or continuous-infusion 5-FU. Some of the oral 5-FU analogs also may concentrate within tumor cells to a greater degree than infusional 5-FU. The toxicity profile of oral 5-FU analogs is similar to that of infusional 5-FU given as a single agent. Most of the available data on oral 5-FU analogs relate to their use as single agents. Published data regarding administration of these agents during either preoperative or postoperative radiation therapy are limited.

Postoperative Adjuvant Chemotherapy

The role of adjuvant chemotherapy in colorectal cancer has been established. Typically, 6 cycles of 5-FU (425 mg/m^2 per cycle) and leucovorin (20 mg/m^2 per cycle) are administered, with the drugs infused over 5 consecutive days every 3 to 5 weeks. The administration of adjuvant chemotherapy has resulted in significant improvements in time to relapse (41% vs 27%) and overall survival (40% vs 28%) compared to outcomes after surgery alone (Tepper et al, 1997). In general, 5-FU analogs remain the primary chemotherapeutic agents used for adjuvant therapy, but a number of other agents have been developed for the treatment of colorectal cancer. Irinotecan and oxaliplatin have mechanisms of action distinct from that of 5-FU and are used in the treatment of 5-FU-refractory disease.

Infusional 5-FU or oral 5-FU with the same pharmacokinetics as infusional therapy should be considered. Other agents, like irinotecan and oxaliplatin, are gaining greater prominence in adjuvant therapy and are under study for use in chemoradiation.

Preoperative Versus Postoperative Chemoradiation

Preoperative chemoradiation avoids the disadvantages of postoperative chemoradiation. The key advantage of preoperative chemoradiation is the potential reduction in tumor size, which increases the chance for a sphincter-preserving surgical procedure. This is especially important for lesions located in the distal rectum. The advantages and disadvantages of preoperative and postoperative chemoradiation are listed in Table 10–5.

Factors that have been studied to see if they can increase the likelihood of tumor regression and the possibility of performing sphincter-sparing surgery include (1) allowing an appropriate interval between the completion of radiation therapy and surgery to maximize tumor regression, (2) administering higher radiation doses, and (3) administering chemotherapy.

A sufficiently long interval between completion of preoperative chemoradiation and surgery is critical to allow maximal tumor regression prior to surgery. In a study by Berger et al (1997), when the interval between preoperative radiation therapy (39 Gy over 3 weeks) and surgery was increased from 2 weeks to 6 to 8 weeks, the downstaging rate also increased, from 10% to 26%. In the Swedish Rectal Cancer Trial (1997), although surgery was to have been performed within 10 days of completion of radiation therapy, the period between radiation therapy and surgery varied widely (from 5 days to 155 days). The downstaging rate

Table 10–5. Advantages and Disadvantages of Preoperative and Postoperative Chemoradiation in Patients with Locally Advanced Rectal Cancer

Preoperative Chemoradiation	Postoperative Chemoradiation
Advantages:	*Advantages:*
May enable sphincter-preserving surgery in patients with distal rectal tumors not otherwise candidates for this approach.	Permits pathologic tumor staging, which indicates whether adjuvant radiation therapy is indicated.
May make inoperable tumors operable.	Permits complete pathologic staging of the primary tumor and lymph nodes and more precise definition of the regions in the radiation portal.
Blood vessels are intact for delivery of chemotherapy.	
Permits assessment of tumor response to chemotherapy, which may have prognostic significance.	Reduced perioperative morbidity since surgery is performed in an unirradiated field.
	Permits prompt surgical intervention in cases with significant bleeding or risk of obstruction.
Disadvantages:	*Disadvantages:*
Two-stage surgical approach: temporary ileostomy required after chemoradiation.	Higher radiation dose required because hypoxia in the operative bed causes relative radiation resistance.
	Microscopic residual disease may grow during postoperative healing.
	Small bowel may be less mobile because of postoperative adhesions; this increases the risk of small-bowel damage.

was only 4% among patients who underwent resection within 10 days after the completion of radiation therapy, whereas the downstaging rate was 45% when more than 10 days elapsed between the completion of radiation therapy and surgery.

Attempts to increase the total radiation dose given during preoperative radiation therapy have not improved rates of tumor regression but have increased the risk of treatment-related side effects. One radiation dose-escalation trial that used doses of up to 61.8 Gy and bolus 5-FU during radiation therapy showed no significant improvements in response parameters, including rates of pathologic complete response, downstaging, and sphincter preservation (Movsas et al, 1998) (Table 10–6).

Just as continuous-infusion 5-FU during postoperative chemoradiation results in improved disease-free and overall survival, so does continuous-

Table 10-6. Results of Published Series of Preoperative Radiation Therapy in Patients with Rectal Cancer

Study	No. of Patients Undergoing Resection	Preoperative XRT Dose	CTX During XRT	Interval between XRT and Resection	Complete Response Rate	Downstaging Rate	Sphincter Preservation Rate
Janjan; 2000	42	45 Gy to the pelvis + 7.5-Gy concomitant boost	CI 5-FU 300 mg/m^2 5 days/wk during pelvic XRT	4–6 wk	31%	86%	79%
Bosset; 2000	60	45 Gy	Bolus 5-FU Week 1: 350–450 mg/m^2 Week 5: 350–370 mg/m^2	3 wk (range, 13–111 days)	15.6%	30%	58%
Pucciarelli; 2000	51	45 Gy	5-day infusion 5-FU 350 mg/m^2 days 1–5 and 29–33	4–5 wk (range, 19–53 days)	15.7%	59%	84%

Study; year	N	XRT	CTX				
Valentini; 1999	40	45 Gy to the pelvis + 5.4-Gy boost	5-day infusion 5-FU 1,000 mg/m² days 1–4 and 29–32 / Cisplatin 60 mg/m² days 1 and 29	6–8 wk	23%	68%	85%
Movsas; 1998	23	45 Gy to pelvis + hyperfractionated boost to total doses of 54.6, 57, or 61.8 Gy	4-day infusion 5-FU 1,000 mg/m² days 1–4 and 29–32	4–6 wk	17.4%	57%	30%
Janjan; 1998	117	45 Gy to pelvis	CI 5-FU 300 mg/m² 5 days/wk during pelvic XRT	4–6 wk	27%	62%	59%
Wagman; 1998	35	46.8 Gy to pelvis + 3.6-Gy boost	None	4–5 wk	14%	63%	77%
Mohiuddin; 1998	70	40–45 Gy + 10- to 15-Gy boost	None	5–10 wk	NR	30%	86%

Abbreviations: XRT, radiation therapy; CTX, chemotherapy; CI, continuous infusion; 5-FU, fluorouracil; NR, not reported.
Reprinted with permission from Janjan NA, Delclos ME, Ballo MT, Crane CH. The colon and rectum. In: Cox JD, Ang KK, eds. *Radiation Oncology: Rationale, Technique, Results.* 8th ed. St. Louis, MO: Mosby; 2003:497–536.

infusion 5-FU during preoperative chemoradiation. With lower total doses of preoperative radiation (45 Gy) and continuous infusion of 5-FU, down-staging rates were similar to those in series that administered higher total radiation doses. When accelerated fractionation (concomitant boost) was used to deliver a total radiation dose of 52.5 Gy with a continuous infusion of 5-FU, the pathologic downstaging rates were approximately 20% higher and the pathologic complete response rates were nearly twice those of other series using the same or higher doses of radiation and bolus or intermittent infusion of 5-FU (Table 10–6).

Besides permitting sphincter-preserving surgery, tumor downstaging may also have prognostic importance. The degree of response to preoperative radiation therapy also has been reported to influence survival rates in patients with locally advanced rectal cancers. Five-year overall survival rates after preoperative radiation therapy were 92% for patients whose tumors were downstaged to Duke's stage 0 or A but only 67% and 26%, respectively, for patients whose tumors were downstaged to Duke's stage B or C (Berger et al, 1997).

Management of Treatment-Related Side Effects

Hematologic and gastrointestinal side effects need to be closely monitored during the course of chemoradiation. Chemotherapeutic agents used in the treatment of rectal cancer, like 5-FU and irinotecan, cause diarrhea. In addition to these side effects, other side effects of chemotherapy include hand-foot syndrome, mucositis, and mucosal superinfection, especially candidiasis. Occasionally mild nausea can occur, so nutritional status and fluid balance must be evaluated. Because radiation effects are well defined, gastrointestinal side effects that occur in the first 2 weeks of radiation therapy are generally attributable to chemotherapy. A pharmacokinetic study showed a wide variation in 5-FU metabolism and showed that these variations were directly correlated with variations in toxicity (Gamelin et al, 1996). Acute side effects correlated with plasma 5-FU levels greater than 3,000 µg/l and not with the 5-FU dose that was administered. Possible infection with *Clostridium difficile* should always be considered in patients with intractable diarrhea. Clinical signs, like fever and blood in the stool, may suggest underlying sepsis and should initiate prompt evaluation. Other etiologies should be considered if the symptoms are not typical or if they are refractory to usual supportive-care strategies.

A 3-step bowel management program has been instituted at M. D. Anderson (Callister et al, 2000) (Table 10–7). At the time of treatment simulation, all patients receive written instructions in bowel management and prescriptions for an antidiarrheal (loperamide) and an antiemetic to be used if symptoms develop. The 3-step program anticipates the development of treatment-related side effects; at the first sign of symptoms, patients proceed to the next step of the bowel management strategy. Under this program, patients should not have more than 3 bowel movements in

Table 10–7. The University of Texas M. D. Anderson Cancer Center 3-Step Bowel Management Program

Step*	Strategy
1	Loperamide (1–2 tablets) as needed.
2	Loperamide (1–2 tablets) 4 times a day on a scheduled basis half an hour before meals and before bedtime.
3	• Continue loperamide (1–2 tablets) 4 times a day and begin opioid analgesics.
	• Loperamide (1–2 tablets) as needed.
	• Add a sustained-release analgesic like morphine or oxycodone and an immediate-release analgesic for breakthrough abdominal cramping or stooling.
	• The analgesics are titrated to effect using the same principles that are used in pain management.
	• Because of difficulties in titration and changing needs over the course of radiation therapy, the use of a fentanyl patch is avoided unless fentanyl is required for primary pain management.
	• The goal is to give sufficient medications to consistently control frequent stooling and abdominal cramping.

* If one step is ineffective, the next step is used. Medications are titrated to effect. The goal is to maintain 3 or fewer stools per day.

a day; it is important to recognize that patients do not need to have watery or loose stools to follow the bowel management guidelines. The goal is to prevent, rather than treat, symptoms like frequent stooling, fluid and electrolyte imbalance, and skin irritation.

In step 1, loperamide is used as needed. In step 2, scheduled administration of loperamide is begun to prevent, rather than treat, symptoms of frequent stooling. In step 3, opioid analgesics are added to the loperamide, to relieve the symptoms of abdominal cramping and to exploit the constipating effects of opioid analgesics. Established principles for pain management are used to titrate the dose to effect. Unlike the case with loperamide, there is no dose limit with opioid analgesics, and usually the doses of opioids required in step 3 are modest. Because the treatment-related changes in the bowel do not resolve during therapy, a sustained-release analgesic is preferred in step 3 to avoid the need for multiple doses of medications during the day. Medications that have a 3-hour duration of effect, like tincture of opium or short-acting analgesics, can result in cycles of symptoms and disrupted sleep if a strict schedule of administration is not followed. Fentanyl patches are usually avoided because of the difficulty in titration and because analgesic needs are not always stable as patients undergo radiation therapy. However, fentanyl in lozenge form is highly effective in relieving incident-related pain, like pain during defecation, in patients with distal rectal cancers.

Results of this bowel management program were prospectively evaluated using a validated bowel assessment survey. With a 95% compliance rate for completion of the survey each week during the course of chemoradiation, no significant differences were documented between the presenting symptoms and the symptoms that were reported at the completion of chemoradiation (Callister et al, 2000).

Cases of secretory diarrhea can be controlled with octreotide. Octreotide prolongs intestinal transit time, promotes absorption of electrolytes in the intestine, and decreases the secretion of fluids and electrolytes. Complete response rates of more than 90% were observed after 3 days of treatment in 2 pilot trials in patients being treated with 5-FU-based chemotherapy regimens (Wadler et al, 1998; Kornblau et al, 2000). In these 2 studies, octreotide was injected subcutaneously at a dose of 100 µg twice a day to 500 µg 3 times a day. In other studies, octreotide has been given as a continuous intravenous infusion. The optimal dose and route of administration of octreotide are currently unknown and have been indexed to the clinical presentation.

Generally, the intergluteal and perianal regions are the only areas that have any skin reaction during chemoradiation. With the first signs of dry desquamation, an emollient that also acts as a barrier for the skin, like Lantiseptic's Skin Protectant (Marietta, GA), is maintained on the skin. When the skin is compromised, routine use of toilet paper can result in irritation, and small regions of moist desquamation in the perianal area can place the patient at risk for a secondary infection due to bacteria in the stool. Soft hydrated wipes are recommended to reduce trauma to the skin and improve hygiene. Sitz baths or warm compresses and Domeboro, an aluminum acetate solution (Bayer Corporation, Pittsburgh, PA), are also used to maintain good hygiene and provide symptomatic relief among patients with moist desquamation in the perineal region. Sulfadiazine (Silvadene) cream is used in areas of moist desquamation to soothe symptoms and as an antibacterial agent. Among patients who develop candidiasis in the perianal region, a compound with nystatin, Desitin ointment (zinc oxide ointment), and lidocaine is beneficial. However, this ointment must be removed at the time of treatment to reduce the effects of scatter radiation.

TREATMENT OF RECURRENT DISEASE

Recurrent rectal cancer can vary significantly in its clinical presentation. Because the morbidity of recurrent disease is so profound, aggressive therapeutic attempts are frequently undertaken to secure local-regional control. Routine follow-up testing and early evaluation of symptoms improves the chance of early detection of recurrent disease and long-term disease-free survival. Complete macroscopic resection of disease can be achieved in 57% of cases of recurrent rectal cancer, and partial resection with gross residual disease is possible in 29%; 14% of recurrent tumors are inoperable. The survival rate is improved with complete or partial resection, and the 5-year disease-free survival rate after complete or partial resection is 23%.

Palliative radiation therapy relieves bleeding in 100% of cases and pain in 65% of cases. A variety of palliative radiation schedules have been used at M. D. Anderson. These have been tailored according to prognosis and to accommodate patients. These radiation schedules include 35 Gy in 14 fractions of 2.5 Gy; 39 Gy in 26 fractions of 1.5 Gy given twice daily; and 30 Gy in 6 fractions of 5 Gy given twice weekly. Disease that recurs in a previously irradiated area necessitates the use of specialized techniques to minimize potential bowel damage. Approaches have included re-irradiation with intensity-modulated radiation therapy, intraoperative radiation therapy, and CT-guided brachytherapy implants. These techniques minimize the dose to the surrounding tissues while concentrating the dose in the tumor. With intraoperative radiation therapy in addition to surgery, overall survival rates were 72% at 1 year, 45% at 2 years, and

KEY PRACTICE POINTS

- For the average-risk individual (someone 50 years of age or older with no risk factors for colorectal cancer except older age), the preferred screening strategy is a colonoscopy every 5 years because it permits evaluation of the entire colon and clears adenomas by polypectomy, reducing the incidence of and deaths from colorectal cancer.

- Combined-modality therapy (surgery, radiation therapy, and chemotherapy) has significantly improved local and distant disease control in colorectal cancer, and it is now the standard of care for locally advanced disease.

- Advances in surgical technique have also been responsible for improvements in the rate of local control of rectal cancer. Total mesorectal excision has reduced the local recurrence rate from 39% to 10% and increased the 5-year survival rate from 50% to 71%.

- At present, the role of local excision in the treatment of rectal cancer depends on stage and other tumor characteristics and is still largely undefined. Patient selection is important. Attempts to maximize sphincter preservation must not result in inferior rates of tumor control or poorer functional outcome.

- Infusional 5-FU or oral 5-FU with the same pharmacokinetics as infusional therapy should be considered. Other agents, like oxaliplatin and irinotecan, are gaining greater prominence in adjuvant therapy and are under study for use in chemoradiation.

31% at 3 years; corresponding local control rates were 71%, 48%, and 31%, respectively (Bussieres et al, 1996).

In all cases, aggressive symptom management is necessary to improve quality of life. When recurrent disease is localized to the pelvis, survival can be prolonged. Treatment of incurable disease should relieve or prevent disease-related morbidity without causing excessive side effects.

Suggested Readings

Berger C, deMuret A, Garaud P, et al. Preoperative radiotherapy (RT) for rectal cancer: predictive factors of tumor downstaging and residual tumor cell density (RTCD): prognostic implications. *Int J Radiat Oncol Biol Phys* 1997;37:619–627.

Blumberg D, Opelka FG, Hicks TC, Timmcke AE, Beck DE. Significance of a normal surveillance colonoscopy in patients with a history of adenomatous polyps. *Dis Colon Rectum* 2000;43:1084–1092.

Bussieres E, Gilly FN, Rouanet P, et al. Recurrences of rectal cancers: results of a multimodal approach with intraoperative radiation therapy. *Int J Radiat Oncol Biol Phys* 1996;34:49–56.

Callister M, Janjan N, Crane C, et al. Effective management of symptoms during preoperative chemoradiation for locally advanced rectal cancer. *Int J Radiat Oncol Biol Phys* 2000;48[suppl]:177 (abstract 60).

Camma C, Giunta M, Fiorica F, Pagliaro L, Craxi A, Cottone M. Preoperative radiotherapy for resectable rectal cancer—a meta-analysis. *JAMA* 2000;284: 1008–1015.

Church TR, Ederer F, Mandel JS. Fecal occult blood screening in the Minnesota study: sensitivity of the screening test. *J Natl Cancer Inst* 1997;89:1440–1448.

Das IJ, Lanciano RM, Movsas B, Kagawa K, SJ Barnes. Efficacy of a belly board device with CT-simulation in reducing small bowel volume within pelvic irradiation fields. *Int J Radiat Oncol Biol Phys* 1997;39:67–76.

DeCosse JJ. Depth of invasion of colon carcinoma, lymphatic spread, and laparoscopic surgery. *Cancer* 1997;80:177–178.

Desch CE, Benson AB, Smith TJ, et al. Recommended colorectal cancer surveillance guidelines by the American Society of Clinical Oncology. *J Clin Oncol* 1999; 17:1312–1321.

Dorrance HR, Docherty GM, O'Dwyer PJ. Effect of surgeon specialty interest on patient outcome after potentially curative colorectal cancer surgery. *Dis Colon Rectum* 2000;43:492–498.

Fisher B, Wolmark N, Rockette H, et al. Postoperative adjuvant chemotherapy or radiation therapy for rectal cancer: results from NSABP R-01. *J Natl Cancer Inst* 1988;80:21–29.

Flanagan FL, Dehdashti F, Ogunbiyi O, Kodner IJ, Siegel BA. Utility of FDG-PET for investigating unexplained plasma CEA elevation in patients with colorectal cancer. *Ann Surg* 1998;227:319–323.

Francois Y, Nemoz CJ, Baulieux J, et al. Influence of the interval between preoperative radiation therapy and surgery on downstaging and on the rate of sphincter-sparing surgery for rectal cancer: the Lyon R90-01 randomized trial. *J Clin Oncol* 1999;17:2396–2402.

Gamelin EC, Danquechin-Dorval EM, Dumesnil YF, et al. Relationship between 5-fluorouracil [5FU] dose intensity and therapeutic response in patients with advanced colorectal cancer receiving infusional therapy containing 5FU. *Cancer* 1996;77:441–451.

Gastrointestinal Tumor Study Group. Prolongation of the disease-free interval in surgically treated rectal carcinoma. *N Engl J Med* 1985;312:1465–1472.

Gastrointestinal Tumor Study Group. Survival after postoperative combination treatment of rectal cancer. *N Engl J Med* 1986;315:1294–1295.

Giess CS, Schwartz LH, Bach AM, Gollub MJ, Panicek DM. Patterns of neoplastic spread in colorectal cancer: implications for surveillance CT studies. *AJR Am J Roentgenol* 1998;170:987–991.

Horton KM, Abrams RA, Fishman EK. Spiral CT of colon cancer: imaging features and role in management. *Radiographics* 2000;20:419–430.

Ikeda Y, Mori M, Yoshizumi T, Sugimachi K. Cancer and adenomatous polyp distribution in the colorectum. *Am J Gastroenterol* 1999;94:191–193.

Janjan NA, Abbruzzese J, Pazdur R, et al. Prognostic implications of response to preoperative infusional chemoradiation in locally advanced rectal cancer. *Radiother Oncol* 1999;51:153–160.

Janjan NA, Breslin T, Lenzi R, Rich TA, Skibber JM. Avoidance of colostomy placement in advanced colorectal cancer with twice weekly hypofractionated radiation plus continuous infusion 5-fluorouracil. *J Pain Symptom Manage* 2000; 20:266–272.

Janjan NA, Crane CH, Feig BW, et al. Prospective trial of preoperative concomitant boost radiotherapy with continuous infusion 5-fluorouracil for locally advanced rectal cancer. *Int J Radiat Oncol Biol Phys* 2000;47:713–718.

Janjan NA, Khoo VS, Abbruzzese J, et al. Tumor downstaging and sphincter preservation with preoperative chemoradiation in locally advanced rectal cancer: the M. D. Anderson Cancer Center experience. *Int J Radiat Oncol Biol Phys* 1999;44:1027–1038.

Janjan NA, Khoo VS, Rich TA, et al. Locally advanced rectal cancer: surgical complications after infusional chemotherapy and radiation therapy. *Radiology* 1998;206:131–136.

Kaminsky-Forrett MC, Conroy T, Luporsi E, et al. Prognostic implications of downstaging following preoperative radiation therapy for operable T3–T4 rectal cancer. *Int J Radiat Oncol Biol Phys* 1998;42:935–941.

Koelbl O, Richter S, Flentje M. Influence of patient positioning on dose-volume histogram and normal tissue complication probability for small bowel and bladder in patients receiving pelvic irradiation: a prospective study using a 3D planning system and a radiobiological model. *Int J Radiat Oncol Biol Phys* 1999;45:1193–1198.

Kornblau S, Benson AB, Catalano R, et al. Management of cancer treatment related diarrhea: issues and therapeutic strategies. *J Pain Symptom Manage* 2000;19: 118–129.

Krook JE, Moertel CG, Gunderson LL, et al. Effective surgical adjuvant therapy for high-risk rectal carcinoma. *N Engl J Med* 1991;324:709–715.

Mellgren A, Sirivongs P, Rothenberger DA, Madoff RD, Garcia-Aguilar J. Is local excision adequate therapy for early rectal cancer? *Dis Colon Rectum* 2000;43: 2064–2074.

Meta-Analysis Group in Cancer. Efficacy of intravenous continuous infusion of fluorouracil compared with bolus administration in advanced colorectal cancer. *J Clin Oncol* 1998;16:301–308.

Mettlin CJ, Menck HR, Winchester DP, Murphy GP. A comparison of breast, colorectal, lung, and prostate cancers reported to the National Cancer Data Base and the Surveillance, Epidemiology, and End Results Program. *Cancer* 1997;79: 2052–2061.

Minsky BD, Coia L, Haller DG, et al. Radiation therapy for rectosigmoid and rectal cancer: results of the 1992–1994 Patterns of Care Process Survey. *J Clin Oncol* 1998;16:2542–2547.

Minsky BD, Conti JA, Huang Y, Knopf K. Relationship of acute gastrointestinal toxicity and the volume of irradiated small bowel in patients receiving combined modality therapy for rectal cancer. *J Clin Oncol* 1995;13:1409–1416.

Mohiuddin M, Marks GM, Lingareddy V, Marks J. Curative surgical resection following reirradiation for recurrent rectal cancer. *Int J Radiat Oncol Biol Phys* 1997;39:643–649.

Movsas J, Hanlon AL, Lanciano R, et al. Phase I dose escalating trial of hyperfractionated pre-operative chemoradiation for locally advanced rectal cancer. *Int J Radiat Oncol Biol Phys* 1998;42:43–50.

Paty PB, Cohen AM. Technical considerations for coloanal anastomosis and J-pouch. *Semin Radiat Oncol* 1998;8:48–53.

Rex DK, Johnson DA, Lieberman DA, Burt RW, Sonnenberg A. Colorectal cancer prevention 2000: screening recommendations of the American College of Gastroenterology. *Am J Gastroenterol* 2000;95:868–877.

Rodriguez-Bigas MA, Boland CR, Hamilton SR, et al. A National Cancer Institute workshop on hereditary nonpolyposis colorectal cancer syndrome: meeting highlights and Bethesda guidelines. *J Natl Cancer Inst* 1997;89:1758–1762.

Royce ME, Medgyesy D, Zukowski TH, Dwivedy S, Hoff PM. Colorectal cancer: chemotherapy treatment overview. *Oncology* 2000;14:40–46.

Salo JC, Paty PB, Guillem J, Minsky BD, Harrison LB, Cohen AM. Surgical salvage of recurrent rectal carcinoma after curative resection: a 10-year experience. *Ann Surg Oncol* 1999;6:171–177.

Swedish Rectal Cancer Trial. Improved survival with preoperative radiotherapy in resectable rectal cancer. *N Engl J Med* 1997;336:980–987.

Tepper JE, O'Connell MJ, Niedzwiecki D, et al. Impact of number of nodes retrieved on outcome in patients with rectal cancer. *J Clin Oncol* 2001;19:157–163.

Wadler S, Benson AB, Engelking C, et al. Recommended guidelines for the treatment of chemotherapy-induced diarrhea. *J Clin Oncol* 1998;16:3169–3178.

Willett CG. Local excision followed by postoperative radiation therapy. *Semin Radiat Oncol* 1998;8:24–29.

Willett CG, Goldberg S, Shellito PC, et al. Does postoperative irradiation play a role in the adjuvant therapy of T4 colon cancer? *Cancer J Sci Am* 1999;5:242–247.

Winawer SJ. Natural history of colorectal cancer. *Am J Med* 1999;106[1A]:3S–6S.

11 METASTATIC CANCER OF THE LIVER

Jean-Nicolas Vauthey

CHAPTER OVERVIEW

Surgical resection remains the only treatment that leads to long-term survival and occasionally cure in patients with colorectal or other metastases of the liver. Five-year survival rates after resection of hepatic colorectal metastases are 30% to 40%. Because of this, a surgeon experienced in hepatic resections should always be consulted to evaluate patients with hepatic colorectal metastases. In recent years, the indications for resection have been extended, and the only absolute contraindications for resection of hepatic colorectal metastases are extrahepatic disease and an anticipated incomplete resection. Complex and extended resection can now be performed using novel techniques such as radiofrequency ablation and portal vein embolization as adjuncts to resection. It is anticipated that the goal of complete resection and ablation with negative margins will be achieved in an increasing number of patients using these combined approaches and novel chemotherapy agents (irinotecan and oxaliplatin).

In patients who have undergone liver resection, close follow-up is important because repeat hepatic resection remains an option in selected patients.

SURGICAL TREATMENT OF COLORECTAL LIVER METASTASES

Colorectal cancer is the most common metastatic cancer occurring in the liver. It is estimated that in the United States approximately 150,000 patients annually are diagnosed with colorectal cancer. Of these, approximately 20% present with metastases confined to the liver or develop such metastases during the course of the disease. Left untreated, hepatic colorectal metastases carry a dismal prognosis. Six studies of the natural history of such metastases reporting on a total of 1,051 patients described 5-year survival rates equal to or less than 3%.

There is now evidence that surgical resection can alter this dismal prognosis. In 1995, Scheele et al reported on 366 patients who underwent complete potentially curative resection of hepatic colorectal metastases and received no adjuvant therapy. The patients in this study were followed prospectively with assessment of carcinoembryonic antigen (CEA) levels, ultrasonography, and chest radiography every 4 to 6 months, allowing for a proper evaluation of disease-free survival and overall survival. Following complete curative resection, some 40% of these patients were still alive at 5 years, and 30% remained disease-free at 5 years. The likelihood of remaining free of colorectal cancer recurrence after a tumor-free period of 1 to 7 years was determined for 350 patients who survived hepatic resection. The likelihood of remaining tumor-free increased as time elapsed following curative liver resection (Figure 11–1). Importantly, after 7 years, no recurrences occurred in 26 patients at risk, and the chance of remaining tumor-free or being cured was 100%, as determined by the ultimate analysis of these long-term survivors. This study has provided the best presumptive evidence that the natural history of hepatic colorectal metastases can be altered and that cure is possible after resection alone. These results have since been confirmed in other large single-institutional series.

CEA for Detection of Colorectal Cancer Recurrence

During the past 3 decades, measurement of the tumor marker CEA has been pivotal in the detection of colorectal cancer recurrence. CEA seems to modulate intercellular adhesion and participates in epithelial cell–collagen interaction. Because of a lack of specificity, the CEA assay cannot be used as a diagnostic test. However, CEA is useful in the postoperative monitoring of patients after resection of primary tumors. A rise in CEA usually predicts recurrence 6 to 8 months before the appearance of clinical signs. CEA is most sensitive for hepatic metastases and is relatively insensitive for local or peritoneal involvement. A slowly rising CEA level

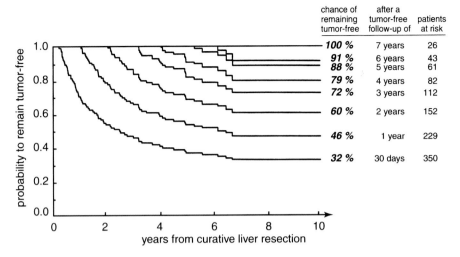

chance of remaining tumor-free	after a tumor-free follow-up of	patients at risk
100 %	7 years	26
91 %	6 years	43
88 %	5 years	61
79 %	4 years	82
72 %	3 years	112
60 %	2 years	152
46 %	1 year	229
32 %	30 days	350

Figure 11–1. Disease-free survival of 350 patients who underwent complete resection of hepatic colorectal metastases. Likelihood of surviving long term is provided by separate analysis of cohorts of patients surviving 30 days or longer after surgery. Reprinted with permission from Scheele et al (1995).

usually indicates local or regional recurrence, while a rapidly rising CEA level suggests hepatic metastases. Overall, 75% to 90% of patients with hepatic colorectal metastases have an elevated CEA concentration.

Wanebo (1986) advocated second-look surgery for patients with elevated postoperative CEA levels without evidence of recurrence. In Wanebo's series, more than 90% of the patients who underwent exploration on the basis of an increased CEA level had recurrence, and 41% underwent curative resection. In another large prospective multicenter series reported by Minton et al (1985), CEA-directed surgery again was correlated with detection of recurrences. However, statistical analysis of the long-term survivors indicated that the 5-year survival rate was 37% in CEA-directed second-look patients and 28% in non-CEA-directed patients ($P > .05$).

Today, CEA level alone is rarely an indication for surgery. Rather, CEA should be part of an algorithm for the management of recurrent colon cancer (Figure 11–2). An elevated CEA level indicates the need for further imaging, including a positron emission tomography (PET) scan, to localize these recurrences with greater accuracy. A finite number of tests are undertaken to maintain cost-effectiveness while reducing the number of unnecessary laparotomies for unresectable disease. The combination of CEA assessment and radiographic imaging helps detect recurrences before they are symptomatic, directly affecting the resectability rate as well as prognosis. The goal of the workup is to offer a potentially curative resection to patients with liver-only or localized disease.

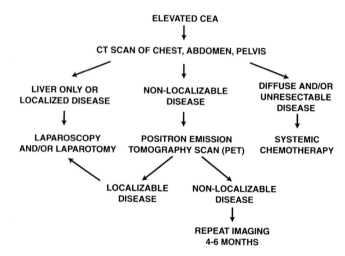

Figure 11–2.   Preoperative management of recurrent colorectal cancer. Modified with permission from Vauthey et al (1996a).

Preoperative Imaging Strategies

Appropriate imaging is the cornerstone of preoperative evaluation. The initial imaging should include helical computed tomography (CT) of the abdomen with thin (5-mm) cuts through the liver and rapid bolus intravenous contrast injection (2 to 5 mL per second) so as to obtain 4 sets of images (precontrast, arterial, portal, and delayed phases). A chest x-ray and CT of the pelvis, if local pelvic recurrence of carcinoma is suspected, should rule out extra-abdominal disease.

Magnetic resonance imaging enhanced with a cell-specific contrast agent is used to further characterize the lesions if doubt exists regarding the diagnosis or the intrahepatic extent of a tumor. The advent of cell-specific contrast agents, such as superparamagnetic iron oxide and manganese-pyridoxal diphosphate, has improved the sensitivity of magnetic resonance imaging in the detection and characterization of hepatic metastases. Superparamagnetic iron oxide particles are taken up by the reticuloendothelial system and cause a reduced T2 signal. In contrast, manganese-pyridoxal diphosphate is taken up by hepatocytes and causes an enhanced T1 signal.

At M. D. Anderson Cancer Center, we do not recommend or routinely perform CT arterial portography (CTAP) in patients with hepatic colorectal metastases. Although CTAP is probably more sensitive than conventional CT with intravenous contrast, the advent of helical CT has provided high-quality imaging, and the CTAP claim of higher sensitivity has become less clear-cut. CTAP is invasive, time consuming, technically demanding, and costly. It is also associated with such artifacts as flow defects (frequent in segments 4 and 5) and overflow (as a result of a replaced hepatic artery), and it is difficult to distinguish lesions from artifacts or simply to define lesions in areas of abnormal contrast. CTAP results in more false-positive results than does helical CT or cell-specific, contrast-enhanced magnetic resonance imaging.

Recently, PET has been used to image liver tumors. Tumor cells have increased levels of membrane glucose transporters and intracellular hexokinase, which converts glucose to glucose-6-phosphate. When the analogue 2-[18F]-fluoro-2-deoxy-D-glucose (FDG) is given to patients, tumor cells accumulate FDG-6-phosphate. FDG can then be used to image malignant tumors. Vitola et al (1996) evaluated the use of PET in patients with hepatic metastases and found PET to be more accurate than CT (93% vs 76%). At M. D. Anderson, PET is performed preoperatively in selected patients with multiple hepatic colorectal metastases or unfavorable biological features before consideration for surgical resection.

Contraindications and Operative Technique

The only true contraindications to resection of hepatic colorectal metastases are the presence of extrahepatic disease and the anticipated inability to achieve complete resection. There are, however, exceptions to this rule. These include local recurrence, isolated lung metastasis, and direct invasion of adjacent organs such as the diaphragm, gallbladder, and colon (Table 11–1).

Current techniques of resection are based on the liver's segmental anatomy, as described by Couinaud (1957). The recommended terms for major resections are right and left hepatectomy and extended right and extended left hepatectomy. Commonly performed anatomic resections are shown in Figure 11–3.

Resection of hepatic colorectal metastases begins with a laparotomy through a bilateral subcostal incision. The abdomen is examined for evidence of extrahepatic disease. Any suspicious nodule is biopsied, and frozen sections are obtained. The liver is then mobilized by sharp dissection of all its supporting ligaments. The liver is palpated to identify lesions not noted on preoperative imaging studies. Intraoperative ultrasonography is a valuable adjunct that can identify nonpalpable lesions and define vascular anatomy, hence aiding in the decision to proceed with a segmental or more traditional resection. The goal of the operation is to elim-

Table 11–1.   Absolute Contraindications to Resection of Hepatic Colorectal Metastases

Extrahepatic tumor—except for local recurrence, isolated lung metastases, or direct invasion of adjacent structures
Lymph node metastases at the liver hilum
Anticipated incomplete resection

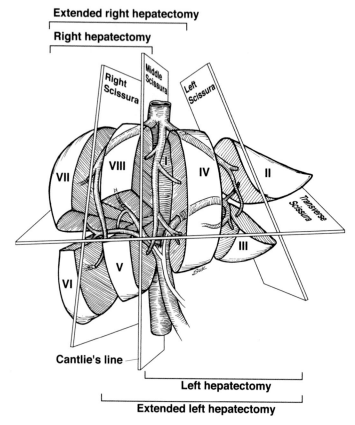

Figure 11–3. The liver is divided into 8 segments on the basis of the anatomic studies of Couinaud (1957). The hepatic veins and the umbilical fissure define the resection lines for major hepatic resections. Reprinted with permission from Vauthey (1998).

inate all metastases with negative resection margins. Under intermittent vascular inflow occlusion (Pringle maneuver), the hepatic parenchyma is divided with an ultrasonic dissector. Small vessels are controlled with electrocautery, while larger vessels and biliary radicals are individually sutured and ligated.

Results of Surgery and Factors Affecting Survival

Liver resection is now a well-controlled procedure, with complications occurring in 30% or less of patients. The perioperative mortality rate for resection of hepatic colorectal metastases at major centers is now approaching zero. Factors affecting recurrence are presented in Table 11–2. Factors most consistently associated with recurrence are a positive resection margin, discovery of liver metastases synchronous with the primary tumor, and a primary tumor with 1 or more positive lymph nodes.

In the past, hepatic colorectal metastases were not resected in patients with more than 3 or 4 lesions or with lesions within 1 cm of major vessels (vena cava or main hepatic veins). Now, however, the number of metastases is not considered to be as important a predictor of long-term survival as it was previously thought to be. Indeed, excision of all demonstrable tumors with clear resection margins has been shown to be of much greater importance. Although a resection margin of 1 cm or more is desirable, occasionally this cannot be achieved for technical reasons. Provided the margin is microscopically tumor-free, long-term survival and cure are also possible (although somewhat reduced) with margins of less than 1 cm (overall 5- and 10-year survival rates of 37% and 21%, respectively, with margins less than 10 mm, vs 43% and 28%, respectively, with margins of at least 10 mm). An anticipated close resection margin therefore does not constitute a contraindication to resection.

Hilar metastasis has traditionally been considered to be extrahepatic disease and therefore a contraindication to surgical intervention. Other factors that may increase the risk of recurrence after liver resection include symptomatic disease, the presence of satellitosis (metastases around the main metastatic nodule within the same segment or within 2 cm and less than 50% of the size of the main metastasis), and a high preoperative CEA value. The performance of an anatomic resection has also been shown to favorably affect overall and tumor-free survival. Performance of such "anatomic resections" has been facilitated by the widespread availability of intraoperative ultrasonography, which allows for precise delineation of the vascular anatomy within individual segments.

Table 11–2.   Predictors of Recurrence after Hepatic Resection of Colorectal Metastases

Study	Positive Margin	Synchronous Tumor	Node-Positive Primary	Size > 10 cm	No. of Metastases	Bilobar Disease
Gayowski, 1994	Yes	Yes	Yes	No	Yes	Yes
Scheele, 1995	Yes	Yes	Yes	Yes	No	No
Jamison, 1997	No	—	No	No	No	—
Jenkins, 1997	Yes	Yes	—	—	No	—
Ambiru, 1999	Yes	—	Yes	—	Yes	—
Fong, 1999	Yes	—	Yes	—	Yes	No

Reprinted with permission from Wayne JD, Vauthey JN. Metastatic cancer of the liver. In: Bland KI, Sarr MG, eds. *The Practice of General Surgery.* Philadelphia, Pa: Harcourt Health Sciences; 2001:643–651.

Results of Repeat Hepatic Resection

The most common sites of recurrence after resection of hepatic colorectal metastases are the liver and lung. Several groups have now reported successful repeat liver resection. In a recent series, the median survival was 34 months and the 5-year survival rate was 32% for 170 consecutive patients who underwent repeat hepatic resection.

For patients with isolated liver and lung metastases, resection of metastases at both sites has been reported with favorable results in small series. DeMatteo et al (1999) reported on 81 patients who underwent both liver and lung resection for metastatic colorectal carcinoma. Most (87%) of the lung resections in this highly selected group were wedge excisions. The median actuarial survival was 3.8 years after a patient had both liver and lung metastases resected.

With repeat liver or lung resection providing an option for cure, follow-up after resection of colorectal metastases is justified. Routine follow-up should include an office visit 2 months after hospital discharge. A CEA value that was elevated preoperatively should return to normal within 6 weeks. Office visits with performance of liver function studies and assessment of CEA levels should thereafter be repeated every 3 months. Patients should undergo abdominal and pelvic CT and chest radiography every 4 to 6 months and colonoscopy the first year after colon resection and every 3 years thereafter if the findings on baseline colonoscopy are negative. This rigorous schedule should be continued for up to 7 years, on the basis of long-term follow-up data on the disease-free survival after liver resection (Figure 11–1).

Adjuvant Hepatic Artery Chemotherapy

Because of the poor response rate to systemic chemotherapy, surgeons and oncologists have explored the use of hepatic artery chemotherapy (HAC) in patients with resectable and unresectable hepatic colorectal metastases. The rationale for regional chemotherapy is that direct delivery should increase the response rate while limiting systemic toxicity. Initially delivered via percutaneous catheters or subcutaneous ports, HAC was advanced by the development of totally implantable infusion pumps in the 1980s. This delivery system allows patients greater freedom of movement and ensures accurate and reliable delivery of chemotherapeutic agents. In a series comparing HAC delivered via ports and pumps, the implantable pump was associated with fewer device-related complications and provided more durable patency (28 months vs 9 months for ports).

Arterial anatomy is defined preoperatively with selective celiac axis and superior mesenteric artery angiography. The abdomen is explored through a subcostal incision to rule out extrahepatic disease. The vascular anatomy is then confirmed. With standard anatomy, control of the common and proper hepatic arteries is obtained, and the catheter is placed in the gastroduodenal artery, which is ligated distally. A cholecystectomy is performed in all patients to prevent chemotherapy-induced cholecystitis. The pump is placed in a subcutaneous pocket made through a separate transverse skin incision. Vascular isolation is confirmed using fluorescein dye injection and a Wood's lamp. An additional baseline evaluation of the pump is obtained 3 or 4 days after the operation by hepatic arterial perfusion of Tc-99m macroaggregated albumin via the side port of the pump.

Four randomized trials utilizing HAC have been reported. In a study by Wagman et al (1990), the addition of HAC to surgery alone increased the mean disease-free survival from 9 to 32 months. However, the 3-year survival did not differ between the 2 groups. Similarly, Lorenz et al (1998) reported a multicenter prospective randomized trial of resection plus HAC with 5-fluorouracil (5-FU) versus resection alone; the addition of HAC failed to show an improvement in survival.

Kemeny et al (1999) published a single-center, randomized study comparing regional floxuridine and dexamethasone via an implantable pump plus systemic 5-FU and leucovorin (combined therapy) with systemic 5-FU and leucovorin alone (monotherapy) after liver resection. The combined therapy provided significantly higher 2-year survival rates (86% vs 72%, $P = .03$) and hepatic disease-free survival rates (90% vs 60%; $P < .001$) compared with monotherapy. The Eastern Cooperative Oncology Group prospective randomized trial (Kemeny et al, 2002) compared 56 patients randomly assigned to hepatic resection alone with 53 patients randomly assigned to hepatic resection followed by HAC with floxuridine for 4 cycles and systemic 5-FU for 12 cycles. This study showed 3-year recurrence-free survival rates of 34% for the surgery-alone group and 58% ($P < .05$) for the patients receiving adjuvant chemotherapy. The 5-year survival rates, however, were not significantly different. The results of these trials show a trend toward increased survival in patients treated with adjuvant HAC. Of note, these studies did not include the use of newer agents (such as irinotecan or oxaliplatin combined with fluoropyrimidines) that have been found to be effective (response rates of greater than 50%) in the treatment of metastatic colorectal carcinoma.

HAC FOR UNRESECTABLE METASTASES

Six randomized studies have compared systemic chemotherapy with HAC for unresectable metastases (Table 11–3). Five of 6 compared sustained-release floxuridine delivered via implantable pumps with systemic 5-FU or floxuridine. All found a greater response rate to HAC than to systemic chemotherapy. In addition, in all 6 studies, HAC was associated with longer median survival than systemic therapy was, but the difference was

Table 11-3. Randomized Studies Comparing Systemic Chemotherapy with HAC for Unresectable Colorectal Metastases

Reference	N	Chemotherapy		Response Rate (%)			Median Survival (months)		
		Systemic	HAC	Systemic	HAC	P	Systemic	HAC	P
Kemeny, 1987	162	5-FU	FUDR	20	50	.001	12	17	NS
Chang, 1987	64	5-FU	FUDR	17	62	.003	15	22	.03*
Hohn, 1989	143	5-FU	FUDR	10	42	.0001	16	17	NS
Martin, 1990	69	5-FU	FUDR	21	48	.02	11	13	NS
Rougier, 1992	163	5-FU	FUDR	9	43	—	11	15	.03
Allen-Mersh, 1994	100	—	FUDR	—	—	—	8	15	.03

Abbreviations: HAC, hepatic artery chemotherapy; 5-FU, 5-fluorouracil; FUDR, floxuridine; NS, not significant.
* Patients with positive portal lymph nodes excluded.
Modified with permission from Vauthey et al (1996b).

significant in only 3 studies (8–16 months vs 13–22 months, respectively). While HAC appears to be a valuable option for the management of unresectable colorectal cancer metastases, none of the studies to date are large enough to permit a valid conclusion. Furthermore, none of the studies used the current standard chemotherapy for colorectal cancer (5-FU plus leucovorin) as systemic treatment. At M. D. Anderson, HAC is currently used in patients with unresectable hepatic colorectal metastases whose disease does not respond to systemic therapy.

SURGICAL TREATMENT OF NONCOLORECTAL LIVER METASTASES

While surgical resection of colorectal liver metastases has gained wide-spread acceptance, the role of hepatic resection for noncolorectal liver metastases is less clear. Until recently, there were no large series to guide clinical decision making. However, the reduction in operative morbidity and mortality with major hepatic resections has allowed for a re-examination of the role of surgery in the treatment of noncolorectal liver metastases.

Liver Metastases from Carcinoid Tumors

Over the past 2 decades, resection of liver metastases from carcinoid tumors has become part of the standard of care for patients with malignant carcinoid syndrome. This is because of the indolent nature of these tumors, which are often slow-growing. In 1961, Moertel et al defined the natural history of carcinoid tumors metastatic to the liver. The mean survival from the onset of symptoms was 8.1 years in a series of 28 patients with malignant carcinoid syndrome. Today, survival may be extended even further with the combination of resection, hormonal therapy with somatostatin analogues (octreotide), and hepatic artery embolization.

Soreide et al (1992) reported a retrospective review of 75 patients who underwent aggressive surgical management of their advanced abdominal carcinoid tumors. Of these patients, 36 underwent 1 or more interventions directed at metastatic disease in the liver: resection, hepatic artery ligation, or embolization. The median survival in this group was 216 months, compared with 48 months for patients who did not undergo hepatic intervention ($P < .001$). Que et al (1995) from the Mayo Clinic reviewed 75 patients, most of whom underwent hepatic resection for symptomatic metastatic neuroendocrine tumors. Fifty (75%) of these tumors were carcinoids. Resections included 38 formal lobectomies or extended resections and 38 nonanatomic resections. Perioperative mortality was 2.4% and morbidity was 24%. The 4-year survival rate was 73%, but perhaps more important, symptomatic response was achieved in 90% of patients, with a mean duration of response of 19.3 months.

Chen et al (1998) reported on a series of 38 patients with liver-only metastases from neuroendocrine tumors. Most tumors (21) were metastatic carcinoid tumors. The 5-year actuarial survival rate was 73% for the 15 patients who were able to undergo complete resection of their disease. This was significantly better than the 29% 5-year actuarial survival rate observed for the 23 patients who had a similar tumor burden but were believed to have unresectable disease. Although not randomized, this small series suggests that hepatic resection may not only provide palliation in these highly symptomatic patients but also improve survival in selected patients.

Finally, orthotopic liver transplantation has been suggested as an alternative therapy for selected patients with neuroendocrine hepatic metastases. Le Treut et al (1997) reported a 4-year survival rate of 69% in a series of 15 patients who underwent orthotopic liver transplantation for metastatic carcinoid tumors. This is in contrast to a 4-year survival rate of 8% reported for 16 patients with noncarcinoid apudomas. Of note, however, were a 19% mortality rate and a 48% incidence of major surgical complications. Further long-term studies are needed to clarify the role of transplantation in the treatment of hepatic metastases from neuroendocrine tumors. Given the scarcity of organ donors and limited resources, it is unlikely that organ transplantation will be available to many patients with metastatic carcinoid tumors in the near future.

Nonneuroendocrine Metastases

The role of hepatic resection for metastases from nonneuroendocrine primary tumors is less well defined. Recently, several institutions have published their experience with noncolorectal, nonneuroendocrine metastases, and this provides some guidelines for selecting patients who will benefit from hepatic resection. The review of patients who underwent surgery at M. D. Anderson indicated a 5-year actuarial survival rate of 44%, with a median survival of 54 months, for 45 patients undergoing resection of noncolorectal liver metastases (Tuttle, 1998). Similarly, Harrison et al (1997) reported a 5-year overall survival rate of 37% for 96 patients undergoing liver resection for noncolorectal, nonneuroendocrine metastases. More than 78% of the primary tumors in this series were genitourinary or soft-tissue tumors. By multivariate analysis, the only predictors of increased survival were a disease-free interval of less than 36 months prior to discovery of liver metastases; curative resection; and primary tumor type (genitourinary > soft tissue > gastrointestinal). These results confirm the findings of Schwartz (1995), who found by a review of the literature that long-term survival was possible for patients with liver metastases from renal tumors (particularly Wilms' tumor) but not for those with soft-tissue or gastrointestinal (noncolorectal, nonneuroendocrine) primary tumors.

Thus, despite the fact that recent survival data for patients undergoing resection of noncolorectal, nonneuroendocrine metastases are encouraging, in most patients disease will eventually recur. Patient selection is critical when opting for resection, and resection should be considered only in the context of a multimodality treatment plan at specialized centers.

NOVEL TREATMENT APPROACHES

Radiofrequency Ablation

Radiofrequency ablation (RFA) is a relatively new technique that is rapidly gaining wide acceptance for local ablation of tumors not amenable to resection. RFA is performed percutaneously as an interventional radiologic procedure or intraoperatively laparoscopically or as part of a laparotomy. An RFA needle is placed within the tumor under CT or ultrasound guidance. The needle array is deployed, and thermal energy is generated. The cell membranes are destroyed, and the intracellular proteins degenerate as the temperature exceeds 45° to 50° (Figure 11–4).

Curley et al (1999) reported on 123 patients with primary or metastatic hepatic malignancies treated with RFA. Half (61) of these patients had hepatic colorectal metastases. Patients with small (<3 cm) peripheral tumors were treated with percutaneous ultrasound-guided RFA (n = 31), while the remaining patients were treated during an open operative procedure. To prevent bile duct injuries, patients with tumors near the main right or left bile ducts were excluded. Patients were still considered for RFA when the tumor abutted a major hepatic branch or the vena cava. In this series, there were no treatment-related deaths, and the complication rate was 2.4%. After a median follow-up of 15 months, only 1.8% of tumors had recurred at the RFA site. Unfortunately, 27.6% of patients had recurrence at distant sites. Two of the 3 local recurrences occurred in patients with tumors less than 6 cm in diameter. The only complications in this series were 1 perihepatic abscess and 1 hemorrhage into the treated tumor.

Solbiati et al (1997) reported on 29 patients with 44 liver metastases, most from colorectal cancer, who were treated with percutaneous RFA. At a median follow-up of 18 months, the disease-free survival rate was 33% and the overall survival rate was 89%. Progression of disease at the RFA site was seen in 34% of treated lesions. This is in contrast to the 1.8% local recurrence rate reported by Curley et al (1999). All patients in Solbiati et al's study were treated percutaneously, whereas only 25% of the patients in the series of Curley et al were treated in this manner. Curley et al used the percutaneous technique only in isolated peripheral lesions, while

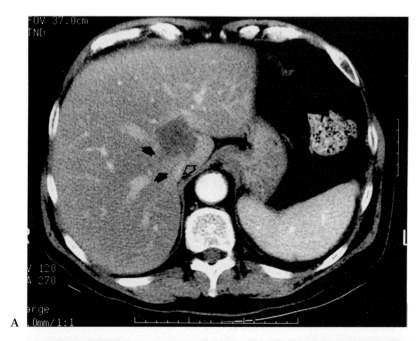

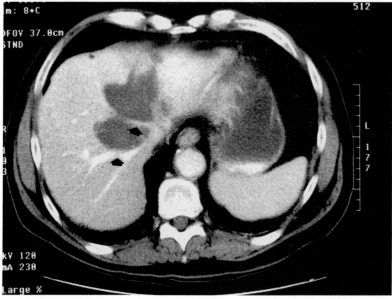

Figure 11–4. Radiofrequency ablation (RFA) of a liver metastasis. Computed tomography scans of liver metastases before (*A*) and 3 months after (*B*) RFA. Reprinted with permission from Curley et al (1999).

Solbiati et al used the percutaneous technique in patients with multiple central lesions. This difference in approach may directly affect the ability to achieve complete tumor destruction.

It appears from preliminary data that RFA can be used as a local ablative technique when the patient is not a candidate for surgery. Unfortunately, the extrahepatic recurrence rate is high because patients remain at risk for systemic failure. RFA should further be investigated as part of prospective studies because current studies provide only short-term follow-up data. At M. D. Anderson, RFA is now being used alone or in combination with resection in patients in whom resection is contraindicated or in whom a complete resection is not possible.

Portal Vein Embolization

Preoperative portal vein embolization (PVE) prior to extended liver resection is an option in selected patients if there is concern regarding possible postoperative liver failure or complications due to a small liver remnant volume. The rationale for this technique is to induce hypertrophy of the future liver remnant (FLR).

The first clinical report demonstrating this technique was by Kinoshita et al in 1986. In this study, 21 patients with a diagnosis of hepatocellular carcinoma underwent preoperative PVE and hepatic artery embolization. Postembolization CT scans and operative findings confirmed hypertrophy of the contralateral liver. Kawasaki et al (1994) reported on 5 patients with metastatic colorectal cancer who underwent preoperative right PVE to allow extended right hepatectomy in conjunction with wedge resections of the left lateral segment. Embolizations were performed between 9 days and 8 months before surgical resection, and the mean survival was 47 months. The procedure is associated with true DNA synthesis of the contralateral liver (nonembolized) and hypertrophy secondary to clonal expansion of the hepatocytes. Clinically, the procedure leads to improved function of the FLR, as demonstrated by studies showing increased biliary excretion of the FLR and improved postoperative liver function tests after resection in patients who have undergone PVE.

At M. D. Anderson, PVE is performed in the interventional radiology department under fluoroscopic guidance. Madoff et al (2003) recently reported on 26 patients who underwent PVE before major hepatic resection for hepatobiliary malignancy. In 25 of the patients, an ipsilateral percutaneous approach was used to access the portal vein, and the embolization material consisted of microspheres and coils. The median length of hospital stay was less than 24 hours, and an increase in FLR occurred in 23 of the 26 patients. PVE is well tolerated and in noncirrhotic livers induces a 25% to 80% increase in the absolute volume of the nonembolized liver (Figure 11–5). Four to 6 weeks are usually required to enable adequate hypertrophy in normal livers. After this period, sur-

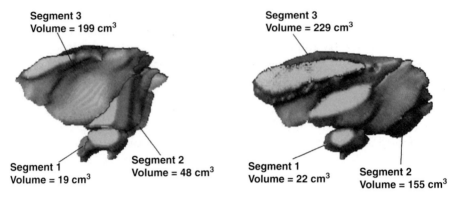

Figure 11–5. Preoperative 3-dimensional reconstruction of the future liver remnant (FLR) prior to extended right lobectomy (segments 1, 2, and 3) before (left) and after (right) portal vein embolization. The FLR increased from 266 cm³ to 406 cm³ in 6 weeks. Reprinted with permission from Vauthey et al, 2000.

KEY PRACTICE POINTS

- Without treatment, median survival of patients with hepatic metastases from colorectal carcinoma is only 12 to 15 months, and the 5-year survival rate is less than 3%.

- Selected patients with hepatic colorectal metastases are candidates for hepatic resection after previous curative colorectal surgery.

- The operative mortality rate after resection of hepatic colorectal metastases is approaching zero, and the 5-year survival rate is 30% to 40%.

- Contraindications include uncontrolled primary disease, hepatic hilar lymph node metastases, and inability to remove all known disease.

- Palliative or curative hepatic resection should be considered in patients with functional and nonfunctional neuroendocrine liver metastases.

- RFA may be useful as an adjunct to resection and in selected patients who are not candidates for resection.

- Percutaneous PVE increases the size and the function of the anticipated FLR preoperatively and may increase the number of patients with advanced metastatic liver cancer who are candidates for curative hepatic resection.

gical resection can be planned. Accessing the ipsilateral lobe minimizes the possibility of damage to the portal vein branches of the FLR.

General indications for PVE are based on the size of the FLR and the extent of the proposed procedure. PVE is particularly useful in patients with multiple hepatic metastases in whom a small liver remnant is anticipated. Typically these patients do not have the compensatory hypertrophy associated with large primary hepatic tumors.

We recently reported on 42 patients who underwent extended hepatectomy for hepatobiliary malignancies (hepatic metastases, hepatocellular carcinoma, and cholangiocarcinoma) at M. D. Anderson. In 18 patients with FLR of 25% or less at presentation, PVE was performed to minimize the potential complications associated with these extended resections. PVE increased the FLR volume from 18% to 23% of the estimated total liver volume prior to resection. Although 31% of patients in the entire series also underwent complex resections (vascular reconstruction, bile duct resection, and caudate lobe resection), there was no perioperative mortality or mortality within 3 months of the resection, and the morbidity rate was 24%. On the basis of this experience, we now perform PVE to optimize hepatic function in patients in whom we anticipate FLR volumes of less than 20% to 25% before resection.

SUGGESTED READINGS

Abdalla EK, Barnett CC, Doherty D, et al. Extended hepatectomy in patients with hepatobiliary malignancies with and without preoperative portal vein embolization. *Arch Surg* 2002;137:675–680.

Abdalla EK, Hicks ME, Vauthey JN. Portal vein embolization: rationale, technique and future prospects. *Br J Surg* 2001;88:165–175.

Adson MA, Van Heerden JA, Adson MH, et al. Resection of hepatic metastases from colorectal cancer. *Arch Surg* 1984;119:647–651.

Allen-Mersh TG, Earlam S, Fordy C, et al. Quality of life and survival with continuous hepatic-artery floxuridine infusion for colorectal liver metastases. *Lancet* 1994;344:1255–1260.

Ambiru S, Miyazaki M, Isono T, et al. Hepatic resection for colorectal metastases: analysis of prognostic factors. *Dis Colon Rectum* 1999;42:632–639.

Chen H, Hardacre JM, Uzar A, et al. Isolated liver metastases from neuroendocrine tumors: does resection prolong survival? *J Am Coll Surg* 1998;187:88–93.

Couinaud C. Le foie. Etudes anatomiques et chirurgicales. Paris, France: Masson; 1957.

Curley SA, Chase JL, Roh MS, et al. Technical considerations and complications associated with the placement of 180 implantable hepatic arterial infusion devices. *Surgery* 1993;114:928–935.

Curley SA, Izzo F, Delrio P, et al. Radiofrequency ablation of unresectable primary and metastatic hepatic malignancies: results in 123 patients. *Ann Surg* 1999;230:1–8.

D'Angelica M, Brennan MF, Fortner JG, et al. Ninety-six five-year survivors after liver resection for metastatic colorectal cancer. *J Am Coll Surg* 1997;185:554–559.

DeMatteo RP, Minnard EA, Kemeny N, et al. Outcome after resection of both liver and lung metastases in patients with colorectal cancer. *Proceedings of the American Society of Clinical Oncology* 1999;18:249a.

Doci R, Bignami P, Quagliuolo V, et al. Continuous hepatic arterial infusion with 5-fluorodeoxyuridine for treatment of colorectal metastases. *Reg Cancer Treat* 1990;3:13–18.

Fong Y, Fortner J, Sun RL, et al. Clinical score for predicting recurrence after hepatic resection for metastatic colorectal cancer: analysis of 1001 consecutive cases. *Ann Surg* 1999;230:309–321.

Gayowski TJ, Iwatsuki S, Madariaga JR, et al. Experience in hepatic resection for metastatic colorectal cancer: analysis of clinical and pathologic risk factors. *Surgery* 1994;116:703–710; discussion 710–711.

Harrison LE, Brennan MF, Newman E, et al. Hepatic resection for noncolorectal, nonneuroendocrine metastases: a fifteen-year experience with ninety-six patients. *Surgery* 1997;121:625–632.

Hohn DC, Stagg RJ, Friedman MA, et al. A randomized trial of continuous intravenous versus hepatic intraarterial floxuridine in patients with colorectal cancer metastatic to the liver: The Northern California Oncology Group Trial. *J Clin Oncol* 1989;7:1646–1654.

Jamison RL, Donohue JH, Nagorney DM, et al. Hepatic resection for metastatic colorectal cancer results in cure for some patients. *Arch Surg* 1997;132:505–510; discussion 511.

Jenkins LT, Millikan KW, Bines SD, et al. Hepatic resection for metastatic colorectal cancer. *Am Surg* 1997;63:605–610.

Kawasaki S, Makuuchi M, Kakazu T, et al. Resection for multiple metastatic liver tumors after portal embolization. *Surgery* 1994;115:674–677.

Kemeny MM, Adak S, Gray B, et al. Combined-modality treatment for resectable metastatic colorectal carcinoma to the liver: surgical resection of hepatic metastases in combination with continuous infusion of chemotherapy—an intergroup study. *J Clin Oncol* 2002;20:1499–1505.

Kemeny N, Daly J, Reichman B, et al. Intrahepatic or systemic infusion of fluorodeoxyuridine in patients with liver metastases from colorectal carcinoma. A randomized trial. *Ann Intern Med* 1987;107:459–465.

Kemeny N, Huang Y, Cohen AM, et al. Hepatic arterial infusion of chemotherapy after resection of hepatic metastases from colorectal cancer. *N Engl J Med* 1999;341:2039–2048.

Kinoshita H, Sakai K, Hirohashi K, et al. Preoperative portal vein embolization for hepatocellular carcinoma. *World J Surg* 1986;10:803–808.

Le Treut YP, Delpero JR, Dousset B, et al. Results of liver transplantation in the treatment of metastatic neuroendocrine tumors. A 31-case French multicentric report. *Ann Surg* 1997;225:355–364.

Lorenz M, Muller HH, Schramm H, et al. Randomized trial of surgery versus surgery followed by adjuvant hepatic arterial infusion with 5-fluorouracil and folinic acid for liver metastases of colorectal cancer. *Ann Surg* 1998;228:756–762.

Madoff DC, Hicks ME, Abdalla EK, Vauthey JN. Portal vein embolization using polyvinyl alcohol particles and coils in preparation for major liver resection for hepatobiliary malignancy: safety and efficacy—a study in 26 patients. *Radiology* 2003;227:251–260.

Martin JK Jr, O'Connell MJ, Wieand HS, et al. Intra-arterial floxuridine vs systemic fluorouracil for hepatic metastases from colorectal cancer. A randomized trial. *Arch Surg* 1990;125:1022–1027.

Minton JP, Hoehn JL, Gerber DM, et al. Results of a 400-patient carcinoembryonic antigen second-look colorectal cancer study. *Cancer* 1985;55:1284–1290.

Moertel CG, Sauer WG, Dockerty MB, et al. Life history of the carcinoid tumor of the small intestine. *Cancer* 1961;14:901–912.

Que FG, Nagorney DM, Batts KP, et al. Hepatic resection for metastatic neuro-endocrine carcinomas. *Am J Surg* 1995;169:36–43.

Rougier P, Laplanche A, Huguier M, et al. Hepatic arterial infusion of floxuridine in patients with liver metastases from colorectal carcinoma: long-term results of a prospective randomized trial. *J Clin Oncol* 1992;10:1112–1118.

Scheele J, Stangl R, Altendorf-Hofmann A, et al. Resection of colorectal liver metastases. *World J Surg* 1995;19:59–71.

Schwartz S. Hepatic resection for noncolorectal nonneuroendocrine metastases. *World J Surg* 1995;19:72–75.

Solbiati L, Ierace T, Goldberg SN, et al. Percutaneous US-guided radio-frequency tissue ablation of liver metastases: treatment and follow-up in 16 patients. *Radiology* 1997;202:195–203.

Soreide O, Berstad T, Bakka A, et al. Surgical treatment as a principle in patients with advanced abdominal carcinoid tumors. *Surgery* 1992;111:48–54.

Tuttle TM. Hepatectomy for noncolorectal liver metastases. In: Curley SA, ed. *Liver Cancer*. New York, NY: Springer; 1998:201–211.

Vauthey JN. Liver imaging: a surgeon's perspective. *Radiol Clin North Am* 1998; 36:445–457.

Vauthey JN, Chaoui A, Do KA, et al. Standardized measurement of the future liver remnant prior to extended liver resection: methodology and clinical associations. *Surgery* 2000;127:512–519.

Vauthey JN, Dudrick PS, Lind DS, Copeland EM. Management of recurrent colorectal cancer: another look at carcinoembryonic antigen-detected recurrence. *Dig Dis* 1996a;14:5–13.

Vauthey JN, Marsh Rde W, Cendan JC, Chu NM, Copeland EM III. Arterial therapy of hepatic colorectal metastases. *Br J Surg* 1996b;83:447–455.

Vitola JV, Delbeke D, Sandler MP, et al. Positron emission tomography to stage suspected metastatic colorectal carcinoma to the liver. *Am J Surg* 1996;171:21–26.

Wagman LD, Kemeny MM, Leong L, et al. A prospective, randomized evaluation of the treatment of colorectal cancer metastatic to the liver. *J Clin Oncol* 1990; 8:1885–1893.

Wanebo HJ. Reoperative surgery for recurrent colorectal cancer: role of carcinoembryonic antigen in patient selection. In: Beahrs OH, Higgins GA, Weinstein JJ, eds. *Colorectal Tumors*. Philadelphia, Pa: Lippincott; 1986:303–313.

12 Staging and Therapeutic Approaches for Patients with Localized, Potentially Curable Pancreatic Adenocarcinoma

Peter W. T. Pisters, Douglas B. Evans,
Robert A. Wolff, and Christopher Crane

Chapter Overview

Pancreatic adenocarcinoma is a significant clinical problem with a cumulative mortality rate almost equal to its incidence. Pancreatic adenocarcinoma is clinically staged as localized, locally advanced, or metastatic disease using computed tomography (CT) and chest radiography. The treatment goals are palliative in patients with locally advanced or metastatic disease. This chapter focuses on evaluation and treatment of localized, potentially resectable pancreatic adenocarcinoma. Although patients with such disease comprise a minority of patients with pancreatic adenocarcinoma, they are the only ones for whom treatment is curative in intent.

Pretreatment evaluation of most patients should include multiphase spiral CT scanning, a chest x-ray, and consideration of outpatient tissue diagnosis using CT- or endoscopic ultrasonography–guided fine-needle aspiration biopsy. Pretreatment biopsy analysis allows the patient and physician to consider referral to a regional center for pancreatectomy with or without chemoradiation. Such referral appears to be well justified on the basis of the established relationship between hospital volume and both short- and long-term outcome in patients with pancreatic cancer.

Given the existing level 1 evidence, the standard of care for localized pancreatic adenocarcinoma is pancreatectomy alone. However, the median survival duration after surgery alone is modest (11 to 12 months), and the 5-year survival rate is low (~10%). Consequently, consideration of investigational approaches such as preoperative and postoperative chemoradiation is easily justified.

INTRODUCTION

Despite advances in diagnosis and new treatment approaches, pancreatic adenocarcinoma remains a significant clinical challenge, accounting for approximately 30,000 deaths per year in the United States (Jemal et al, 2003). In particular, appropriate management of tumor-associated biliary obstruction and accurate staging are major challenges in the pretreatment assessment of these patients. This chapter focuses on the pretreatment staging and therapeutic approaches used for patients with localized pancreatic adenocarcinoma at M. D. Anderson Cancer Center.

PRETREATMENT STAGING

Staging for all patients who present with pancreatic adenocarcinoma includes baseline laboratory evaluation with serum tumor markers and a multiphase, multidetector helical computed tomography (CT) scan.

For optimal staging and assessment of resectability, a CT report for a patient with suspected periampullary cancer should include the following information: (1) the presence or absence of peritoneal and visceral metastases; (2) the patency of the portal vein and superior mesenteric vein and the relationship between these veins and the tumor; (3) the relationship between the tumor and important regional arteries, including the superior mesenteric artery, celiac axis, and hepatic artery; and (4) the presence or absence of aberrant vascular anatomy.

A substantial majority of the patients referred to M. D. Anderson for suspected pancreatic adenocarcinoma have undergone CT scanning that is of insufficient quality to permit evaluation of these issues. Consequently, our general practice is to repeat a baseline multiphase, multidetector helical CT scan for all new patients with suspected periampullary neoplasms.

The specific objective radiographic criteria outlined above are used to assess resectability (Fuhrman et al, 1994). Using these criteria, we and others have reported resectability rates of 75% to 80% using a single, relatively inexpensive imaging study. Consequently, we do not routinely use other types of pretreatment imaging, such as magnetic resonance imaging (except in patients allergic to the intravenously administered CT contrast medium) and angiography, for assessment of resectability.

Measurement of Serum CA 19-9 Level

The baseline pretreatment serum CA 19-9 level is measured in all patients with suspected pancreatic adenocarcinoma. In interpreting this level, it is important to bear in mind that it may be elevated in cases of other malignant conditions and mildly elevated in cases of certain benign conditions, such as pancreatitis. In addition, the serum CA 19-9 level is influenced by the presence of jaundice and the patient's Lewis blood-group phenotype. Because many patients undergo initial serum CA 19-9 evaluation soon after presentation with clinical jaundice, repeat evaluation should be performed after successful palliation of the jaundice. As with most tumor markers, the serum CA 19-9 level may optimally be used as supporting evidence in the clinical diagnosis and staging of pancreatic cancer, as a variable in the assessment of biochemical response to therapy, and for posttreatment follow-up evaluation in clinical trials.

Staging Laparoscopy

Staging laparoscopy is used selectively at M. D. Anderson based on the understanding that it detects helical CT–occult disease in 4% to 15% of patients presenting with ostensibly localized pancreatic cancer (Pisters et al, 2001b). Routine staging laparoscopy is believed to be a relatively expensive, potentially morbid approach that has a relatively low rate of detection of CT-occult disease. However, in the absence of high-quality CT or in the presence of equivocal CT findings suggestive of metastatic disease, staging laparoscopy should be considered.

The criteria used to select patients for staging laparoscopy include the presence of (1) a small, low-density liver lesion or low-volume ascites suggestive of metastatic disease; (2) clinical features suggestive of more advanced disease—such as weight loss, pain, and compromised performance status—that appear to be out of proportion with the CT findings; or (3) a significant elevation in the serum CA 19-9 level. With regard to the third criterion, it is difficult to assign a specific CA 19-9 level threshold at which there should be substantial concern about the possibility of occult metastatic disease. Analysis of large cohorts of patients has suggested that an elevation in the serum CA 19-9 level above 750 U/mL is associated with a high probability of locally advanced or metastatic disease (Tian et al, 1992). A threshold in the range of 500 U/mL to 1,000 U/mL therefore appears to be reasonable.

Pretreatment Biopsy

At M. D. Anderson, we advocate reasonable efforts to achieve a pretreatment tissue diagnosis for patients presenting with what we believe to be a localized, resectable periampullary neoplasm. This approach is designed to separate the diagnostic and therapeutic phases of pancreatic cancer treatment, and such an approach has advantages for both patients and physicians. For patients in particular, a pretreatment biopsy-based diagnosis allows them to consider referral to a regional center that specializes in pancreatic cancer treatment. This appears to be quite reasonable in view of the established relationship between institutional pancreatectomy volume and both short-term operative mortality and long-term cancer outcome.

We have used endoscopic ultrasonography (EUS)- and CT-guided fine-needle aspiration (FNA) for tissue diagnosis of suspected pancreatic neoplasms. In recent years, EUS-guided FNA has often been combined with endoscopic retrograde cholangiopancreatography (ERCP) and endobiliary stent placement. This combination allows for relief of jaundice and tissue diagnosis in a 2-step procedure.

Our current use of EUS-guided FNA for tissue diagnosis is based on significant experience using this technique. We recently reported our experience with a series of 233 patients with suspected but undiagnosed periampullary neoplasms (Raut et al, 2003). Among 216 patients with a final diagnosis of carcinoma, EUS-guided FNA cytology findings consistent with malignancy were obtained in 197 (sensitivity, 91%). In comparison, all 15 patients with a final diagnosis of a benign disorder had no malignant cells or had cytology findings considered to be inconclusive for malignancy (specificity, 100%). Four patients experienced complications of the pretreatment EUS-guided biopsies (2 duodenal perforations and 1 case each of pancreatitis and abdominal pain). On the basis of our recent experience, we believe that EUS-FNA is a safe, reliable way to establish a tissue diagnosis before treatment, allowing consideration of investigational treatment approaches that generally require a pretreatment tissue diagnosis.

Management of Tumor-Associated Jaundice

The majority of the patients who present with adenocarcinoma of the pancreatic head present with clinical jaundice. Internal biliary drainage via retrograde placement of an endobiliary stent is the preferred method of biliary drainage in these patients. ERCP with internal biliary drainage can be performed safely and generally with less short- and long-term morbidity compared with percutaneous transhepatic approaches to biliary drainage. Accordingly, patients at M. D. Anderson with clinical evidence of jaundice undergo ERCP with endobiliary stent placement and EUS with EUS-guided FNA in the same sedation period. This allows for relief of jaundice and tissue diagnosis in a single, 2-step procedure.

There is also a subset of patients who present with persistent or progressive jaundice following failed attempts at endobiliary stent placement before referral. Many of these patients can undergo successful biliary decompression when ERCP is attempted again under optimal conditions in more experienced hands. If the second ERCP is unsuccessful, we generally palliate jaundice using percutaneous transhepatic means. This provides early relief of jaundice and access to the biliary tree for subsequent therapeutic procedures. A percutaneous transhepatic catheter (PTC) can be advanced into the duodenum and capped off to facilitate internal biliary drainage. Alternatively, many patients with transhepatic biliary drains can undergo successful retrograde endobiliary stent placement performed as a secondary procedure after initial percutaneous transhepatic drainage. When this approach is used, a wire is advanced through the existing PTC, which is then withdrawn, leaving the wire extended through the PTC tract and across the ampulla into the duodenum. Immediate endoscopy is then performed, and the wire is used to guide an endobiliary stent retrograde across the stricture. This strategy often allows for removal of the PTC, which, even when capped off, causes discomfort for the patient and can be associated with significant morbidity.

Consideration of Therapeutic Options

Following complete staging, including medical history, physical examination, serum CA 19-9 assessment, CT staging, and tissue diagnosis with EUS-guided FNA, in most patients disease is sufficiently staged to permit discussion of therapeutic options.

Evidence-based interpretation of the literature suggests that the standard of care for patients with localized pancreatic adenocarcinoma remains pancreatectomy alone (Pisters et al, 2003). Unfortunately, the long-term outcome for patients with pancreatic adenocarcinoma treated using surgery alone is poor, with a median survival duration of 11 to 12 months and a 5-year survival rate of approximately 10% (Gastrointestinal

Tumor Study Group, 1987; Bakkevold et al, 1993; Klinkenbijl et al, 1999; Neoptolemos et al, 2001). Consequently, there is still considerable interest in investigational strategies for patients with localized pancreatic adenocarcinoma. Indeed, we are currently studying 2 separate lines of investigational treatment in these patients: preoperative and postoperative combined-modality therapy.

Preoperative Combined-Modality Treatment

Preoperative treatment of localized pancreatic adenocarcinoma has several practical and theoretical advantages. Foremost among the latter is the ability to administer immediate systemic treatment for a disease that is systemic at diagnosis in virtually all patients. Other potential advantages of preoperative treatment include (1) improved rates of R0 (gross and microscopic margin-negative) resection; (2) improved patient selection for pancreaticoduodenectomy (patients with progressive disease in preoperative staging studies are spared the morbidity of this procedure); (3) the ability to administer combined-modality treatment in a greater proportion of patients who have had surgical resection than is possible with postoperative adjuvant therapy, where prolonged postpancreatectomy recovery may delay or prevent planned postoperative chemoradiation; and (4) reduction in the pancreaticojejunal anastomotic leak rate owing to radiation-related pancreatic fibrosis and decreased exocrine output.

Our recent pilot and phase II studies of preoperative chemoradiation have used short-course, higher-dose-per-fraction radiation regimens (termed rapid fractionation). Our experience with a preoperative regimen at a dose of 30 Gy demonstrates that this treatment is generally well tolerated, with a toxicity profile that appears to depend mostly on the radiation sensitizer used. The hospital admission rate, which is frequently used as a surrogate endpoint of cumulative toxicity, was 4%, 11%, and 43% in patients who underwent preoperative irradiation at 30 Gy and concurrent administration of 5-fluorouracil (5-FU), paclitaxel, and gemcitabine, respectively (Pisters et al, 1998, 2002; Wolff et al, 2002). Also, in a retrospective review of the M. D. Anderson experience with preoperative chemotherapy (5-FU, paclitaxel, or gemcitabine) and irradiation (30.0 or 45.0 to 50.4 Gy) in 132 patients with localized and subsequently resected pancreatic cancer, the median survival duration was 21 months (Breslin et al, 2001). This median survival compares favorably with the median survival duration of 11 to 12 months after pancreatectomy alone described above. In the absence of randomized clinical trials that directly compare preoperative chemoradiation and pancreatectomy with pancreatectomy alone, however, it is impossible to say whether these apparent differences in median survival are related to patient selection, treatment, or both.

Our current preoperative phase II study of patients with localized pancreatic adenocarcinoma involves induction chemotherapy with cisplatin

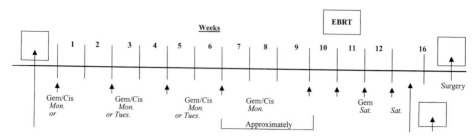

Figure 12–1. Treatment schema for the M. D. Anderson phase II study of preoperative chemotherapy (gemcitabine and cisplatin) and gemcitabine-based chemoradiation in patients with resectable adenocarcinoma of the pancreas. Gem, gemcitabine; Cis, cisplatin; EBRT, external-beam radiation therapy.

and gemcitabine followed by gemcitabine-based chemoradiation. The schema and details of this treatment are outlined in Figure 12–1. This therapeutic approach is based on data suggesting that the use of gemcitabine doublet combinations such as gemcitabine and cisplatin may improve response rates in patients with advanced pancreatic adenocarcinoma (Colucci et al, 2002) as well as encouraging results of a prior phase II study of concurrent gemcitabine-based chemoradiation that we performed (Wolff et al, 2002). In our prior study, 58 patients who underwent preoperative gemcitabine-based chemotherapy and concurrent radiation therapy (30 Gy in 10 fractions) followed by surgical resection had a median survival duration in excess of 30 months. These encouraging phase II study results were the basis for our current phase II trial, which builds upon our prior experience with preoperative treatment of localized pancreatic cancer.

Postoperative Combined-Modality Treatment

We also offer investigational options for patients with pancreatic adenocarcinoma who choose to undergo up-front pancreatectomy or are referred following pancreatectomy. The approach in our current postoperative trial involves interferon-alpha-based chemoradiation. This trial is a confirmatory, single-institution phase II study designed to evaluate the preliminary results of this approach observed at the Virginia Mason Clinic (Nukui et al, 2000; Picozzi et al, 2000).

Investigators at the Virginia Mason Clinic recently completed a phase II trial of cisplatin (30 mg/m^2/week), interferon-alpha (3 million U administered subcutaneously every other day), 5-FU (200 mg/m^2/day delivered via continuous infusion over 5 weeks), and radiation therapy (50 Gy in 25 fractions) after surgery for pancreatic adenocarcinoma (Nukui et al, 2000; Picozzi et al, 2000). The patient population (n = 53) was at high risk, as the incidence of lymph node positivity was 85% and one third of the patients had microscopically positive resection margins. The 2-year overall survival rate in the initial 17 patients was 84%, which compares favorably with the 3-year overall survival rate of 54% seen in a historical cohort of patients who underwent postoperative 5-FU–based chemoradiation at the same institution. Updated results of this trial were presented at the 2003 annual meeting of the American Society of Clinical Oncology (Picozzi et al, 2003). The toxicity of this regimen was significant—37 (70%) of 53 patients required interruption of chemoradiation, and 23 patients (43%) were hospitalized, almost exclusively because of gastrointestinal toxic effects occurring during chemoradiation. However, all but 3 hospitalizations were for non-grade-IV events, and 50 patients (84%) completed the full radiation course. With a median follow-up of 33 months, overall median survival was 46 months. The 1-, 2-, and 5-year overall survival estimates were 88%, 53%, and 49%, respectively.

These encouraging results have prompted 2 confirmatory single-institution phase II trials (at M. D. Anderson and Washington University) as well as a cooperative-group phase II trial (American College of Surgeons Oncology Group [ACOSOG] Z05031). These confirmatory studies use minor modifications of the original Virginia Mason Clinic regimen—specifically, a smaller radiation field and slight changes in the chemotherapy dose or schedule—which are designed to make the regimen easier to deliver. The single-institution and ACOSOG Z05031 trials will be important secondary confirmatory assessments of the toxicity profile and relapse-free survival associated with this regimen.

PANCREATECTOMY FOR LOCALIZED
PANCREATIC ADENOCARCINOMA

Pancreatectomy is the cornerstone of local therapy for localized pancreatic adenocarcinoma. At M. D. Anderson, we use a standard form of pancreaticoduodenectomy for resection of tumors that arise in the right pancreas. A recent review of our experience demonstrated that our mortality rate for pancreaticoduodenectomy in a series of 300 patients was 1.4% (Pisters et al, 2001a). This rate compares quite favorably with those in other high-volume centers, which have been reported to range from 2% to 5%, and is considerably lower than those reported in comprehensive analyses of surgical outcome in institutions that perform a relatively low number of complex pancreatic surgeries (10% or higher).

The relatively low operative mortality rate at M. D. Anderson is a consequence of a standardized approach to the technical aspects of pancreaticoduodenectomy (Figure 12–2) and is also most likely related to the concentration of pancreatic tumor surgery in the hands of 4 surgeons. This reflects a departmental policy of using an organ-specific approach to

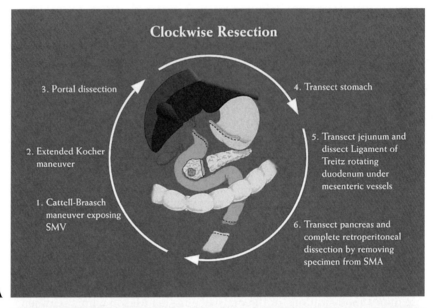

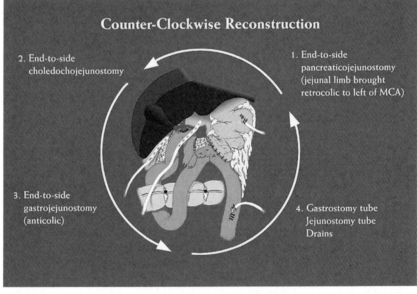

Figure 12–2. Step-wise approach to (*A*) pancreatic resection and (*B*) gastrointestinal reconstruction as part of pancreaticoduodenectomy. SMV, superior mesenteric vein; SMA, superior mesenteric artery; MCA, middle colic artery. Reprinted with permission from Evans DB, Lee JE, Pisters PWT. Pancreaticoduodenectomy (Whipple operation) and total pancreatectomy for cancer. In: Nyhus LM, Baker RJ, Fischer JF, eds. *Master of Surgery.* 3rd ed. Boston: Little, Brown and Co.; 1997: 1233–1249.

cancer surgery. We also believe that the use of clinical pathways of care for patients undergoing pancreatectomy and readily available interventional radiology for the management of postoperative complications have contributed to a reduction in morbidity and overall length of hospital stay in patients who undergo pancreaticoduodenectomy.

Pancreaticoduodenectomy with Vascular Resection and Reconstruction

A substantial subpopulation of patients referred for evaluation of pancreatic adenocarcinoma have radiographically detected involvement of the superior mesenteric or portal vein. This patient population comprises approximately 30% of patients who undergo pancreatic resection at M. D. Anderson. This percentage is larger than that reported for pancreatic tumor surgery by other regional centers and may reflect changes in referral patterns that have arisen because of our published experience with vascular resection and reconstruction.

Independent of the technical surgical issues related to this topic, the primary oncologic issue is appropriate patient selection. Patients who are considered candidates for potentially curative pancreaticoduodenectomy with vascular resection and reconstruction have tumor abutment or involvement of the superior mesenteric or portal vein *without* involvement of the superior mesenteric artery or celiac axis (Figure 12–3). Such patients can undergo R0 pancreaticoduodenectomy with vascular resection and reconstruction with R0 resection rates similar to those in patients who undergo pancreaticoduodenectomy without vascular resection.

Postoperative Care

Our approach to the postoperative care of patients who undergo pancreatectomy is based on established pathways of care. These are clinical care guidelines that outline the physician orders and general treatment goals for each day of the patient's postpancreatectomy hospital stay. Comparative reviews of our experience before and after the introduction of these clinical pathways have demonstrated that their use reduces length of hospital stay and financial costs of care (Porter et al, 2000).

More recently, we have endeavored to streamline the postoperative care for many of these patients with the selective use of enteral (gastrostomy and jejunostomy) tubes and abdominal drains by some surgeons. Our clinical impression is that this may further decrease length of hospital stay and postoperative morbidity.

CONCLUSIONS

Our general therapeutic approach for patients with localized, potentially curable periampullary malignancies involves state-of-the-art staging and pretreatment tissue diagnosis. Over the past several years, helical CT and

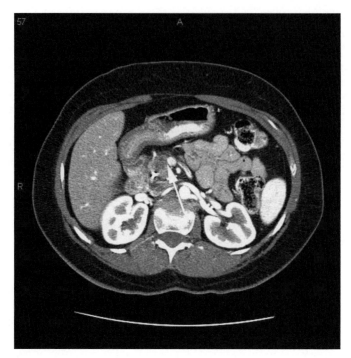

Figure 12–3. Contrast-enhanced spiral computed tomography (CT) scan of the abdomen showing a low-density tumor of the pancreatic head with abutment or involvement of the superior mesenteric vein. The arrow marks the area of tumor-vein abutment. This patient underwent a margin-negative (R0) pancreaticoduodenectomy. Pathologic examination revealed a 2.5-cm node-negative adenocarcinoma with histologic involvement of the resected vein. Patients with CT scans such as this one have radiographically resectable tumors if en bloc superior mesenteric vein resection and reconstruction are performed along with pancreatectomy. The R0 resection rate and long-term survival in appropriately selected patients who undergo pancreatectomy with vascular resection and reconstruction appear to be similar to those in patients who do not require vein resection.

EUS-guided FNA have formed the cornerstone of this approach. The disease in the vast majority of these patients can be accurately staged with an established tissue diagnosis using this approach.

There remains considerable variation in the treatment approaches used for localized pancreatic adenocarcinoma. On the basis of current level 1 evidence, it appears that pancreatectomy alone remains the standard of care. However, given the relatively poor outcome in patients who undergo surgery alone, reasonable investigational approaches that should be considered for these patients include preoperative and postoperative chemoradiation.

KEY PRACTICE POINTS

- Contemporary staging of pancreatic adenocarcinoma involves contrast-enhanced multidetector helical CT, chest radiography, and evaluation of serum CA 19-9 level.

- Pretreatment tissue diagnosis is performed using EUS- or CT-guided FNA.

- Pretreatment palliation of jaundice is achieved using ERCP with endobiliary stent placement.

- Referral to a regional center for pancreatectomy is associated with improved short- and long-term survival and therefore should be considered for all patients with potentially curable disease.

- Pancreatectomy alone remains the standard of care for patients with localized disease.

- The median survival duration with pancreatectomy alone is 11 to 12 months, and the 5-year survival rate is approximately 10%.

- Investigational approaches include preoperative and postoperative chemoradiation. Such approaches are quite reasonable in view of the poor outcome associated with surgery alone.

SUGGESTED READINGS

Bakkevold KE, Arnesjo B, Dahl O, et al. Adjuvant combination chemotherapy (AMF) following radical resection of carcinoma of the pancreas and papilla of Vater—results of a controlled, prospective, randomised multicentre study. *Eur J Cancer* 1993;29A:698–703.

Breslin T, Hess KR, Harbison DB, et al. Neoadjuvant chemoradiation for adenocarcinoma of the pancreas: treatment variables and survival duration. *Ann Surg Oncol* 2001;8:123–132.

Colucci G, Giuliani F, Gebbia V, et al. Gemcitabine alone or with cisplatin for the treatment of patients with locally advanced and/or metastatic pancreatic carcinoma: a prospective, randomized phase III study of the Gruppo Oncologia dell'Italia Meridionale. *Cancer* 2002;94:902–910.

Fuhrman GM, Charnsangavej C, Abbruzzese JL, et al. Thin-section contrast-enhanced computed tomography accurately predicts the resectability of malignant pancreatic neoplasms. *Am J Surg* 1994;167:104–111.

Gastrointestinal Tumor Study Group. Further evidence of effective adjuvant combined radiation and chemotherapy following curative resection of pancreatic cancer. *Cancer* 1987;59:2006–2010.

Jemal A, Murray T, Samuels A, et al. Cancer statistics, 2003. *CA Cancer J Clin* 2003; 53:5–26.

Klinkenbijl JH, Jeekel J, Sahmoud T, et al. Adjuvant radiotherapy and 5-fluorouracil after curative resection of cancer of the pancreas and periampullary region: phase III trial of the EORTC gastrointestinal tract cancer cooperative group. *Ann Surg* 1999;230:776–782.

Neoptolemos JP, Dunn JA, Stocken DD, et al. Adjuvant chemoradiotherapy and chemotherapy in resectable pancreatic cancer: a randomised controlled trial. *Lancet* 2001;358:1576–1585.

Nukui Y, Picozzi VJ, Traverso LW. Interferon-based adjuvant chemoradiation therapy improves survival after pancreaticoduodenectomy for pancreatic adenocarcinoma. *Am J Surg* 2000;179:367–371.

Picozzi VJ, Kozarek RE, Jacobs AD, et al. Adjuvant therapy for resected pancreas cancer (PC) using alpha-interferon (IFN)-based chemoradiation: completion of a phase II trial. Proc Am Soc Clin Oncol 2003;22:265a.

Picozzi VJ, Kozarek R, Rieke JW, et al. Adjuvant combined modality therapy for resected, high-risk adenocarcinoma of the pancreas using cisplatin (CDDP), 5 FU, and alpha-interferon (IFN) as radiosensitizing agents: update of a phase II trial. *Proc Am Soc Clin Oncol* 2000;19:266a.

Pisters PW, Abbruzzese JL, Janjan NA, et al. Rapid-fractionation preoperative chemoradiation, pancreaticoduodenectomy, and intraoperative radiation therapy for resectable pancreatic adenocarcinoma. *J Clin Oncol* 1998;16: 3843–3850.

Pisters PW, Hudec W, Hess KR, et al. Effect of preoperative biliary decompression on pancreaticoduodenectomy-associated morbidity in 300 consecutive patients. *Ann Surg* 2001a;234:47–55.

Pisters PW, Lee JE, Vauthey JN, et al. Laparoscopy in the staging of pancreatic cancer. *Br J Surg* 2001b;88:325–337.

Pisters PW, Picozzi VJ, Abrams R. Therapy for localized pancreatic adenocarcinoma: one, two, or three modalities? In: Perry MC, ed. *ASCO Educational Book*. Alexandria, Va: American Society of Clinical Oncology; 2003:397–418.

Pisters PW, Wolff RA, Janjan NA, et al. Preoperative paclitaxel and concurrent rapid-fractionation radiation for resectable pancreatic adenocarcinoma: toxicities, histologic response rates, and event-free outcome. *J Clin Oncol* 2002;20: 2537–2544.

Porter GA, Pisters PW, Mansyur C, et al. Cost and utilization impact of a clinical pathway for patients undergoing pancreaticoduodenectomy. *Ann Surg Oncol* 2000;7:484–489.

Raut C, Grau A, Staerkel G, et al. Diagnostic accuracy of endoscopic ultrasound-guided fine-needle aspiration in patients with presumed pancreatic cancer. *J Gastrointest Surg* 2003;7:118–128.

Tian F, Appert HE, Myles J, et al. Prognostic value of serum CA 19-9 levels in pancreatic adenocarcinoma. *Ann Surg* 1992;215:350–355.

Wolff RA, Evans DB, Crane CH, et al. Initial results of preoperative gemcitabine (GEM)-based chemoradiation for resectable pancreatic adenocarcinoma. *Proc Am Soc Clin Oncol* 2002;21:130a.

13 TREATMENT OF PRIMARY LIVER CANCER

Steven A. Curley

CHAPTER OVERVIEW

The advent of modern liver surgery correlates with the development of new diagnostic imaging modalities in the 1970s, when computed tomography, magnetic resonance imaging, and transcutaneous ultrasonography quickly supplanted liver colloid scans and hepatic angiography, the only liver diagnostic radiographic tests available to surgeons previously. The ongoing refinements over the last 30 years in these imaging modalities have provided more precise anatomic definition of tumor size, location, and number, thereby aiding surgeons in planning the extent of hepatic resection. Furthermore, more detailed and accurate anatomic scans of extrahepatic sites have reduced the proportion of patients who undergo an unnecessary laparotomy with no liver resection performed because of a finding of unsuspected extrahepatic spread of malignant disease. Recent use of portal vein embolization at M. D. Anderson Cancer Center and other centers has increased the proportion of patients who are candidates for surgical treatment. New surgical techniques have reduced blood loss, transfusion requirements, and operation time and have improved patient outcomes. There is a glaring need to develop better agents for neoadjuvant and adjuvant therapy in attempts to improve patient survival.

Diagnosis and Staging

The development of high-speed helical computed tomography (CT) and organ-specific scanning protocols has markedly improved preoperative CT staging of liver tumors. Three-dimensional reconstruction and arterial and venous imaging without invasive arterial angiography can be accomplished with currently available equipment and software programs. For hepatocellular carcinoma (HCC), the helical CT detection rate for small tumors (40% to 60%) is less than that for hepatic metastases, owing to the difficulty of detecting small tumors in cirrhotic livers and particularly of distinguishing HCC from macroregenerative nodules. Further improvements in morphologic CT imaging over the next 5 years will include rapid data acquisition during a single breath-hold, rapid scan sections with thinner individual sections, multidetector systems, and multiplanar 3-dimensional reconstructions and volume rendering with even more detailed image resolution.

Magnetic resonance (MR) imaging is more sensitive than helical CT in the detection of early HCC and in distinguishing between HCC and macroregenerative nodules. The development of liver-specific MR imaging contrast agents has further improved the diagnostic accuracy in both primary and metastatic liver malignancies, and such agents can also help establish the probability of a benign versus a malignant liver tumor.

Paralleling the improvements in CT and MR imaging, ultrasonography equipment and image detail have continued to improve. Transcutaneous ultrasonography has been used to detect liver tumors, to guide percutaneous biopsies of liver tumors, and to guide therapy for selected tumors with direct injection or ablation techniques. Ultrasonography is rarely used as a screening or follow-up evaluation tool in patients with metastatic liver tumors, but because it is a readily available and relatively inexpensive technology, ultrasonography is commonly used in programs that screen high-risk populations for the development of HCC. In studies from the United States and Europe, ultrasonography has been shown to be superior to serum alpha fetoprotein measurement for the detection of early HCC in patients with chronic viral hepatitis.

The most important use of ultrasonography in hepatobiliary surgery is intraoperative ultrasonography, which is particularly helpful in cirrhotic patients with HCC. Intraoperative ultrasonography has become the gold standard against which all other diagnostic imaging modalities are compared for detecting the number and extent of tumors and the association of tumors with intrahepatic blood vessels in both primary and metastatic liver tumors.

Rapid progress in the 1990s in laparoscopic surgery included the development of laparoscopic ultrasound probes. Laparoscopy provides the advantage of a visual inspection to exclude the presence of extrahepatic disease on the peritoneal surfaces in the abdominal cavity, and laparoscopic ultrasonography can be performed on the liver and spleen and, in selected instances, on retroperitoneal structures such as the kidneys, adrenal glands, and pancreas. Laparoscopic evaluation and laparoscopic ultrasonography have further reduced the rate of unnecessary exploratory laparotomy and thus increased the proportion of patients who undergo successful hepatic resection at the time of laparotomy. Like intraoperative ultrasonography, laparoscopic ultrasonography reveals small primary or metastatic liver tumors not visualized on preoperative CT or MR imaging studies in up to 15% of patients.

Positron emission tomography (PET) is a nuclear medicine study that is being widely evaluated in patients with malignant disease. PET does not provide the anatomic detail and definition of modern CT or MR imaging, but it does offer the potential advantages of whole-body imaging and the ability to detect subclinical disease in the liver and at extrahepatic sites. PET has been less useful in the evaluation of HCC, as many of these tumors do not have a significantly higher uptake of the radioisotope compared with the surrounding hepatic parenchyma. Novel radioisotopes and combinations of these radioactive compounds are being studied to further improve imaging sensitivity and specificity in patients with HCC and hepatic metastases.

RESECTION OF MALIGNANT LIVER TUMORS

Improved preoperative imaging studies, routine use of intraoperative ultrasonography, an understanding of the vascular and segmental anatomy of the liver, application of new surgical instruments and technology, and improved perioperative anesthesia management have combined to increase the number of patients undergoing successful hepatic resection as treatment for primary liver tumors.

Indications for Resection

The indications for resection of HCC have recently been reevaluated. Studies from the 1980s and early 1990s suggested that cirrhosis and multiple tumor nodes were harbingers of poor outcome after resection of HCC. However, these studies were performed when operative mortality rates in cirrhotic HCC patients were 6% to 15% and the need for intraoperative and postoperative blood transfusion was common. Current studies that have compared the outcome of patients undergoing surgery utilizing modern hepatic resection techniques with the outcome of patients operated on in the 1980s or early 1990s have demonstrated improved outcome for patients treated with modern techniques. Specifically, perioperative blood transfusion rates fell from 69% to 87% in the 1980s and early 1990s to 23% to 39% in the later period. The operative and hospital death rate was reduced from 13.2% to under 2%, and 5-year survival rates improved from 19% to 32% to 25% to 49%. All of the patients in these series had pathologic cirrhosis, and with the advent of better surgical technique, including a significant reduction in intraoperative blood loss, long-term survival rates and surgical outcome were improved even in patients with multiple tumor nodules.

Screening programs for patients who have chronic hepatitis B or C virus infection and are at high risk of developing HCC may be able to increase the proportion of patients diagnosed with early-stage disease. Such programs will also increase the proportion of HCC patients who can be treated surgically.

The quality of life of patients who undergo resection for HCC is significantly better than that of patients treated nonsurgically, even among patients who develop recurrent HCC after resection. Some differences in quality of life may be related to the severity of underlying liver disease in patients treated surgically versus those treated medically, but definitive surgical treatment also improves patients' sense of well-being. Surgical therapy for HCC should be considered in all patients with potentially resectable lesions; even those with biliary tumor thrombi that can be treated with resection of the tumor and thrombectomy through a choledochotomy have a median survival of 2.3 years and a 5-year survival rate of 28%.

Stapling Devices in Liver Resection

Vascular staplers can be used to reduce operative time and intraoperative blood loss in properly selected patients. Hepatic inflow and outflow control can be achieved with stapling devices. However, these techniques should be applied judiciously and should not be used if tumor is near the vascular pedicle to be divided because of the significant negative prognostic effect of a positive-margin resection. When a hepatic tumor is near the main right or left portal vein branches, the surgeon should use the traditional technique of extrahepatic dissection in the porta hepatis, with ligation of the portal vein, hepatic artery, and bile duct branch to the affected lobe.

A major advantage of stapling techniques is intrahepatic ligation and division of the vascular inflow to a lobe. A key point in the safe use of staplers for hepatic resection is that complete mobilization of the lobe to be resected is required. This is true whether staplers are used to achieve inflow control of the portal pedicles or outflow control of the major hepatic veins. A vascular gastrointestinal anastomosis (GIA) stapler can be used to divide the hepatic right lobe blood supply after cholecystectomy is performed to establish the inferior liver surface landmarks. The stapler is introduced at the junction of segments IVB and V and exits posteriorly in segment VII; this maneuver is safe only if the right lobe of the liver has first been fully mobilized and the direct venous branches from the posterior aspect of the liver into the vena cava have been individually ligated and divided. The vascular GIA stapler can also be used to ligate and divide the inflow blood supply during left hepatic lobectomy or during resection of segments II and III of the liver (a so-called left lateral segmentectomy).

The low profile, flexible neck, and long handle of a vascular laparoscopic flexible-neck GIA stapler make it ideal for outflow control with ligation and division of the hepatic veins. This technique is used most commonly for the right hepatic vein, but with proper hepatic mobilization and division of the parenchyma around the vessels, the middle and left hepatic vein can also be divided using this device.

At M. D. Anderson Cancer Center, 254 major liver resections using vascular staplers for inflow and outflow control have been performed since 1998 (Table 13–1). The median operative time and blood loss have been significantly reduced by the use of stapling devices; the perioperative blood transfusion rate has been reduced from 36% in our experience from the early 1990s to less than 6% currently. Postoperative morbidity and mortality rates are unchanged by the use of staplers to attain hepatic

Table 13–1. **Hepatic Resections Performed Using Stapling Devices for Inflow and Outflow Vascular Control at M. D. Anderson, 1998–2001**

Procedure	Number of Patients	Median Blood Loss, ml	Number of Patients Transfused, %*	Ischemia Time,† min	Median LOS, days
Right lobectomy	56	594	8 (14%)	16	6.8
Left lobectomy	50	378	1 (2%)	17	6.8
Segment II–III resection	30	161	0	5	7.3
Extended right hepatectomy	24	713	3 (12%)	17	9.6
All patients	160	472	12 (8%)	15	8.4

Abbreviation: LOS, length of hospital stay.

* Perioperative or postoperative transfusion of packed red blood cells.

† Median time of vascular inflow occlusion (Pringle maneuver) during transection of the hepatic parenchyma.

inflow and outflow control, but median hospital time has been significantly reduced because of shorter operating time and reduced blood transfusion requirements.

Repeat Hepatectomy for Recurrent Malignant Tumors

The long-term disease-free survival rates for patients undergoing surgical resection of primary liver tumors are usually below 40% in the most optimistic reports and may be below 20% in others. Clearly, most patients develop recurrent malignant disease after hepatic resection. In a subset of these patients, the only recurrence will be new tumor deposits in the liver. A further subset of these patients may have undergone significant hepatic regeneration and have tumors in locations amenable to repeat liver resection.

Repeat hepatic resection may help selected patients with HCC. Intrahepatic recurrence as the only site of disease is more common in patients with HCC than those with metastatic liver tumors, but fewer than 10% of patients who develop recurrent disease are candidates for repeated surgical treatments. Patients who develop hepatic recurrence of HCC after hepatic resection of their primary tumor may not be candidates for repeat resection because of multifocality, vascular invasion by tumor, or the severity of underlying cirrhosis. In properly selected patients, however, repeat hepatic resection for HCC can be performed and results in long-term survival rates of up to 30%. The incidence of postresection liver failure is no higher in patients who undergo a second hepatic resection, indicating the importance of carefully selecting patients who will have adequate functional hepatic reserve after a second operation.

Portal Vein Embolization

Direct tumor invasion of a lobar portal vein branch may lead to ipsilateral hepatic lobe atrophy and contralateral lobe hypertrophy. The development of compensatory hypertrophy of a lobe or segments of the liver after tumor occlusion of contralateral portal venous branches led to the concept of planned portal vein embolization (PVE) to initiate hypertrophy in segments of the liver that would remain following a major liver resection. PVE as a potentially useful treatment to induce hepatic hypertrophy before liver resection was first reported in a small group of HCC patients in 1986. These patients also underwent hepatic arterial embolization of their primary liver tumor, but the PVE was noted to induce hypertrophy rarely seen with hepatic arterial embolization alone. Interest in preoperative PVE has increased because extended hepatectomy (resection of 5 or more hepatic segments) is now more frequently considered an appropriate and safe treatment option for patients with hepatobiliary malignancies.

Indications for PVE

In patients with normal hepatic parenchyma, preservation of a perfused section of liver comprising 25% of the total hepatic volume is usually sufficient to prevent major postoperative complications and hepatic insufficiency. This 25% value has been determined somewhat empirically, and there is a paucity of data regarding the exact volume of liver that can be resected safely without postoperative liver failure when the remaining liver parenchyma is completely normal. In a recent series of 20 patients with normal liver parenchyma who underwent an extended right hepatic lobectomy, a future liver remnant of 25% or less of the total liver volume was associated with increased severity of postoperative liver insufficiency, longer hospital stay, and complications. We reviewed our experience with extended liver resection in 55 patients with normal hepatic parenchyma. On the basis of preoperative calculation of a future liver remnant that was 25% or less of the total liver volume, 18 of these patients underwent preoperative PVE. The median increase in the percentage of future liver remnant was 8%. As a result of this increase, there was no significant difference in the immediate preoperative percentage of future liver remnant between the PVE group (median 23% future liver remnant) and the group that did not undergo preoperative PVE (median 25% future liver remnant). Importantly, there was no difference in major postoperative complications or length of hospital stay between the 2 groups. Preoperative PVE allowed a safe liver resection in 18 patients who otherwise would not have been candidates for an extended hepatic resection, and the median survival time after liver resection in the patients treated with PVE was not significantly different from that in the patients who did not require PVE.

The functional capacity of liver compromised by cholestasis, acute or chronic inflammation, steatosis, or cirrhosis is variable. A larger future liver remnant is required to avoid posthepatectomy hepatic insufficiency or failure in patients with diseased hepatic parenchyma. Two recent studies suggest that at least 40% of the total hepatic volume should remain in order to minimize postoperative complications in patients who have underlying chronic liver disease or who have received high-dose chemotherapy. In addition to requiring preoperative PVE, patients with underlying chronic liver disease may also require careful assessment of functional hepatic reserve before and after PVE to assess the risk of postoperative liver failure.

Preoperative Volumetric Determination of the Future Liver Remnant

Rapid-sequence, thin-section helical CT is used to directly measure total liver volume, volume of the liver to be resected, and volume of the future liver remnant (Figure 13–1). The total liver volume can also be estimated on the basis of the described association between body surface area and the total liver volume, where total liver volume = 706.2 × body surface area

+2.4. The future liver remnant volume (for example, the volume of segments I, II, and III in a patient undergoing an extended right hepatectomy) can be directly measured on helical CT images and then divided by the total estimated liver volume to calculate the percentage of future liver remnant. If the future liver remnant is estimated to be too small when the

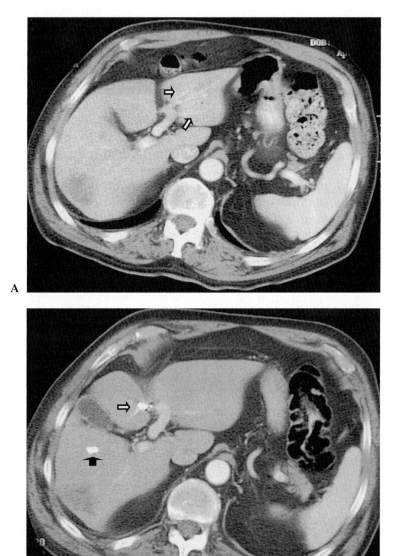

A

B

presence or absence of chronic liver disease is also considered, PVE may be considered to increase the size of the future liver remnant.

Preoperative estimates of the volume of liver to be resected, tumor volume, and future liver remnant based on CT volumetric analysis correlate well with resected specimen volume. The improved resolution and refinement of CT technique have minimized errors in CT volume calculation related to partial volume effect, respiratory phase, and interobserver variation. Volumetric accuracy for the entire liver or portions of the liver is reproducible within ±5%.

Approach and Materials for PVE

A percutaneous transhepatic approach has become the standard technique for PVE. The principal advantage of this technique is that it allows direct access to the portal venous branches of the lobe and segments to be embolized via an ipsilateral approach. This technique minimizes the risk of main trunk portal vein thrombosis and vascular injury to the portal venous branches supplying the future liver remnant. The side effects are minor and transient and include pain from the transhepatic approach and low-grade fever.

It is important to embolize not only the main right portal vein but also the portal venous branches to segment IV if an extended right hepatic lobectomy is planned. Systematic embolization of segment IV branches is imperative for 2 reasons. First, all segments of the liver bearing tumor are embolized to minimize the risk of accelerated tumor growth. Accelerated tumor growth has been reported after incomplete right trisectoral embolization. Second, embolization of segment IV portal vein branches in addition to the main right portal vein may contribute to better hypertrophy of segments I, II, and III prior to the extended right hepatic lobectomy.

Figure 13–1. Portal vein embolization (PVE). (*A*) Computed tomography (CT) scan of a patient with right-lobe and medial left-lobe (segment IV) involvement by a colorectal cancer liver metastasis. An extended hepatic resection would be necessary to surgically excise all of the malignant disease; however, the lateral segment of the left lobe (arrows) comprises less than 20% of the total hepatic volume, and the risk of postoperative liver failure would be excessive. (*B*) CT scan from the same patient 4 weeks after PVE. There has been significant compensatory hypertrophy of the left lateral segment, which on volumetric CT analysis now makes up between 25% and 30% of the total hepatic volume. The metallic coils used to embolize portal vein branches to the right lobe of the liver (black arrow) and the medial segment of the left lobe of the liver (white arrow) are clearly evident. Reprinted with permission from Curley SA, Cusack JC Jr, Tanabe KK, Stoelzing O, Ellis LM. Advances in the treatment of liver tumors. *Curr Probl Surg* 2002;39:449–571.

A variety of materials have been used for PVE. These include cyano-acrylate, ethiodized oil (Ethiodol), Gelfoam (absorbable gelatin sponge), thrombin, metal coils, polyvinyl alcohol, microspheres, and absolute ethanol. Cyanoacrylate has been shown to produce reliable portal vein occlusion that persists 4 weeks after PVE, whereas Gelfoam and thrombin may produce only transient PVE with recanalization of the vessels. Cyano-acrylate produces a 90% increase in the volume of the future liver remnant 30 days after embolization, compared with a 53% increase in volume when thrombin and Gelfoam are used. However, a marked inflammatory reac-tion is associated with cyanoacrylate PVE, and peribiliary fibrosis and casting of the portal vein may increase operative technical difficulty. Polyvinyl alcohol produces minimal periportal inflammation and creates durable portal vein occlusion when used in combination with metal coils. Polyvinyl alcohol, microspheres, and Gelfoam seem to occlude small outflow vessels in the tumor-bearing segments, whereas the metal coils occlude large inflow vessels. PVE with absolute ethanol may be particu-larly useful in treating patients with HCC because the hypertrophy induced with this substance may be greater than that produced with other embolic materials. PVE with absolute ethanol produces a transient increase in hepatocellular inflammation as measured by serum transami-nase levels and may produce substantial periportal fibrosis, but recana-lization of the embolized branches is rare.

RADIOFREQUENCY ABLATION

Background and Basics of Radiofrequency Tissue Ablation

In general, thermal injury to cells begins at 42°C, with the time of exposure to low-level hyperthermia needed to achieve cell death ranging from 3 to 50 hours, depending on the tissue type and conditions. As the temperature increases above 42°C, the exposure time necessary to kill cells decreases exponentially. For example, at 46°C only 8 minutes is needed to kill malignant cells, and 51°C can be lethal after only 2 minutes. At temperatures above 60°C, intracellular proteins become denatured, lipid bilayers melt, DNA and RNA are destroyed, and cell death is inevitable. Interestingly, malignant cells are more resistant to lethal damage from freezing but more sensitive to hyperthermic damage than are normal cells.

The use of radiofrequency (RF) energy to produce tissue destruction has been the focus of increasing research and practice for the past several years. During the application of RF energy, a high-frequency alternating current moves from the tip of an electrode into the tissue surrounding that electrode. As the ions within the tissue attempt to follow the change in the direction of the alternating current, their movement results in frictional heating of the tissue (Figure 13–2). As the temperature within the tissue becomes elevated above 60°C, cells begin to die, resulting in a region of

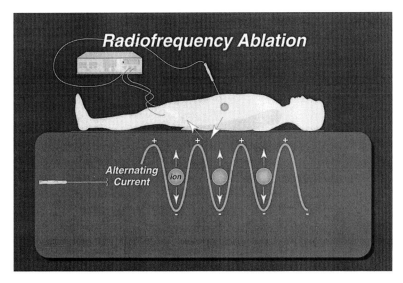

Figure 13–2. Radiofrequency (RF) ablation of a malignant liver tumor. The multiple-array RF needle electrode is inserted into the liver tumor with the intent of producing complete coagulative necrosis of the tumor and a surrounding zone of nonmalignant hepatic parenchyma. The RF needle electrode and grounding pads from the patient are attached to an RF generator. The lower portion of the diagram illustrates the ionic agitation that occurs around the multiple-array RF needle electrode when alternating current from the RF generator is applied. Ionic agitation produces frictional heating in the tissue, which results in coagulative necrosis of tissue around the electrode. Reprinted with permission from Curley SA, Cusack JC Jr, Tanabe KK, Stoelzing O, Ellis LM. Advances in the treatment of liver tumors. *Curr Probl Surg* 2002;39:449–571.

necrosis surrounding the electrode. A typical RF ablation (RFA) treatment produces local tissue temperatures that exceed 100°C, resulting in coagulative necrosis of the tumor tissue and surrounding hepatic parenchyma. The tissue microvasculature is completely destroyed, and thrombosis of hepatic arterial, portal venous, and hepatic venous branches less than 3 mm in diameter occurs. The tissue temperature falls rapidly with increasing distance away from the electrode, and reliable production of cytotoxic temperatures can be expected only within 5 to 10 mm of the multiple-array hook electrodes.

An RF needle electrode is advanced into the liver tumor to be treated via a percutaneous, laparoscopic, or open (laparotomy) route. With transcutaneous or intraoperative ultrasonography used to guide placement, the needle electrode is advanced to the targeted area of the tumor, and then the individual wires or tines of the electrode are deployed into the tissues. Once the tines have been deployed, the needle electrode is attached to an RF generator, and 2 dispersive electrodes (return or grounding pads) are placed on the patient, 1 on each thigh (Figure 13–2). The RF energy is then applied following an established treatment algorithm. Tumors 2.5 cm or less in their greatest diameter can be ablated with the placement of a needle electrode with an array diameter of 3.5 to 4.0 cm when the electrode is positioned in the center of the tumor. Tumors larger than 2.5 cm require more than 1 deployment of the needle electrode. For larger tumors, multiple placements and deployments of the electrode array may be necessary to completely destroy the tumor (Figures 13–3 and 13–4). Treatment is planned such that the zones of coagulative necrosis overlap to ensure complete destruction of the tumor. To mimic a surgical margin in these unresectable tumors, the needle electrode is used to produce a thermal lesion that incorporates not only the tumor but also nonmalignant liver parenchyma in a zone 1 cm wide surrounding the tumor. CT scans obtained after RFA of primary or metastatic liver tumors

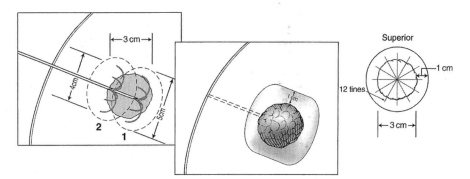

Figure 13–3. Use of a multiple-array radiofrequency (RF) needle electrode to treat a 3-cm-diameter malignant liver tumor. The left panel demonstrates the use of a needle electrode with a multiple-array diameter of 4 cm. The RF needle is first guided into the deepest portion of the tumor, and the multiple array is deployed at the interface of the posterior aspect of the tumor and normal hepatic parenchyma (area 1). This area is treated with RF energy until coagulative necrosis of the tumor and surrounding liver is complete. The multiple array is then retracted into the needle tip, and the tip is withdrawn approximately 1.5 cm. The multiple array is then again deployed to treat the more superficial interface of tumor and normal parenchyma (area 2). The center panel shows that an ideal ablation destroys not only the tumor but a 1-cm margin of surrounding hepatic parenchyma to ensure destruction of any microscopic extension of the tumor mass. The right panel shows an idealized superior view looking directly down on the tumor, again indicating the needle track placement centrally into the tumor with the multiple-array tines radiating out through the tumor into the surrounding hepatic parenchyma to produce thermal ablation of the tumor and a 1-cm zone of surrounding hepatic parenchyma. Reprinted with permission from Curley SA, Cusack JC Jr, Tanabe KK, Stoelzing O, Ellis LM. Advances in the treatment of liver tumors. *Curr Probl Surg* 2002;39:449–571.

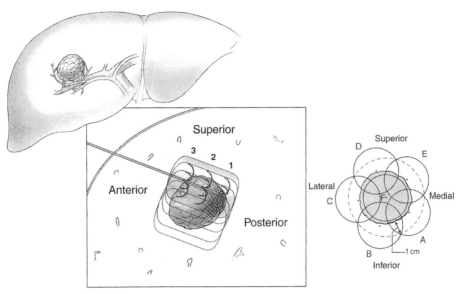

Figure 13–4.   Use of a multiple-array radiofrequency (RF) needle electrode to treat
a 5-cm-diameter malignant tumor in the right lobe of the liver. The upper illustration shows the tumor in relation to the portal venous and hepatic arterial inflow
blood supply to the tumor and the surrounding hepatic parenchyma. The inset
illustration is a sagittal view showing the multiple overlapping cylinders of RF-
induced thermal ablation that must be created to ensure complete destruction of
the tumor and a surrounding zone of normal hepatic parenchyma. The first areas
treated are the more medial aspects of the tumor (*A* and *B*, far right panel [supe-
rior view]) to destroy this region of the tumor and its inflow blood supply. The
needle electrode is placed sequentially at the margin of the tumor in the normal
parenchyma so that part of the secondary multiple array is opened within the
tumor and part is in the surrounding hepatic parenchyma. As demonstrated in the
inset illustration, the needle is first placed at the posterior interface of tumor and
normal parenchyma (area 1); after this area has been completely treated, the array
is retracted and the needle is pulled back to area 2, and the array is deployed again
and treatment performed. Finally, the more anterior or superficial interface
between tumor and parenchyma is treated (area 3) to produce a cylinder-shaped
zone of coagulative necrosis. The far right illustration shows an idealized view
looking directly down on the tumor to emphasize the RF treatment planning.
Overlapping cylinders of thermal ablation are created to destroy the entire tumor
and a 1-cm zone of surrounding hepatic parenchyma; included is the sequence of
needle electrode placements (*A* to *F*). Reprinted with permission from Curley SA,
Cusack JC Jr, Tanabe KK, Stoelzing O, Ellis LM. Advances in the treatment of liver
tumors. *Curr Probl Surg* 2002;39:449–571.

initially demonstrate a cystic-density lesion larger than the original tumor; the size of this cystic area decreases slightly over time.

Indications for RFA of Liver Tumors

RF energy to produce coagulative necrosis in hepatic malignancies has been used in patients who did not meet the criteria for resectability of HCC and metastatic liver tumors and yet were candidates for a liver-directed procedure because of the presence of liver-only disease. The selection of patients to be treated with RFA is based on rational principles and goals. Any local therapy for malignant hepatic tumors, be it surgical resection, RFA, or some other tumor-ablative technique, is generally performed with curative intent, but a significant proportion of patients will subsequently develop clinically detectable hepatic or extrahepatic recurrence of their coexistent micrometastatic disease.

RFA can be used to treat patients with a solitary hepatic tumor in a location that precludes a margin-negative hepatic resection, such as a tumor nestled between the inferior vena cava and the entrance of the 3 hepatic veins into the inferior vena cava (Figure 13–5). Our group has successfully

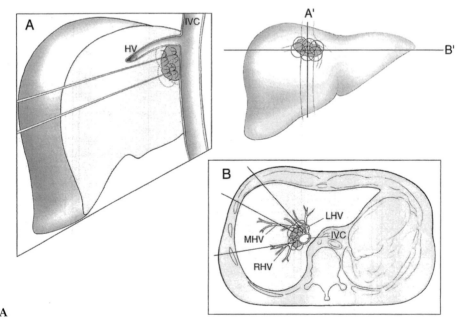

A

Figure 13–5. (*A*) Radiofrequency ablation (RFA) of a malignant hepatic tumor abutting the inferior vena cava (IVC) and nestled under the right, middle, and left hepatic veins (RHV, MHV, LHV, respectively). **A**, Sagittal view of the tumor lying on the IVC and abutting a hepatic vein. Multiple insertions of the RFA needle electrode are required, with the secondary multiple array opened just outside the IVC and then sequentially withdrawn to treat the more anterior aspects of the tumor.

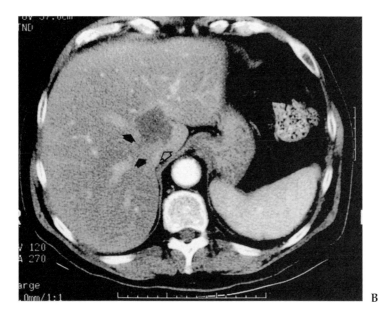

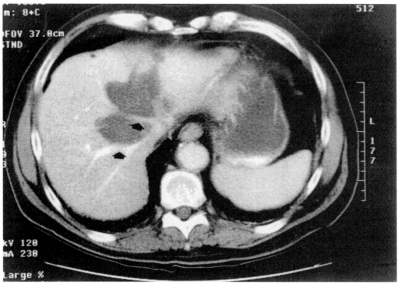

Figure 13–5. *Continued*, **B**, Axial view with lines indicating the multiple placements of the RF needle electrode to produce thermal ablation of the entire tumor and a surrounding zone of hepatic parenchyma. Blood flow in the IVC and hepatic veins prevents thermal destruction or thrombosis of these major vessels. (*B*) Computed tomography (CT) scan of a malignant liver tumor abutting the IVC (open arrow) and hepatic veins (closed arrows). (*C*) CT scan 6 months after RFA of the tumor shown in panel B indicates no evidence of viable tumor and patent right and middle hepatic veins (arrows). The cavitary lesion produced by RFA is larger than the original tumor. Reprinted with permission from Curley SA, Cusack JC Jr, Tanabe KK, Stoelzing O, Ellis LM. Advances in the treatment of liver tumors. *Curr Probl Surg* 2002;39:449–571.

treated tumors abutting major hepatic or portal vein branches because the blood flow acts as a heat sink that protects the vascular endothelium from thermal injury while allowing complete coagulation of tissue immediately surrounding the blood vessel wall. The only area of the liver to avoid when treating a tumor with RFA is the hilar plate, where the portal vein and hepatic arterial branches enter the liver. While these blood vessels can tolerate RFA, the large bile ducts coursing with them do not tolerate heat, and biliary fistulae or strictures will occur after RFA. RFA-induced biliary injury can be minimized by excluding patients with tumors involving the perihilar region. RFA is ideally suited to treat small HCCs in cirrhotic patients who may not be candidates for resection because of the severity of their liver dysfunction. Currently, our group is conducting a randomized, prospective trial comparing resection, RFA, and percutaneous ethanol injection in cirrhotic HCC patients to determine the efficacy, safety, and long-term survival rate after treatment with these 3 techniques.

Given the limitations of currently available RFA equipment, RF treatment for tumors greater than 5.0 cm in diameter must be applied judiciously, if at all. The local recurrence rate in larger tumors is much higher and represents incomplete coagulative necrosis of malignant cells near the tumor periphery. New RFA equipment is being developed to treat larger hepatic tumors; obviously, this equipment must be assessed over time to determine the adequacy of treatment.

RFA Treatment Approaches

RFA of liver tumors can be performed percutaneously, using laparoscopic guidance, or as part of an open surgical procedure. The treatment approach is tailored to the individual patient. In general, patients with 1 to 3 small (<3.0 cm in diameter) tumors located in the periphery of the liver are considered for ultrasound-guided percutaneous RFA. Lesions located high in the dome of the liver near the diaphragm are not always accessible by a percutaneous approach. Furthermore, general anesthesia or monitored sedation is required for most patients treated percutaneously because of pain associated with the heating of tissue near the liver capsule. Patients treated percutaneously are usually discharged within 24 hours of RFA. A percutaneous approach has been used in our patients with small, early-stage HCCs with coexistent cirrhosis and in patients with a limited number of small metastases from other organ sites.

A laparoscopic approach offers the advantages of laparoscopic ultrasonography, which provides better information than transcutaneous ultrasonography regarding the number and location of liver tumors, and permits a survey of the peritoneal cavity to exclude the presence of extrahepatic disease. Using laparoscopic ultrasound guidance, the RFA needle electrode is advanced percutaneously into the target tumors for treatment. Laparoscopic ultrasonography permits more precise positioning of the multiple-array RF needle near major blood vessels. A laparoscopic approach may be ideal for patients with no history of extensive abdominal operations and with 1 or 2 liver tumors less than 4.0 cm in diameter located centrally in the liver near major intrahepatic blood vessels. Laparoscopic RFA has also been used to treat patients with symptomatic (i.e., hormone-releasing), neuroendocrine-tumor liver metastases.

The majority of patients in our studies underwent RFA of hepatic tumors during an open surgical procedure. This is the preferred approach in patients with large tumors (>4.0 to 5.0 cm diameter) or multiple tumors, in patients with tumor abutting a major intrahepatic blood vessel, and when a laparoscopic approach is impractical because of dense post-surgical adhesions. In contrast to the situation with percutaneous RFA, temporary occlusion of hepatic inflow can be performed during intraoperative RFA. Hepatic inflow occlusion facilitates RFA of large or hypervascular tumors and tumors near blood vessels. The amount of blood flow to a tumor is a critical determinant of temperature response to a given increment of heat. Because heat loss or cooling effect is principally dependent on blood circulation in a given area, temperature response and blood flow are inversely related. By temporary occlusion of hepatic inflow during RFA, the cooling effect of blood flow on perivascular tumor cells is minimized. The inflow occlusion increases the size of the zone of coagulative necrosis and enhances the likelihood of complete tumor cell kill, even if the tumor abuts a major intrahepatic blood vessel. Prior preclinical work demonstrated that RFA combined with vascular inflow occlusion can produce complete circumferential necrosis of tissue around major portal or hepatic vein branches without damaging the integrity of the vessel wall. Another advantage of an open approach is the ability to combine resection of tumors too large to ablate in 1 lobe with RFA of smaller tumors in the opposite lobe. At M. D. Anderson, 172 patients have undergone partial hepatic resection of dominant tumors with RFA of smaller contralateral or adjacent segmental lesions. There have been no deaths following treatment in these patients, and the postoperative complication rate is identical to that for patients treated with resection alone.

RFA of Primary Liver Tumors

RFA has recently been used to treat primary liver tumors in patients at M. D. Anderson and the G. Pascale National Cancer Institute in Naples, Italy (Curley et al, 2000). The HCCs treated with RFA in this patient population ranged from 1 to 7 cm in greatest dimension. As the size of the tumor increased, the number of deployments of the multiple-array needle electrode and the total time of applying RF energy increased. Primary liver tumors tend to be highly vascular, so a vascular heat sink phenomenon may contribute to the extended ablation times.

All 110 HCC patients in the recent study were followed for a minimum of 12 months after RFA, with a median follow-up of 19 months. Percutaneous RFA was performed in 76 patients (69%), and intraoperative RFA was performed in 34 patients (31%), with 149 discrete HCC tumor nodules treated with RFA. The median diameter of tumors treated percutaneously (2.8 cm) was smaller than the median diameter of lesions treated during laparotomy (4.6 cm). Four patients of the 110, all with tumors less than 4.0 cm in diameter, had local tumor recurrence at the RFA site; all 4 patients subsequently developed recurrent HCC in other areas of the liver. New liver tumors or extrahepatic metastases developed in 50 patients (45.5%), but 56 patients (50.9%) had no evidence of recurrence. Clearly, a longer follow-up period is required to establish long-term disease-free and overall survival rates.

In this study, procedure-related complications were minimal in patients with HCC. There were no treatment-related deaths, but 12.7% of the HCC patients had complications, including symptomatic pleural effusion, fever, pain, subcutaneous hematoma, subcapsular liver hematoma, and ventricular fibrillation. In addition, 1 patient with Child's class B cirrhosis developed ascites, and another with Child's class B cirrhosis developed bleeding in the ablated tumor 4 days after RFA, necessitating hepatic arterial embolization and transfusion of 2 units of packed red blood cells. All patient events resolved with appropriate clinical management within 1 week after RFA, with the exception of the development of ascites, which resolved with the use of diuretics within 3 weeks after RFA. No patient developed thermal injury to adjacent organs or structures, hepatic insufficiency, renal insufficiency, or coagulopathy following the application of RF energy to the target tumors. The overall complication rate after RFA for HCC was low, which is particularly notable because 50 Child's class A, 31 class B, and 29 class C cirrhotic patients were treated.

Imaging Studies after RFA

Ideally, the size of the necrotic cavitary lesion created by RFA of a hepatic tumor as seen on posttreatment images should be larger than the size of the malignant tumor as seen on pretreatment images. However, interpretation of CT scans, MR images, or sonograms after RFA to determine complete destruction of tumor and to evaluate for local recurrence (incomplete treatment) may be difficult, particularly if the tumor abuts a large intrahepatic blood vessel or the inferior vena cava. Dynamic MR imaging or multiphasic helical CT performed in the first 1 to 3 months after RFA may demonstrate a hypervascular rim of inflammatory tissue around the RFA defect. This inflammatory response may be asymmetric and is impossible to distinguish from a rim of vascularized residual tumor. In our experience at M. D. Anderson, this inflammatory response noted on early scans resolves and is not evident on images obtained 6 months or more after RFA.

The peripheral inflammatory reaction that shows itself as an enhancing halo at the boundary of the necrotic area can be distinguished from local tumor recurrence by serial dynamic MR imaging or helical CT. An enhancing rim of strictly inflammatory tissue seen during the arterial phase on dynamic MR images or helical CT scans will be stable or progressively reduced in intensity on subsequent scans. Conversely, a local recurrence at the edge of a necrotic RFA zone may be detected as progressive ingrowth of vascularized tissue into the necrotic area or as vascularized outgrowth away from the zone of necrosis. The arterial phase of dynamic MR imaging or helical CT is best able to reveal possible areas of local recurrence because washout of the contrast agent during the portal venous phase may result in residual tumor tissue that is isodense with the surrounding hepatic parenchyma.

Regional (Intra-arterial) Chemotherapy

In patients with HCC, uncontrolled tumor in the liver is the most significant cause of morbidity and mortality, although extrahepatic metastases are apparent in up to 25% of patients at the time of diagnosis and up to 90% on autopsy. Thus, effective local chemotherapy would have a significant clinical effect. Administration of the drug into the hepatic artery could theoretically increase local drug delivery to the tumor tissue and possibly lower systemic toxicity. An ideal pharmacologic profile would be a high degree of hepatic extraction, high systemic clearance, rapid biotransformation to less toxic metabolites, and a steep dose-response relationship with respect to tumor cell kill.

Numerous studies have been performed of single agents as well as combinations of drugs. Systemic comparisons of the intra-arterial with the systemic route of administration have not been performed. Many of the studies performed suffer from some degree of selection bias in that only patients with a good performance status were included. Catheters may be placed via laparotomy or percutaneously, and reports of therapy should include an account of complications of catheter placement.

Floxuridine in particular exhibits nearly complete hepatic extraction when administered by hepatic arterial infusion. Although partial response rates in HCC patients treated with hepatic arterial floxuridine infusion exceed 50%, the effect on survival is modest. Doxorubicin has been administered intra-arterially to treat unresectable HCC. Because doxorubicin has a relatively low systemic clearance and is primarily eliminated by hepatic metabolism and biliary excretion, regional hepatic perfusion results in an

---

KEY PRACTICE POINTS

- Intraoperative ultrasonography has become the gold standard against which all other diagnostic imaging modalities are compared for detecting the number and extent of tumors and the association of tumors with intrahepatic blood vessels in both primary and metastatic liver tumors.

- The quality of life of patients with HCC who undergo resection is significantly better than that of patients treated nonsurgically; thus surgical therapy for HCC should be considered in all patients with potentially resectable lesions.

- In resection of HCC, vascular stapling devices can be used to reduce operative time and intraoperative blood loss in properly selected patients. However, these devices should not be used if tumor is near the vascular pedicle to be divided.

- In properly selected patients, repeat hepatic resection for HCC is appropriate and results in long-term survival rates of up to 30%.

- In patients with normal hepatic parenchyma, a liver remnant consisting of 25% of the total liver volume is usually sufficient to prevent major postoperative complications and hepatic insufficiency. In patients with a smaller predicted future liver remnant, PVE may make hepatic resection possible.

- In patients with HCC who are not candidates for resection but who have liver-only disease, RFA is a potential treatment approach.

- Systemic therapy remains investigational and is of minimal benefit in patients with unresectable HCC. Regional therapy, especially hepatic arterial chemoembolization, may have palliative potential.

---

approximately 2-fold pharmacologic advantage. However, an obvious therapeutic benefit has not been reported.

Other drugs, including cisplatin, also have been administered intraarterially to treat HCC, but there appears to be minimal pharmacologic advantage. Drug combinations that have been administered intraarterially include mitomycin C plus 5-fluorouracil; floxuridine, doxorubicin, and mitomycin C; mitomycin C, 5-fluorouracil, vinblastine, vincristine, doxorubicin, and cisplatin; and floxuridine, doxorubicin, leucovorin, and cisplatin.

HEPATIC ARTERIAL CHEMOEMBOLIZATION

Hepatic artery occlusion has been used alone or in combination with intra-arterial chemotherapy. Hepatic artery occlusion may be permanent, accomplished with surgical ligation or inert particle embolization, or it may be intermittent, accomplished with balloon occlusion or chemoembolization with degradable microspheres.

Attempts have been made to increase the activity of locoregionally administered treatments by prolonging the duration of contact between tumor tissue and the chemotherapeutic agent. Intra-arterially administered contrast medium (iodized oil [Lipiodol] or ethiodized oil) is deposited selectively with HCCs, in which it remains for several months. These substances also may act as carriers for chemotherapeutic agents or radioactive iodine (^{131}I). A variety of chemotherapeutic agents have been coadministered with iodized oil, including doxorubicin, floxuridine, mitomycin C, epirubicin, cisplatin, and styrene maleic acid neocarzinostatin (SMANCS). In most of the trials, 50% to 90% of the patients had a decrease in serum alpha fetoprotein levels, with median survival durations ranging from 2 to 14 months and 1- and 2-year survival rates ranging from 33% to 55%.

In summary, despite numerous studies, systemic therapy remains investigational and is of minimal benefit to patients with unresectable HCC. Regional therapy, especially hepatic arterial chemoembolization, may have palliative potential. At M. D. Anderson, hepatic arterial chemoembolization is used to palliate pain or other symptoms in patients with unresectable large or multifocal HCC.

Suggested Readings

Abdalla EK, Barnett CC, Doherty D, et al. Extended hepatectomy in hepatobiliary malignancies with and without preoperative portal vein embolization. *Arch Surg* 2002;137:675–680.

Ahmad SA, Bilimoria MM, Wang X, et al. Hepatitis B or C virus serology as a prognostic factor in patients with hepatocellular carcinoma. *J Gastrointest Surg* 2001; 5:468–476.

Barnett CC, Curley SA. Ablation techniques, ethanol injection, cryoablation, and radiofrequency ablation. In: Pinson CW, ed. *Operative Techniques in General Surgery*. Philadelphia, Pa: W. B. Saunders Company; 2002;4:65–75.

Bilimoria MM, Lauwers GY, Doherty DA, et al. Underlying liver disease, not tumor factors, predicts long-term survival after hepatic resection of hepatocellular carcinoma. *Arch Surg* 2001;136:528–535.

Choi H, Loyer EM, Dubrow RA, et al. Radiofrequency ablation (RFA) of liver tumors: assessment of therapeutic response and complications. *Radiographics* 2001;21:S41–S54.

Curley SA, Cusack JC, Tanabe KK, et al. Advances in the treatment of liver tumors. *Curr Probl Surg* 2002;39:449–571.

Curley SA, Izzo F, Ellis LM, et al. Radiofrequency ablation of hepatocellular cancer in 110 cirrhotic patients. *Ann Surg* 2000;232:381–391.

Esnaola NE, Lauwers GY, Mirza NQ, et al. Predictors of microvascular invasion in patients with hepatocellular carcinoma who are candidates for orthotopic liver transplantation. *J Gastrointest Surg* 2002;6:224–231.

Izzo F, Cremona F, Ruffolo F, et al. Outcome of 67 hepatocellular cancer patients detected during screening of 1,125 patients with chronic hepatitis. *Ann Surg* 1998;227:513–518.

Meric F, Patt YZ, Curley SA, et al. Surgery after downstaging of unresectable hepatic tumors with intra-arterial chemotherapy. *Ann Surg Oncol* 2000;7: 490–495.

Vauthey JN, Lauwers GY, Esnaola NF, et al. Simplified staging for hepatocellular carcinoma. *J Clin Oncol* 2002;20:1527–1536.

Watkins KT, Curley SA. Liver and bile ducts. In: Abeloff MD, Armitage JO, Lichter AS, Niederhuber JE, eds. *Clinical Oncology.* 2nd ed. New York, NY: Churchill Livingstone; 2000:1681–1748.

Wayne JD, Lauwers GY, Ikai I, et al. Preoperative predictors of survival after resection of small hepatocellular carcinomas. *Ann Surg* 2002;235:722–730.

14 GASTRIC CANCER

James C. Yao, Peter W. T. Pisters,
Christopher Crane, and Jaffer A. Ajani

CHAPTER OVERVIEW

While gastric cancer remains one of the most common malignancies diagnosed worldwide, its incidence continues to decrease in Western countries. This change has been accompanied by a proximal migration in cancer localization. Postoperative chemotherapy plus chemoradiation therapy, in the Gastrointestinal Cancer Intergroup 0116 trial, prolonged overall and disease-free survival of patients after a complete resection with negative margins (R0 resection). This treatment should be considered the new standard of care for patients with gastric cancer who have undergone potentially curative R0 resection for stage Ib-IV disease. Preoperative therapy may increase the likelihood of R0 resection, and it remains an area of active investigation. Gastric cancer is incurable when metastases are present. The median survival for patients with stage IV disease remains under 1 year in phase III trials. The development of more active agents is needed for the treatment of metastatic tumors.

Introduction

Gastric cancer remains one of the most commonly diagnosed malignancies worldwide. However, its incidence is on the decline in many countries. The United States, over the last century, has led this decline. It is estimated that 22,400 cases of gastric cancer will be diagnosed and 12,100 people will die of gastric cancer in 2003 (Jemal et al, 2002).

Regional differences in the incidence and anatomic location of gastric cancer exist. In Asia, a significant proportion of gastric cancers are located in the distal stomach. In the United States, a trend of increasing incidence of proximal gastric and gastroesophageal junction carcinoma is clear. Recent analyses of patients who sought treatment at M. D. Anderson Cancer Center between 1995 and 1998 showed that 41% of upper gastrointestinal carcinomas involved the gastroesophageal junction. Several large studies have shown that proximal gastric cancer portends an unfavorable prognosis. Our own data show that the adverse effect of gastric cancer localization is limited in patients with locoregional disease.

These changes in gastric cancer are most likely due to multiple factors. Much of the decline in the incidence of gastric cancer can be attributed to the increased use of refrigeration in the industrialized world. This has led to increased consumption of fresh foods and decreased use of salt and pickling as methods of food preservation. The recent recognition of *Helicobacter pylori* as a cause of peptic ulcer disease and a cocarcinogen have led to treatments that may further decrease the incidence of gastric cancer.

The cause of the rising incidence of proximal gastric and gastroesophageal junction carcinoma is a subject of active investigation. Several large studies have found an association between obesity and proximal gastric cancer (Vaughan et al, 1995; Chow et al, 1998; Lagergren et al, 1999). Tobacco use may also play a role. Although gastroesophageal reflux disease and Barrett's metaplasia are associated with esophageal adenocarcinoma, their associations with gastric cancer are less clear. A Swedish study (Lagergren et al, 1999) reported an association between gastric cardia cancer and reflux. However, this study included in its definition of gastric cancer some cancers located above the gastroesophageal junction.

Proximal gastric cancer localization is most prominent among white men. The percentage of gastric cancers that were proximal among 1,242 M. D. Anderson patients was significantly higher for white men (57%) than for white women (37%), who had a pattern of gastric cancer localization similar to that of nonwhite men (36% of cancers proximal) and nonwhite women (31% of cancers proximal).

Survival rate and tumor characteristics also differ by sex. In 2 large surgical series, 1 from Korea (Kim et al, 1998) and 1 from the United States

(Hundahl et al, 2000), the 5-year survival rates were higher for women than for men. In our series, women were also more likely to have mucin-producing histologic subtypes and peritoneal dissemination.

DIAGNOSIS

The symptoms of gastric cancer are often nonspecific, leading to diagnosis at an advanced disease stage. This is largely because both the stomach and the abdominal cavity are large and compliant to distention. The most common symptoms at diagnosis are abdominal pain and weight loss. Other symptoms may vary by the location of the primary lesion. Dysphagia occurs predominantly among patients with proximal gastric cancer; in contrast, nausea, vomiting, and early satiety are more prominent among patients with nonproximal gastric cancer.

An upper gastrointestinal series is commonly performed as an initial part of the workup for symptoms. Diagnosis is definitively established by esophagogastroduodenoscopy in nearly all cases. Patients with linitis plastica do not always have obvious mucosal disease. Some patients may present with peritoneal carcinomatosis or with ovarian masses. Multiple deep biopsies are encouraged in these situations. Occasionally, endoscopic ultrasonography and surgical biopsy are needed to establish the diagnosis.

STAGING

At M. D. Anderson, we perform a history, physical examination, complete blood cell count (including platelet count), electrolyte measurements, renal and liver function tests, chest roentgenography, and computed tomography of the abdomen and pelvis as part of the standard workup. More extensive staging studies are performed for patients with potentially resectable disease. Endoscopic ultrasonography is helpful in determining the depth of invasion and the extent of nodal involvement and in ruling out involvement of adjacent organs.

The peritoneal cavity is one of the most common sites of metastasis for gastric cancer. These metastases often grow as small plaques and are difficult to detect by radiologic imaging. We perform laparoscopy to rule out occult metastases prior to resection. At laparoscopy, peritoneal lavage is done for cytologic analysis. If a patient is to undergo preoperative therapy, a jejunostomy tube is placed for nutritional support. Among patients who have enrolled in preoperative chemotherapy trials, these strategies have helped to reveal occult metastases and have significantly reduced the number of nontherapeutic laparotomies.

Table 14–2. Selected Chemotherapy Regimens for Advanced Gastric Cancer

5-FU, cisplatin, docetaxel: 28-day cycle
  5-FU 750 mg/m^2/day CIV infusion days 1–5
  Cisplatin 75 mg/m^2/day IV day 1 only
  Docetaxel 75 mg/m^2 IV over 1 hour day 1 only
5-FU, cisplatin: 28-day cycle
  5-FU 750 mg/m^2/day CIV infusion days 1–5
  Cisplatin 20 mg/m^2/day IV days 1–5
5-FU, epirubicin, cisplatin: 21-day cycle
  5-FU 200 mg/m^2/day CIV infusion days 1–21
  Epirubicin 50 mg/m^2 IV day 1
  Cisplatin 60 mg/m^2 IV day 1
5-FU, cisplatin, paclitaxel: 28-day cycle
  5-FU 750 mg/m^2/day CIV infusion days 1–5
  Cisplatin 15 mg/m^2/day IV days 1–5
  Paclitaxel 200 mg/m^2 IV over 3 hours day 1 only
5-FU, carboplatin, paclitaxel: 28-day cycle
  5-FU 600 mg/m^2/day CIV infusion days 1–5
  Carboplatin AUC = 5 day 1 only
  Paclitaxel 175 mg/m^2 IV over 3 hours day 1 only
Irinotecan, cisplatin: 42-day cycle (alternatively, 21-day cycle)
  Irinotecan 50 mg/m^2 IV days 1, 8, 15, 22 (or days 1, 8)
  Cisplatin 30 mg/m^2 IV days 1, 8, 15, 22 (or days 1, 8)

Abbreviations: 5-FU, 5-fluorouracil; CIV, continuous intravenous; IV, intravenous; AUC, area under the curve.

leucovorin (ELF), and 5-fluorouracil plus doxorubicin plus methotrexate (FAMTX). The median survival is 7 months for all 3 groups (Vanhoefer et al, 2000). Epirubicin plus cisplatin plus 5-fluorouracil (ECF) provided a more favorable survival duration than did FAMTX (9 months vs 6 months; $P < .05$) (Waters et al, 1999). ECF, however, has not been compared with FUP or ELF. Patients undergoing treatment with FAMTX must be closely monitored and hospitalized. FAMTX is currently not widely used.

Fluorouracil- or cisplatin-based chemotherapy should be considered the standard. Selected regimens are listed in Table 14–2. Trials of these regimens have shown that the median survival of patients with advanced gastric cancer is less than 1 year with standard chemotherapy. Recently, a phase III trial comparing 5-fluorouracil and cisplatin to 5-fluorouracil, cisplatin, and docetaxel has completed accrual. Interim analysis showed improved response rate, time to progression, and overall survival in patients receiving docetaxel. The 5-fluorouracil, cisplatin, and docetaxel combination should be considered in the front-line setting in patients with adequate performance status.

Second-line chemotherapy for patients with adequate performance status should be tailored to include agents without potential cross-resistance to previous treatments. In one study, the combination of irinotecan and cisplatin (days 1, 8, 15, and 22 of a 42-day cycle) as second-line chemotherapy was studied (Baker et al, 2001). Patients who previously underwent cisplatin-based chemotherapy without success were included. Of 29 evaluable patients, 9 patients (31%) had objective responses. More recently, we used the same dose of chemotherapy on days 1 and 8 of a 21-day schedule, with improved tolerance.

Single-agent chemotherapy should be considered for patients with suboptimal performance status who desire systemic therapy. Consideration should be given to avoiding cisplatin in patients with symptomatic ascites due to problems with fluid accumulation.

Efforts at predicting response to chemotherapy are under way. Several studies retrospectively correlated low intratumoral excision-repair cross-complementing gene *(ERCC1)* mRNA expression with response after platinum-based chemotherapy. Studies also evaluated the relationship between the expression levels of thymidylate synthase *(TS)* and dihydropyrimidine dehydrogenase and the objective response after fluoropyrimidine treatment. However, several studies yielded conflicting results regarding TS, most likely owing to the complexity of multiple factors determining chemotherapy responsiveness. The combination of *TS* and *ERCC1* expression was evaluated as a predictor of response to 5-fluorouracil and cisplatin chemotherapy. In cases in which both *TS* expression and *ERCC1* expression were low, 11 patients of 13 (85%) responded to chemotherapy (Metzger et al, 1998). In cases in which both *TS* and *ERCC1* expression were high, only 2 patients of 10 (20%) responded. Further multivariate analysis with larger study cohorts incorporating other markers will be helpful.

Radiation Therapy

Unresectable Locoregional Disease

The addition of radiation therapy to chemotherapy in patients with locally advanced disease has been studied in a number of trials, which have shown that concurrent 5-fluorouracil-based chemotherapy and radiation therapy at a dose of 35 to 50 Gy is feasible. Chemoradiation therapy provides a survival advantage similar to that seen with chemotherapy alone.

At M. D. Anderson, we have found concurrent 5-fluorouracil, paclitaxel, and radiation therapy at a dose of 45 to 50 Gy to be feasible (Table 14–3). Aggressive nutritional support is important with a combined-modality approach. Gastrostomy feeding tubes are suboptimal in the setting of gastric irradiation. The use of a feeding jejunostomy and a 3-dimensional conformal technique can greatly enhance tolerance.

Table 14–3.   Treatment with 5-Fluorouracil, Paclitaxel, and Radiation Therapy for Locally Advanced Gastric Cancer

5-fluorouracil 300 mg/m^2/day continuous intravenous infusion 5 days per week for 5 weeks
Paclitaxel 45 mg/m^2 IV 1 day per week for 5 weeks
External-beam radiation therapy 1.8 Gy/day 5 days per week to 45–50 Gy

Abbreviation: IV, intravenously.

Metastatic Disease

In patients with disseminated disease, the role of radiation therapy is limited to palliation of symptoms. The role of radiation therapy for brain and spinal cord metastases is well established. Irradiation of areas of painful soft-tissue disease may enhance pain control. Gastric irradiation helps to treat bleeding from primary tumor and gastric outlet obstruction.

Other Palliative Therapies

The role of surgical palliation for advanced gastric cancer is limited because patients with metastatic disease have relatively short survival durations. The operative morbidity and mortality rates are also higher for patients who undergo palliative surgery than for those who undergo curative surgery. Surgery is especially difficult in patients with peritoneal carcinomatosis. Thus, gastrectomy should be considered for intractable bleeding or in cases in which the patient has a dramatic systemic response to chemotherapy with residual local tumor. A combination of gastrostomy for drainage and jejunostomy for enteral nutrition can often offer effective palliation for bowel obstruction.

FUTURE PERSPECTIVES

Despite the advances and research efforts over the last decade, the outcome for patients with gastric cancer remains poor, largely because many gastric cancers are diagnosed at a late stage. The relatively low incidence of the disease in the United States makes large-scale screening unfeasible. Efforts should be directed toward improving therapeutic strategies.

Large, comprehensive database efforts, such as those under way at M. D. Anderson, will help to better define the natural history of this disease and to generate new hypotheses for translational research. Gastric cancer is likely to include distinct subtypes, with different risk factors, patterns of spread, and underlying molecular biologic characteristics. As we enter the era of targeted therapy, it is very important for us to understand these differences.

KEY PRACTICE POINTS

- In Western countries, the overall incidence of gastric cancer continues to decrease, whereas the incidence of proximal gastric and gastroesophageal junction cancer continues to increase.

- Gastric cancer is frequently diagnosed at a late stage. Relapse after curative surgery is common.

- Postoperative chemotherapy followed by chemoradiation therapy is the standard of care in cases in which patients undergo curative resection for stage Ib-IV disease.

- It is important to select treatment on the basis of results of phase III trials. Higher response rates have not always led to improved survival.

- Participation in promising clinical trials should be encouraged.

In the postoperative setting, combined-modality chemoradiation therapy is effective. Preoperative strategies are under investigation. The incorporation of knowledge about individual clinical, pathologic, and molecular profiles of gastric cancer into novel therapeutic strategies remains a challenge for the 21st century.

For patients with more advanced disease, ongoing translational research may in the future allow chemotherapeutic agents to be selected on the basis of molecular predictors. The incorporation of novel biological agents directed at epidermal growth factor receptor and other angiogenic pathways also holds promise.

SUGGESTED READINGS

Ajani JA, Fodor M, Van Cutsem E, et al. Multinational randomized phase II trial of docetaxel (T) and cisplatin (C) with or without 5-fluorouracil (FU) in patients (Pts) with advanced gastric or GE junction adenocarcinoma (AGC-AGEJC) [abstract]. *Proceedings of the American Society of Clinical Oncology* 2000;19:247a.

Ajani JA, Mansfield PF, Janjan N, et al. Preoperative chemoradiation therapy (Ctrt) in patients (Pts) with potentially resectable gastric carcinoma (Prgc): a multi-institutional pilot [abstract]. *Proceedings of the American Society of Clinical Oncology* 1998;17:1089a.

Baker JJ, Ajani JA, Ho L, et al. CPT-11 plus cisplatin as second line therapy of advanced gastric or GE junction adenocarcinoma (AGC-AGEJC) [abstract]. *Proceedings of the American Society of Clinical Oncology* 2001;63.

Bonenkamp JJ, Hermans J, Sasako M, van de Velde CJ. Extended lymph-node dissection for gastric cancer. Dutch Gastric Cancer Group. *N Engl J Med* 1999;340: 908–914.

Chow WH, Blot WJ, Vaughan TL, et al. Body mass index and risk of adenocar-cinomas of the esophagus and gastric cardia. *J Natl Cancer Inst* 1998;90:150–155.

Cullinan SA, Moertel CG, Fleming TR, et al. A comparison of three chemothera-peutic regimens in the treatment of advanced pancreatic and gastric carcinoma. Fluorouracil vs fluorouracil and doxorubicin vs fluorouracil, doxorubicin, and mitomycin. *JAMA* 1985;253:2061–2067.

Cuschieri A, Weeden S, Fielding J, et al. Patient survival after D1 and D2 resec-tions for gastric cancer: long-term results of the MRC randomized surgical trial. Surgical Co-operative Group. *Br J Cancer* 1999;79:1522–1530.

Esaki Y, Hirayama R, Hirokawa K, et al. A comparison of patterns of metastasis in gastric cancer by histologic type and age. *Cancer* 1990;65:2086–2090.

Hundahl SA, Phillips JL, Menck HR. The National Cancer Data Base Report on poor survival of U.S. gastric carcinoma patients treated with gastrectomy: fifth edition American Joint Committee on Cancer staging, proximal disease, and the "different disease" hypothesis. *Cancer* 2000;88:921–932.

Huntsman DG, Carneiro F, Lewis FR, et al. Early gastric cancer in young, asymptomatic carriers of germ-line E-cadherin mutation. *N Engl J Med* 2001;344:1904–1909.

Jemal A, Thomas A, Murray T, et al. Cancer statistics, 2002. *CA Cancer J Clin* 2002;52:23–47.

Kim JP, Lee JH, Kim SJ, Yu HJ, Yang HK. Clinicopathologic characteristics and prognostic factors in 10783 patients with gastric cancer. *Gastric Cancer* 1998;1: 125–133.

Lagergren J, Bergstrom R, Nyren O. Association between body mass and adeno-carcinoma of the esophagus and gastric cardia. *Ann Intern Med* 1999;130:883–890.

Lowy AM, Mansfield PF, Leech SD, Pazdur R, Dumas P, Ajani JA. Response to neoadjuvant chemotherapy best predicts survival after curative resection of gastric cancer. *Ann Surg* 1999;229:303–308.

Macdonald JS, Smalley SR, Benedetti J, et al. Chemoradiotherapy after surgery compared with surgery alone for adenocarcinoma of the stomach or gastroe-sophageal junction. *N Engl J Med* 2001;345:725–730.

Maehara Y, Moriguchi S, Kakeji Y, et al. Pertinent risk factors and gastric carci-noma with synchronous peritoneal dissemination or liver metastasis. *Surgery* 1991;110:820–823.

Metzger R, Leichman CG, Danenbery RD, et al. ERCC1 mRNA levels complement thymidylate synthase mRNA levels in predicting response and survival for gastric cancer patients receiving combination cisplatin and fluorouracil chemotherapy. *J Clin Oncol* 1998;16:309–316.

Schnirer II, Komaki R, Yao JC, et al. Pilot study of concurrent 5-fluorouracil/pacli-taxel plus radiotherapy in patients with carcinoma of the esophagus and gas-troesophageal junction. *Am J Clin Oncol* 2001;24:91–95.

Vanhoefer U, Rougier P, Wilke H, et al. Final results of a randomized phase III trial of sequential high-dose methotrexate, fluorouracil, and doxorubicin versus etoposide, leucovorin, and fluorouracil versus infusional fluorouracil and cis-platin in advanced gastric cancer: trial of the European Organization for Research and Treatment of Cancer Gastrointestinal Tract Cancer Cooperative Group. *J Clin Oncol* 2000;18:2648–2657.

Vaughan TL, Davis S, Kristal A, et al. Obesity, alcohol, and tobacco as risk factors for cancers of the esophagus and gastric cardia: adenocarcinoma versus squamous cell carcinoma. *Cancer Epidemiol Biomarkers Prev* 1995;4:85–92.

Waters JS, Norman A, Cunningham D, et al. Long-term survival after epirubicin, cisplatin, and fluorouracil for gastric cancer: results of a randomized trial. *Br J Cancer* 1999;80:269–272.

15 ESOPHAGEAL CARCINOMA

Stephen G. Swisher, Ritsuko Komaki,
Patrick M. Lynch, and Jaffer A. Ajani

CHAPTER OVERVIEW

Esophageal carcinoma affects a heterogeneous population of patients whose treatment decisions are determined by patient performance status, clinical disease stage, and tumor location. The overall survival rate for patients with esophageal cancer is poor (5% to 30%) because of the high risk of both locoregional and metastatic recurrence. Nevertheless, some patients can be cured. In patients with early-stage disease, surgery alone may be curative. In selected patients with locally advanced disease, a multidisciplinary approach that involves surgery, chemotherapy, and radiation therapy for selected subsets of patients offers the best chance for cure. The treatment decision is in part based on the location and stage of the cancer. Combined chemotherapy and radiation therapy (chemoradiation) or radiation therapy alone may be used to treat both patients with early-stage disease and those with locally advanced cancer of the upper esophagus, to avoid laryngectomy. Surgery may be performed alone (in cases of early-stage disease) or with neoadjuvant (preoperative) chemotherapy and radiation therapy (in cases of locally advanced disease) to treat patients with cancer of the middle or lower esophagus. Chemotherapy may be used to treat patients with metastatic disease. Palliative care for patients with locally advanced and metastatic disease includes radiation therapy and endoscopic stent placement. Multimodality treatment regimens require careful coordination between specialists in medical oncology, radiation therapy, surgery, and interventional gastroenterology to maximize therapeutic benefits and minimize treatment-related morbidity.

INTRODUCTION

Carcinoma of the esophagus accounts for approximately 12,500 new cancer cases and 11,500 deaths in the United States each year. The incidence of esophageal cancer varies worldwide more than the incidence of any other cancer does. In the United States, esophageal cancer incidence is approximately 7 cases per 100,000 people, while in high-risk areas of China, Iran, and Russia, it can be more than 100 cases per 100,000 people. The 2 major pathologic subtypes worldwide are squamous cell carcinoma and adenocarcinoma. In the United States and Europe, adenocarcinoma has become the most common histologic subtype, whereas in other areas of the world, squamous cell carcinoma still predominates. Squamous cell carcinoma is also the predominant histologic subtype in areas in which esophageal carcinoma is endemic.

Although esophageal cancer is curable at an early stage, the overall 5-year survival rate for esophageal cancer is only 13%, primarily because the disease is usually advanced at presentation. The survival rate is very stage dependent (Table 15–1). Many patients with early-stage (stage I) localized disease can be cured with surgery alone; the 5-year survival rate of these patients approaches 70% to 75% with surgery alone (Swisher et al, 1995). Unfortunately, these patients represent the minority of patients; most patients with esophageal cancer present with locally advanced (stage

Table 15–1.   Five-Year Survival Rates for Patients with Esophageal Cancer, by Stage

Stage	TNM Grouping*	Approximate 5-Year Survival Rate, %
0	Tis, N0, M0	100
I	T1, N0, M0	75
IIA	T2, N0, M0	40
	T3, N0, M0	25
IIB	T1, N1, M0	15
	T2, N1, M0	
III	T3, N1, M0	10
	T4, Any N, M0	
IVA	Any T, Any N, M1a	5–10
IVB	Any T, Any N, M1b	<5

* Definitions of TNM are given in Table 15–2.

II–IVA) or metastatic (stage IVB) disease. This chapter focuses on the role of multimodality treatment of patients with esophageal cancer and the algorithms followed at M. D. Anderson Cancer Center to maximize the chance for long-term cure while minimizing the overall risks of treatment.

INITIAL ASSESSMENT

The initial evaluation of a patient with suspected esophageal cancer consists of 4 phases. The first phase involves obtaining a diagnosis; the second, accurately clinically staging and locating the tumor with noninvasive imaging studies; the third, determining the patient's physiologic status and ability to tolerate available treatment modalities; and the fourth, determining the appropriate treatment options on the basis of the individual patient's physiologic status, symptoms, and clinical stage of disease. In patients with advanced cancer, in whom the risk of locoregional and distant recurrence is quite high, maximal benefit can be obtained by a multidisciplinary approach in which patients are seen by surgeons, radiation therapists, medical oncologists, and interventional gastroenterologists and their cases are discussed individually at a multidisciplinary forum.

The diagnostic phase is initiated upon presentation. The most common presenting symptom of patients with esophageal cancer is dysphagia. Patients notice that foods, especially solids, intermittently "stick" in the esophagus. Over time, the dysphagia progresses to occur with liquids as well and can result in vomiting with meals. These symptoms should elicit a diagnostic evaluation with a barium swallow and endoscopy. In most cases, these procedures allow the diagnosis of an esophageal cancer that is causing these symptoms. The other common presenting symptom is anemia.

Once the tumor is diagnosed, the second phase of assessment, clinical staging and anatomic localization of the tumor, begins. This involves obtaining a careful history and physical examination and performing computed tomography (CT) of the chest and abdomen, barium swallow, endoscopic ultrasonography, and positron emission tomography (PET). Because a bone scan and CT or magnetic resonance imaging of the brain yield little diagnostic information in asymptomatic patients, these tests are performed only if symptoms (i.e., new onset of bone pain or neurologic changes, such as headaches or visual disturbances) are present.

Once the disease has been staged (Table 15–2) and the location of the cancer has been determined, a physiologic assessment should be performed to determine the patient's ability to tolerate different therapeutic modalities. Not only should the patient's overall medical condition be evaluated, but also specific attention should be paid to the cardiovascular

Table 15–2.   TNM Definitions for Esophageal Cancer

Primary Tumor (T)

TX	Primary tumor cannot be assessed
T0	No evidence of primary tumor
Tis	Carcinoma in situ
T1	Tumor invades lamina propria or submucosa
T2	Tumor invades muscularis propria
T3	Tumor invades adventitia
T4	Tumor invades adjacent structures

Regional Lymph Nodes (N)

NX	Regional lymph nodes cannot be assessed
N0	No regional lymph node metastasis
N1	Regional lymph node metastasis

Distant Metastasis (M)

MX	Distant metastasis cannot be assessed
M0	No distant metastasis
M1	Distant metastasis

Tumors of the lower thoracic esophagus

M1a	Metastasis in celiac lymph nodes
M1b	Other distant metastasis

Tumors of the midthoracic esophagus

M1a	Not applicable
M1b	Nonregional lymph nodes and/or other distant metastasis

Tumors of the upper thoracic esophagus

M1a	Metastasis in cervical nodes
M1b	Other distant metastasis

Used with permission of the American Joint Committee on Cancer (AJCC), Chicago, IL. The original source for this material is the AJCC Cancer Staging Manual Sixth Edition (2002), published by Springer-Verlag New York, www.springer-ny.com

and respiratory systems. Cardiovascular screening should include a history and physical examination as well as chest roentgenography and electrocardiography. Patients with signs and symptoms of significant cardiac disease should undergo further noninvasive testing, including exercise testing, echocardiography, or a nuclear perfusion scan. Significant reversible cardiac problems should be addressed before therapy (i.e., chemotherapy, radiation therapy, or surgery) is initiated. The pulmonary reserve of patients with esophageal cancer can be estimated by simple spirometry. A forced expiratory volume in 1 second of less than 0.8 liters or less than 35% of predicted value is associated with an increased risk of complications, respiratory insufficiency, and treatment-related death (Ferguson and Durkin, 2002).

Treatment of Early-Stage (Stage I) Esophageal Cancer

One of the problems with esophageal cancer has traditionally been the inability to accurately assess the stage preoperatively. Endoscopic ultrasonography, however, has revolutionized our ability to assess depth of penetration and involvement of regional lymph nodes. Additionally, the combination of CT and PET has allowed a more accurate determination of metastatic spread. These noninvasive modalities have allowed us to more accurately stage esophageal cancers before treatment is initiated. They also have increased the confidence level in determining that patients with endoscopic sonographic evidence of early-stage disease and no evidence of metastatic cancer on PET and CT of the chest and abdomen truly have localized cancer. This is important because it allows treatment to be focused on the primary tumor without concern for distant or micrometastatic cancer. Consequently, patients with early-stage esophageal cancer, as documented by endoscopic ultrasonography, can be treated with esophagectomy for cancers in the middle esophagus (i.e., those occurring between the aortic arch and inferior pulmonary ligament) or lower esophagus (i.e., those occurring between the inferior pulmonary ligament and gastroesophageal junction [GEJ]) or combined chemotherapy and radiation therapy (chemoradiation) for cancers in the upper esophagus (those occurring between the thoracic inlet and aortic arch, <20 cm from the incisors).

At M. D. Anderson, the modality of treatment used in a particular case is determined by the tumor location and the patient's physiologic status (Figures 15–1 and 15–2). Early-stage upper esophageal cancers are treated with chemoradiation because in most cases, surgery requires a laryngectomy. For cases in which the cancer is in the middle or lower esophagus or the GEJ, surgery is typically performed because the morbidity rate is acceptable and a laryngectomy is not required (Figure 15–2). Patients who cannot tolerate surgery, however, are treated with chemoradiation or radiation therapy alone, often with curative results.

The anatomic location of esophageal cancer makes surgical resection a formidable procedure. The esophagus originates at the lower border of the cricoid cartilage and descends into the thorax posterior to the trachea, heart, and great vessels to the esophageal hiatus, where it enters the stomach through the GEJ. The vital structures and posterior location of the esophagus make radical resection of the esophagus difficult. Surgical resection requires several choices, including the type of conduit to be used, the location of the anastomosis, and the anatomic route of the conduit. At M. D. Anderson, resection of the esophagus is approached either transthoracically from the right chest (Ivor-Lewis resection) or transabdominally (transhiatally) by blunt dissection through the hiatus without a thoracotomy. After esophageal resection, a conduit or neoesophagus is created out of the stomach (most common), colon, or jejunum, and an anastomosis is

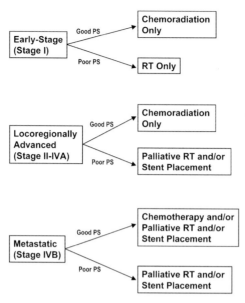

Figure 15–1. Algorithm for treatment of upper esophageal tumors based on physiologic status and clinical stage. PS, performance status; RT, radiation therapy.

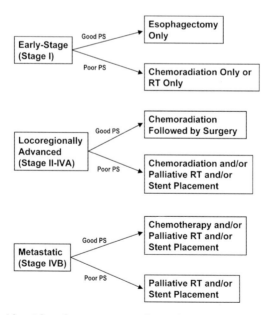

Figure 15–2. Algorithm for treatment of esophageal tumors in the middle or lower esophagus or in the gastroesophageal junction (GEJ) based on physiologic status and clinical stage. PS, performance status; RT, radiation therapy.

created with the residual esophagus in the chest or neck, using a sutured or stapled technique. The conduit is placed in the bed of the resected esophagus (posterior chest), although in some instances, if the esophagus cannot be removed, a substernal or subcutaneous route is chosen.

All esophagectomies begin with a thorough abdominal exploration for evidence of metastases. The most common sites of metastatic esophageal cancer in the abdomen are the liver and nonregional lymph nodes. In cases in which metastatic cancer is identified, surgical resection is not performed because of the short life expectancy associated with metastatic disease. After a complete abdominal exploration, the stomach is mobilized by dividing the gastrocolic ligament, short gastric vessels, and left gastric artery. The vascular supply of the gastric conduit requires that the right gastroepiploic, gastroduodenal, and common hepatic arteries be preserved. A pyloroplasty or pyloromyotomy is performed to avoid gastric stasis that can result from division of the vagus nerves during esophageal transection. Once mobilized, the gastric conduit can easily reach to the neck or chest, as needed, and is vascularly well supplied by blood from the right gastroepiploic artery, which originates from the gastroduodenal and common hepatic arteries. The celiac, perigastric, and periesophageal lymph nodes also are resected and submitted as a separate specimen.

Surgical resection of early-stage esophageal cancers provides a 5-year cure rate of 75% because the cancer is localized to the specific area, with a low likelihood of distant metastatic spread. The operation is complex and associated with high morbidity and mortality rates if performed at a center in which surgeons are inexperienced with the procedure (one study found mortality rates of 20% at low-volume centers vs 2% at high-volume centers [Swisher et al, 2000]). For this reason, if surgical resection is chosen as the treatment modality, it is essential that the operation be performed at a high-volume center that specializes in esophageal resection to minimize the risk of surgery-related morbidity and death.

Many patients with early-stage esophageal cancers have no swallowing disorders before they undergo resection but experience difficulty swallowing after surgery. It is essential to warn patients that they may develop long-term changes in swallowing, with possible dumping syndrome, reflux, and early satiety. These symptoms improve with time but in some cases can persist for a long time.

Patients who have early-stage esophageal cancers located in the upper esophagus require laryngectomy in addition to esophagogastrectomy to attain a complete surgical resection. This disfiguring procedure leaves the patient unable to speak. Furthermore, morbidity and mortality rates (11% to 18%) are significantly higher for these patients than for those who undergo resection of tumors in the body of the esophagus. For these reasons, at M. D. Anderson, patients who have upper esophageal cancer or who cannot tolerate surgical resection are treated with concomitant chemotherapy and radiation therapy rather than surgery (50.4 Gy over 5 weeks; 1.8 Gy/fraction/day, 5 days a week, with concurrent cisplatin and 5-fluorouracil [5-FU]) or are treated with radiation therapy alone (60 Gy over 6 weeks) if they cannot tolerate chemotherapy (Figure 15–1). In cases of early-stage esophageal tumors, chemotherapy serves as a radiosensitizing agent to improve local control from radiation therapy. If the patient's physical condition is too weak, however, radiation therapy alone can be administered. Although chemoradiation is better than radiation therapy alone, the latter has a palliative effect and may be considered for some patients.

Treatment of Locoregionally Advanced (Stage II–IVA) Esophageal Cancer

Although early-stage esophageal cancer is curable, most patients present with locoregionally advanced esophageal cancer (TNM classification of T2–4, N1, or M1a). One reason patients present with late-stage esophageal cancer is that the distensibility of the esophagus often prevents symptoms until the tumor is quite large. Usually, obstruction of 70% or more of the esophageal lumen is required before symptoms develop. Because the average size of the tumor at presentation is greater than 4 cm (Swisher et al, 1995) and more than 1×10^9 cells are required to achieve a size of 1 cm, it is clear that locoregionally advanced cancer has already grown for a long time (2 to 12 years) before detection (Mizuno et al, 1984). In many patients with locoregionally advanced cancer, the cancer has already spread beyond regional lymph nodes to distant sites. This was demonstrated in a study from Germany (Thorban et al, 1996) in which investigators who used monoclonal antibodies to epithelial cell–associated antigens detected cancer cells in the bone marrow of more than 40% of patients undergoing esophageal resection for locoregionally advanced esophageal cancer.

Because patients with esophageal cancer so often present with advanced-stage disease, management of esophageal cancer consists of not only attempting to cure the patients but also palliating their symptoms. Symptoms of dysphagia are progressive and if left untreated lead to the inability to handle even oral secretions. These symptoms are attributable to the primary cancer and can be debilitating if not managed aggressively. Therefore, even though many patients have systemic micrometastatic spread at the time of presentation, control of the primary tumor is essential to avoid the significant problems associated with progressive esophageal obstruction. For patients with good performance status, we at M. D. Anderson have focused on an aggressive multidisciplinary approach to maximize the chance of curing the cancer and palliating the symptoms of patients with locoregionally advanced esophageal cancer. The approach in each case is based in part on the tumor location.

Upper esophageal cancers are relatively rare. The histologic subtype in this region is usually squamous cell carcinoma. Surgical resection in this group of patients is associated with increased morbidity, and lymph node involvement is common (Vigneswaran et al, 1994). The cancers can be treated with surgery, chemotherapy, or radiation therapy depending on the clinical disease stage and the patient's status. For patients with locoregionally advanced cervical esophageal cancers that require laryngectomy in addition to esophagogastrectomy for complete resection, the 2-year survival rate is only 20% even with radical surgery. Because chemoradiation offers similar survival rates without the disability created by radical surgery, concurrent chemotherapy and radiation therapy is used at M. D. Anderson to treat patients with cancer of the cervical esophagus (50.4 Gy over 6 weeks, 1.8 Gy/fraction/day, with concurrent cisplatin and 5-FU) (Figure 15–1).

Locoregionally advanced esophageal cancer in the middle or lower esophagus or the GEJ is treated aggressively at M. D. Anderson, with preoperative chemoradiation and surgical resection, in patients with good performance status (Figure 15–2). Middle esophageal tumors are near the tracheobronchial tree and are associated with direct extension into the membranous portion of the trachea, aorta, or azygos vein. Injury to the posterior membranous wall or mediastinal vessels by blunt dissection during transhiatal resection can lead to catastrophic results (Orringer et al, 1993). Because of these risks, all patients who are considered for surgical resection in this anatomic region should undergo preoperative bronchoscopy to rule out extension into the tracheobronchial tree. Lower esophageal tumors are most commonly adenocarcinoma and are amenable to surgery, chemotherapy, and radiation therapy. The presence of large celiac lymph nodes is associated with decreased overall survival rates.

The treatment of locoregionally advanced esophageal cancers with surgery alone or chemoradiation alone is associated with a 5-year survival rate of only 20%. This is due in large part to locoregional and distant recurrences from microscopic disease remaining at the completion of therapy. In attempts to improve these outcomes, investigational therapies at our institution have involved the combination of all 3 modalities, with neoadjuvant (preoperative) concurrent chemotherapy and radiation therapy followed by surgery (50.4 Gy over 6 weeks, 1.8 Gy/fraction/day with concurrent cisplatin and 5-FU). Postoperative chemotherapy and radiation therapy regimens have been poorly tolerated compared with preoperative regimens and have shown no survival advantages over surgery alone (Ajani et al, 1990). At M. D. Anderson, we therefore have focused on neoadjuvant chemotherapy and radiation therapy. These aggressive approaches have resulted in the pathologic downstaging of disease in a subset of patients with locoregionally advanced esophageal carcinoma. Careful coordination of gastrointestinal oncology care, radiation therapy, and surgery have led to low treatment-related morbidity rates.

Our studies have confirmed that the subset of patients with the best outcomes comprises patients who have a pathologic complete response to neoadjuvant therapy (Swisher et al, 1996). In an attempt to increase the number of patients who respond to neoadjuvant therapy, at M. D. Anderson, we have evaluated the role of additional paclitaxel- or irinotecan-based chemotherapy administered prior to concurrent chemoradiation and surgery (Ajani et al, 2001). This novel 3-step approach allows additional chemotherapy to be given without dose-limiting chemoradiation toxicity. A preliminary review of this 3-step approach has demonstrated an encouraging overall survival rate, which was higher than expected (3-year survival rate, 65%). This is especially encouraging because these results were obtained with a low morbidity rate in a population in which 87% of patients were shown by endoscopic ultrasonography to have advanced tumor extending through the esophageal wall (T classification of T3). Whether these encouraging results can be repeated at centers whose surgeons are less experienced with esophageal cancer remains to be determined.

The treatment of locoregionally advanced esophageal cancers in patients with poor performance status, regardless of the esophageal location of the cancer, is less encouraging because aggressive multimodality approaches are often associated with much higher treatment-related morbidity and mortality rates. Patients who are physiologically unfit for surgery often cannot tolerate aggressive chemoradiation regimens either. Alternative treatment modalities focus on palliation (usually of dysphagia) as their main goal. The prognosis in cases of esophageal cancer treated with radiation therapy alone is poor (Okawa et al, 1989). Nevertheless, significant palliation can be achieved in a large number of patients. At the University of California at San Francisco, the symptoms of 60% of patients improved for longer than 2 months (Wara et al, 1976). In these critically ill patients, 2 months of palliation may be all that is required. The addition of other modalities, such as intraluminal brachytherapy, laser therapy, and endoesophageal stent placement, can offer additional help (Simsek et al, 1996). If treatment worsens the quality of life, it should be abandoned in favor of a completely palliative approach focusing on alleviation of dysphagia and pain. Some patients with poor physiologic status cannot tolerate concurrent chemoradiation and should be treated with palliative radiation therapy with or without endoscopic stent placement. Our current chemoradiation regimens are often not selective enough for the tumor and many times cannot be tolerated by patients with poor performance status.

Treatment of Metastatic (Stage IVB) Esophageal Cancer

Noninvasive studies are quite helpful in identifying patients with metastatic disease. At presentation, 25% of patients with esophageal cancer have metastatic cancer. At autopsy, the most frequent locations of metastatic cancer, in decreasing order of incidence, are the lymph nodes (73%), lung (52%), liver (42%), adrenal glands (20%), bronchus (17%), and bone (14%) (Anderson and Lad, 1982). The presence of metastatic cancer is the worst prognostic factor in terms of long-term survival (Table 15–1). The median survival time of patients with metastatic esophageal cancer is less than 7 months. Because of this short survival, surgical resection is seldom performed, even for palliative purposes, in patients with metastatic cancer.

Metastatic esophageal cancer (M classification of M1b) is seldom cured, although systemic treatment with chemotherapy may allow some palliative and short-term survival benefits and should be considered for patients with good performance status (Figures 15–1 and 15–2). Patients whose disease is symptomatic may also require palliative treatment for the primary tumor. Palliation can be accomplished with radiation therapy, endoscopic stent placement, or both in most patients (Raijman et al, 1998). Advances in chemotherapy, radiation therapy, and endoscopic stents have allowed palliation of obstruction without the need to resort to surgical bypass. These advances have allowed improvements in the quality of life for patients with metastatic esophageal cancer, although long-term survival rates have not been markedly changed.

Metastatic esophageal cancer that is symptomatic (i.e., obstruction) can be treated with radiation therapy alone (30 Gy over 2 weeks) or in combination with chemotherapy. The placement of expandable metal stents with Silastic coverings can also palliate dysphagia in patients with metastatic esophageal cancer (Raijman et al, 1998). The endoscope is used to localize the obstructing tumor. A contrast agent is then injected submucosally to delineate the cephalad and caudad extension of cancer, and a wire is passed through the obstruction under direct endoscopic observation. The esophagoscope is then removed, and an expandable wire stent (diameter, 18 mm; length, 10 or 15 cm) with Silastic covering is placed under fluoroscopic guidance. Expandable metal stents with Silastic coverings can also be used to palliate tracheoesophageal fistulas and avoid the need for high-risk surgery in patients with a limited life expectancy.

Asymptomatic metastatic esophageal cancer in patients with good performance status can be treated with chemotherapy alone. A standard regimen given at M. D. Anderson is cisplatin 100 mg/m^2 intravenous piggyback (IVPB) over 1 to 3 hours on day 1 and 5-FU 1,000 mg/m^2/day administered by continuous infusion on days 1 to 5. The cycle is repeated every 4 weeks, and response is evaluated after 2 cycles. An alternative regimen is cisplatin 15 mg/m^2/day IVPB over 1 hour on days 1 to 5, 5-FU 750 mg/m^2/day as a continuous infusion on days 1 to 5, and paclitaxel 175 mg/m^2 IVPB over 3 hours. This alternative regimen is repeated every 4 weeks and can be evaluated for response after 2 cycles. In both of these strategies, the emphasis is on palliation, and a lack of response or worsening physiologic status is a reason to stop therapy. Other supportive agents to consider are agents that stimulate erythropoiesis and granulopoiesis.

CONCLUSIONS

Even though the overall survival rates are still low for patients with esophageal cancer, significant improvements have been made in reducing the morbidity and mortality rates associated with treatment. Treatment should be tailored to the anatomic site of the cancer, clinical stage, and the patient's physiologic status. Early-stage esophageal cancer can be cured in a large percentage of patients with surgery alone or with chemoradiation in those unable to tolerate surgery. Locoregionally advanced esophageal

---

KEY PRACTICE POINTS

- Esophageal cancer is heterogeneous; it can be early-stage (T1N0), locoregionally advanced (T2-4, N1, and M1a), or metastatic (any T, any N, and M1b) at diagnosis.

- The initial assessment of patients with suspected esophageal cancer should focus on obtaining a diagnosis, determining the location and clinical stage of the tumor, and evaluating the physiologic status of the patient.

- Noninvasive tests that are used to assess the clinical stage before treatment include barium swallow, endoscopic ultrasonography, thoracic and abdominal CT, and PET scan. Bone scan and magnetic resonance imaging of the brain should be performed for any symptoms of suspected metastasis.

- In patients with good performance status, surgical resection alone is used for early-stage esophageal cancer; preoperative chemoradiation followed by surgical resection is used for locoregionally advanced disease; and chemotherapy with or without palliative stenting or radiation therapy is used for metastatic esophageal cancer.

- In patients with poor performance status, radiation or chemoradiation is used for early-stage and locoregionally advanced esophageal cancer, and palliative care with stenting or radiation therapy is used for metastatic esophageal cancer.

cancer can be cured in subsets of patients who respond to neoadjuvant chemoradiation followed by surgery or chemoradiation alone in patients unable to tolerate surgery. Metastatic esophageal cancer is seldom cured but can be palliated in many instances by chemotherapy with or without palliative radiation therapy or endoscopic stent placement. Multimodality treatment regimens have provided some hope of survival even in patients with advanced cancer, but this treatment strategy requires careful coordination between specialists in medical oncology, radiation therapy, surgery, and interventional gastroenterology to maximize treatment benefit and minimize treatment-related morbidity. These achievements give hope that further research in the field will yield new strategies to combat this aggressive malignancy.

ACKNOWLEDGMENT

The authors are grateful to Debbie Smith for her assistance in the preparation of this chapter.

SUGGESTED READINGS

Ajani JA, Komaki R, Putnam JB, et al. A three-step strategy of induction chemotherapy then chemoradiation followed by surgery in patients with potentially resectable carcinoma of the esophagus or gastroesophageal junction. *Cancer* 2001;92:279–286.

Ajani JA, Roth JA, Ryan B, et al. Evaluation of pre- and postoperative chemotherapy for resectable adenocarcinoma of the esophagus or gastroesophageal junction. *J Clin Oncol* 1990;8:1231–1238.

Anderson L, Lad TE. Autopsy findings in squamous cell carcinoma of the esophagus. *Cancer* 1982;50:1587–1590.

Ferguson MK, Durkin AE. Preoperative prediction of the risk of pulmonary complications after esophagectomy for cancer. *J Thorac Cardiovasc Surg* 2002;123: 661–669.

Mizuno T, Masaoka A, Ichimura H, et al. Comparison of actual survivorship after treatment with survivorship predicted by actual tumor-volume doubling time from tumor diameter at first observation. *Cancer* 1984;53:2716–2720.

Okawa T, Kita M, Tanaka M, et al. Results of radiotherapy for inoperable locally advanced esophageal cancer. *Int J Radiat Oncol Biol Phys* 1989;17:49–54.

Orringer MB, Marshall B, Stirling MC. Transhiatal esophagectomy for benign and malignant disease. *J Thorac Cardiovasc Surg* 1993;105:265–277.

Raijman I, Siddique I, Ajani J, Lynch P. Palliation of malignant dysphagia and fistulae with coated expandable metal stents: experience with 101 patients. *Gastrointest Endosc* 1998;148:172–179.

Simsek H, Oksuzoglu G, Akhan O. Endoscopic Nd-YAG laser therapy for esophageal wallstent occlusion due to tumor ingrowth. *Endoscopy* 1996;28:400.

Swisher SG, DeFord L, Merriman KW, et al. Effect of operative volume on morbidity, mortality, and hospital use after esophagectomy for cancer. *J Thorac Cardiovasc Surg* 2000;119:1126–1134.

Swisher SG, Holmes C, Hunt KK, et al. The role of neoadjuvant therapy in surgically resectable esophageal cancer. *Arch Surg* 1996;131:819–825.

Swisher SG, Hunt KK, Holmes EC, et al. Changes in the surgical management of esophageal cancer from 1970 to 1993. *Am J Surg* 1995;169:609–614.

Thorban S, Roder JD, Nekarda H, et al. Immunocytochemical detection of disseminated tumor cells in the bone marrow of patients with esophageal carcinoma. *J Natl Cancer Inst* 1996;88:1222–1227.

Vigneswaran WT, Trastek VF, Pairolero PC, et al. Extended esophagectomy in the management of carcinoma of the upper thoracic esophagus. *J Thorac Cardiovasc Surg* 1994;107:901–907.

Wara WM, Mauch PM, Thomas AN, et al. Palliation for carcinoma of the esophagus. *Radiology* 1976;121:717–720.

16 ANAL CANCER

Nora A. Janjan, John M. Skibber,
Miguel A. Rodriguez-Bigas, Christopher Crane,
Marc E. Delclos, Edward H. Lin, and Jaffer A. Ajani

CHAPTER OVERVIEW

Anal cancer is a relatively rare tumor. Despite this, anal cancer has provided a model for organ preservation and combined-modality therapy. Previously, an abdominoperineal resection was the only therapeutic option for anal cancer. Advances in radiation techniques and clinical studies of combined chemotherapy and radiation therapy led to the establishment of chemoradiation as definitive treatment for anal cancer. Surgery is now reserved for recurrent or persistent disease. Functional outcome and quality of life are key issues in anal cancer treatment. Although the total number of patients with anal cancer is small, innovations in the treatment of this disease established therapeutic principles that have been applied in the treatment of nearly every type of cancer.

EPIDEMIOLOGY

Anal cancer is a rare neoplasm, accounting for less than 2% of all cancers of the digestive tract. Despite its rarity, specific risk factors for anal cancer development have been identified. High rates of human papillomavirus (HPV) infection have been observed in anal cancer, and an increased risk of anal HPV infection has been demonstrated in HIV-seropositive patients. An inverse relationship has been shown between the CD4 count and HPV infection. Immunosuppression from other causes, like organ transplantation, increases the risk of anal cancer by a factor of 100. Smoking increases the risk of anal cancer by a factor of 2 to 5; conversely, a prior diagnosis of anal cancer increases the risk of lung cancer by a factor of 2.5.

ANATOMY AND PATTERNS OF DISEASE SPREAD

Anal cancers may arise around the anus or in the anal canal. The anal canal is about 3 to 4 cm long. The anatomy of the anal region is shown in Figure 16–1. A conventional definition classifies cancers that arise above the

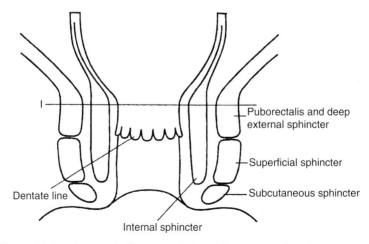

Figure 16–1.   Anatomic diagram of the sphincter muscles of the anus.

dentate (pectinate) line as anal canal tumors and tumors that arise below the dentate line as cancers of the anal margin. The dentate line is a histologic transition zone between squamous and columnar epithelium and designates the location of the anal valves. The anorectal ring is the palpable muscle bundle formed by the upper portion of the internal sphincter, the deep or subcutaneous part of the external sphincter, the puborectalis muscle, and the distal longitudinal muscle from the large bowel. Perianal cancers (cancers of the anal margin) are located within a 5-cm radius around the anal verge in the buttock and the perineal region.

Direct invasion into the sphincteric muscles and perianal connective tissue occurs early. About half of patients will have tumor invasion of the rectum or perianal region. Extensive tumors may infiltrate the sacrum or pelvic sidewalls. Extension to the vagina is common, but invasion of the prostate gland is uncommon.

Both the vascular and lymphatic drainage of the anus is extensive. The arterial supply above the dentate line is from the superior and middle rectal arteries, which are branches of the inferior mesenteric and hypogastric arteries, respectively. Venous drainage is to the portal system. Below the dentate line, the arterial supply is to the middle and inferior rectal arteries, and venous drainage is to the inferior rectal vein.

Although hematogenous dissemination of anal cancer occurs, local and lymphatic extension of disease is more common. Tumors proximal to the dentate line drain to the perirectal, external iliac, obturator, hypogastric, and para-aortic nodal regions. At abdominoperineal resection, about 30% of patients with tumors in the anal canal have pelvic lymph node metastases and 16% have inguinal node metastases. Tumors in the distal anal canal drain to the inguinal-femoral and external and common iliac nodal regions. About 15% to 20% of patients have clinical evidence of inguinal lymph node involvement at presentation, and it is usually unilateral. Inguinal node metastases are evident in 30% of superficial and 63% of deeply infiltrating or poorly differentiated tumors. The inguinal nodes are located within an anatomic region bounded by defined anatomic landmarks (Figure 16–2). The most medial location for the inguinal lymph nodes is 3 cm from the pubic symphysis or midline. From there, they extend to the lateral aspect of the femoral head. The most inferior location is 2.5 cm caudal to the inferior pubic ramus, and the most superior extent is the superior aspect of the femoral head.

Pathology

Two epithelial transition zones occur at the anal region. The first area of transitional epithelium exists between the glandular mucosa of the rectum and the squamous mucosa of the anal region. This transitional epithelium

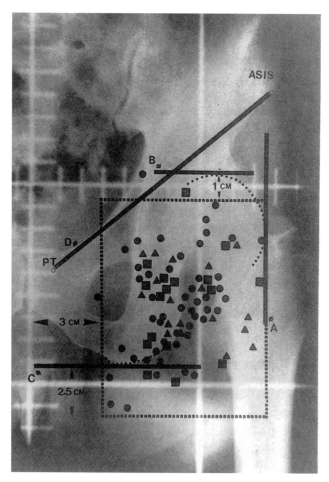

Figure 16–2. X-ray image indicating the anatomic location of the inguinal lymph nodes. Eighty-six percent of the nodes lie within the defined rectangle. PT, pubic tubercle; ASIS, anterior superior iliac spine. Reprinted with permission from Janjan NA, Ballo MT, Delclos ME, Crane CH. The anal region. In: Cox JD, Ang KK, eds. *Radiation Oncology: Rationale, Technique, Results.* 8th ed. St. Louis, MO: Mosby; 2003:537–556.

extends for about 6 to 20 mm and incorporates rectal, urothelial, and squamous elements. The second area of transitional epithelium exists between the squamous epithelium in the anal canal and the skin around the anus; this is a region of modified squamous epithelium, called the pecten. The pectinate (dentate) line is the superior aspect of the pecten. The skin of the perianal region is similar to skin located elsewhere and contains apocrine glands.

Keratinizing squamous cell carcinoma is the most common type of anal cancer in the region distal to the pectinate line. Cancers that develop in the transition zone between squamous and columnar epithelium around the dentate line are usually nonkeratinizing squamous cell carcinomas, and these are often referred to as basaloid or cloacogenic cancers. Both squamous cell carcinomas and cloacogenic tumors should be treated with definitive chemoradiation.

Other histologic subtypes include adenocarcinoma of the anus, small cell carcinoma, and melanoma. All of these histologic subtypes are associated with high rates of local recurrence and disseminated disease. A 1997 National Cancer Data Base report (Myerson et al, 1997) described the differences in anal cancer recurrence rates by histologic subtype and disease stage. Over one fourth of patients with adenocarcinoma develop distant metastases. The risk of local or distant recurrence was twice as high for squamous cell cancers as for adenocarcinomas, but the risk of distant metastasis was more than twice as high for adenocarcinomas as for squamous cell carcinomas (Table 16–1).

CLINICAL PRESENTATION

Bleeding and anal discomfort are the most common symptoms of anal cancer, and they occur in about half of patients. Other complaints include the sensation of a mass in the anus, pruritis, and anal discharge. Although obstructive symptoms can occur with proximal tumors, such symptoms are unusual when the tumor involves the distal anus. Fewer than 5% of patients have sphincteric destruction resulting in fecal incontinence. Vaginal or other fistulas are uncommon. Only 10% of patients are found to have distant metastases at the time of diagnosis. Local relapse is more common than the development of extrapelvic disease. When distant metastases occur, they most commonly are found in the liver and the lungs.

STAGING

The American Joint Committee on Cancer clinical staging system (Table 16–2) is the system most commonly used for carcinomas of the anal canal. Cancers that arise in the anal margin are staged according to the system used for skin cancers.

Table 16-1. Recurrence by Site and "Combined" Stage for 1988 Anal Carcinoma Cases

	Type of Recurrence (%)*			No Recurrence (%)*	Never Disease Free (%)	Total (%)	Total No. of Cases
	Local	Regional	Distant				
All cases	9.2	6.4	16.4	48.7	19.3	100.0	347
Histology							
Epidermoid carcinoma	10.5	7.7	11.8	51.8	18.2	100.0	247
Adenocarcinoma	5.6	3.4	28.1	41.6	21.3	100.0	89
"Combined" stage†							
Stage I	9.8	3.3	8.2	68.9	9.8	100.0	61
Stage II	9.8	16.4	16.4	42.6	14.8	100.0	61
Stage III	4.5	11.1	33.3	20.0	31.1	100.0	45
Stage IV	3.2	0.0	16.1	42.0	38.7	100.0	31

* Recurrence status was unknown for 703 cases, reducing the total number of cases from 1,050 to 347.
† Pathologic stage, augmented by clinical stage where pathologic stage was not available.
Meyerson RJ, Karnell LH, Menck HR. *Cancer*, 80:805–815, 1997. Copyright © 1997 American Cancer Society. Reprinted by permission of John Wiley & Sons, Inc.

Table 16–2. AJCC Staging System for Anal Cancer

	Primary Tumor (T)
TX	Primary tumor cannot be assessed
T0	No evidence of primary tumor
Tis	Carcinoma in situ
T1	Tumor 2 cm or less in greatest dimension
T2	Tumor more than 2 cm but not more than 5 cm in greatest dimensions
T3	Tumor more than 5 cm in greatest dimension
T4	Tumor of any size invades adjacent organs(s), e.g., vagina, urethra, bladder (Note: Direct invasion of the rectal wall, perirectal skin, subcutaneous tissue, or the sphincter muscle[s] is not classified as T4.)

	Regional Lymph Nodes (N)
NX	Regional lymph nodes cannot be assessed
N0	No regional lymph node metastasis
N1	Metastasis in perirectal lymph node(s)
N2	Metastasis in unilateral internal iliac and/or inguinal lymph node(s)
N3	Metastasis in perirectal and inguinal lymph nodes and/or bilateral internal iliac and/or inguinal lymph nodes

	Distant Metastasis (M)
MX	Distant metastasis cannot be assessed
M0	No distant metastasis
M1	Distant metastasis

	Stage Grouping		
Stage 0	Tis	N0	M0
Stage I	T1	N0	M0
Stage II	T2	N0	M0
	T3	N0	M0
Stage IIIA	T1	N1	M0
	T2	N1	M0
	T3	N1	M0
	T4	N0	M0
Stage IIIB	T4	N1	M0
	Any T	N2	M0
	Any T	N3	M0
Stage IV	Any T	Any N	M1

Used with permission of the American Joint Committee on Cancer (AJCC), Chicago, IL. The original source for this material is the AJCC Cancer Staging Manual, Sixth Edition (2002), published by Springer-Verlag New York. www.springer-ny.com.

PROGNOSTIC FACTORS

Tumor size and differentiation and nodal status are the most important prognostic factors in anal cancer. This relationship holds when anal cancer is treated with radiation therapy alone and with chemoradiation. In a study conducted by Grabenbauer et al (1998), disease-free and colostomy-free survival rates after definitive chemoradiation were 87% and 94%, respectively, for T1 and T2 disease versus 59% and 73%, respectively, for T3 and T4 disease. The same trend was seen among 132 patients who underwent abdominoperineal resection (Frost et al, 1984). Five-year survival rates after abdominoperineal resection were 78% for tumors 1 to 2 cm in size, 55% for tumors 3 to 5 cm, and 40% for tumors 6 cm or larger. Nodal disease also influences survival and disease-free survival; the 5-year overall survival rates were 44% among node-positive patients and 74% among node-negative patients (Frost et al, 1984).

COMBINED-MODALITY THERAPY

Combined-modality therapy in the past was defined as the sequential use of surgery, radiation therapy, and chemotherapy. Trials in patients with anal cancer that demonstrated the radiation-sensitizing effects of chemotherapy led to the paradigm of administering chemotherapy during radiotherapy.

Regimens with Radiation plus 5-Fluorouracil and Mitomycin C

The initial experience with combined-modality therapy for anal cancer began in 1974, when Nigro and associates administered radiation with 5-fluorouracil (5-FU) and mitomycin C in 3 patients prior to abdominoperineal resection. The surgical pathology reports in 2 of these patients confirmed a complete response with no evidence of residual tumor; the third patient refused surgery and remained disease free. Subsequent studies with 5-FU and mitomycin C showed durable primary tumor control in 75% to 95% of patients (Table 16–3).

Subsequent trials were conducted by the United Kingdom Coordinating Committee for Cancer Research and the European Organization for Research and Treatment of Cancer. In these studies, summarized in Table 16–4, patients were randomly assigned to radiation therapy alone or combined-modality therapy. The results showed significant improvements in control of the primary tumor and in the colostomy-free survival rate among patients who underwent radiation therapy and chemotherapy, but no improvement in overall survival was observed.

The issue of the most effective combination of chemotherapy with radiation was explored in a Radiation Therapy Oncology Group (RTOG)/Eastern Cooperative Oncology Group (ECOG) prospective randomized trial that compared chemoradiation with 5-FU alone with chemoradiation with 5-FU plus mitomycin C (Flam et al, 1996). Advantages were seen at 4 years' follow-up for the combination chemotherapy arm in terms of the colostomy rate (9% vs 23%), the colostomy-free survival rate (71% vs 59%), and the disease-free survival rate (73% vs 51%). However, no improvement was observed in overall survival, primarily because of

Table 16-3. Selected Studies of Radiation Therapy plus 5-Fluorouracil and Mitomycin C for Anal Cancer

Study	Chemotherapy Dosages 5-Fluorouracil*	Chemotherapy Dosages Mitomycin C	Radiation Therapy (Dose/Fractions/Time)†	Primary Tumor Control Smaller Tumors	Primary Tumor Control Larger Tumors	Serious Complications‡	5-Year Survival Rate
Leichman et al, 1985	1,000 mg/m²/24h IVI days 1–4, 29–32	15 mg/m² IVB day 1	30 Gy/15/days 1–21	31/34 (91%) (≤5 cm)	7/10 (70%) (>5 cm)	NS	80%, crude
Sischy et al, 1989	1,000 mg/m²/24h IVI days 2–5, 28–31	10 mg/m² IVB day 1	40.8 Gy/24/days 1–35	22/26 (85%) (<3 cm)	32/50 (5%) (≥3 cm)	2/79 (3%)	73%, 3-year actuarial
Cummings et al, 1991	1,000 mg/m²/24h IVI days 1–4, 43–46	10 mg/m² IVB days 1 and 43	48 Gy/24/days 1–58 (split course)	15/17 (88%) (≤5 cm)	13/16 (81%) (>5 cm or T4)	1/33 (3%)	65%, actuarial
Cummings et al, 1984	1,000 mg/m²/24h IVI days 1–4, 43–46	10 mg/m² IVB days 1 and 43	50 Gy/20/days 1–56 (split course)	10/10 (100%) (≤5 cm)	3/4 (75%) (>5 cm or T4)	5/14 (36%)	65%, actuarial
Schneider et al, 1992	1,000 mg/m²/24h IVI days 1–4, 29–32	10 mg/m² IVB days 1 and 29	50 Gy/25–28/days 1–35 ± boost	21/22 (95%) (≤5 cm)	14/19 (74%) (>5 cm or T4)	3/41 (7%)	77%, actuarial
Tanum et al, 1991	1,000 mg/m²/24h IVI days 1–4	10–15 mg/m² IVB day 1	50–54 Gy/25–27/days 1–35	28/30 (93%) (≤5 cm)	42/56 (75%) (>5 cm or T4)	14/89 (16%)	72%, actuarial
Cummings et al, 1984	1,000 mg/m²/24h IVI days 1–4	10 mg/m² IVB day 1	50 Gy/20/days 1–28	3/3 (100%) (≤5 cm)	11/13 (85%) (>5 cm or T4)	10/16 (63%)	75%, actuarial
Doci et al, 1996	750 mg/m²/24h IVI (120h) days 1–5, 43–47, 85–89	15 mg/m² IVB days 1, 43, 85	54–60 Gy/30–33/days 1–53 (split course)	28/38 (74%) (≤5 cm)	9/17 (53%) (>5 cm)	2/56 (4%)	81%, actuarial
Papillon et al, 1987	600 mg/m²/24h IVI (120h) days 1–5	12 mg/m² IVB day 1	42 Gy/10/days 1–19 DPF plus interstitial boost 20 Gy day 78	—	57/70 (81%) (≥4 cm)	<5%	NS

Abbreviations: IVI, continuous intravenous infusion; IVB, intravenous bolus injection; NS, not stated; T4, invading adjacent organs; DPF, direct perineal field.

* All infusions were for 96 hours except where otherwise indicated.

† All series except the Papillon et al series used pelvic fields tangential to perineum.

‡ Serious complications were defined as those necessitating surgery or grade 3 or greater.

Reprinted with permission from Cummings (1998).

Table 16–4. Randomized Phase III Trials of Radiation Therapy plus 5-Fluorouracil and Mitomycin C for Anal Cancer

Study Group, First Author, and Year	Treatment Groups	Radiation Dose	Chemotherapy	No. of Eligible Patients	Colostomy-Free Survival Rate	Local Recurrence Rate	Overall Survival Rate
EORTC, Bartelink, 1997	Radiation alone	45 Gy + 15–20 Gy boost if CR or PR	None	103 total	22%	69%	56% (all patients)
	Radiation + 5-FU and Mit C	45 Gy + 15–20 Gy boost if CR or PR	5-FU, 750 mg/m² days 1–5 and 29–33 Mit C, 15 mg/m² day 1	103 total	41% (P = .002)	42% (P = .02)	56% (all patients) NS
UKCCCR, UKCCCR, 1996	Radiation alone	45 Gy + 15–25 Gy boost if CR or PR	None	285	N/A	59%	58% (3-year)
	Radiation + 5-FU and Mit C	45 Gy + 15–25 Gy boost if CR or PR	5-FU, 1,000 mg/m² days 1–4 and 29–32, or 750 mg/m² days 1–5 and 29–33 Mit C, 12 mg/m² day 1	292	N/A	36% (P < .0001)	65% (3-year) NS
RTOG/ECOG, Flam, 1996	Radiation + 5-FU	45 Gy	5-FU 1,000 mg/m² days 1–4 and 28–31	145	59%	36%	67%
	Radiation + 5-FU and Mit C	45 Gy	5-FU 1,000 mg/m² days 1–4 and 28–31 Mit C 10 mg/m² days 1 and 29	146	71% (P = .0019)	18% (P = .0001)	76% (P = .18)

Abbreviations: EORTC, European Organization for Research and Treatment of Cancer; 5-FU, 5-fluorouracil; Mit C, mitomycin C; CR, complete response; PR, partial response; UKCCCR, United Kingdom Coordinating Committee for Cancer Research; N/A, not available; NS, not significant; RTOG, Radiation Therapy Oncology Group; ECOG, Eastern Cooperative Oncology Group.
Modified from Chawla and Willett (2001). Reprinted with permission.

deaths due to hematologic toxicity in the 5-FU/mitomycin C arm (Table 16–4). This trial also showed that interruptions in radiation treatment were associated with lower rates of local control and disease-free survival.

Regimens with Radiation plus 5-Fluorouracil and Cisplatin

Because of concerns regarding severe hematologic and other side effects of mitomycin C, including long-term effects on the lungs, kidneys, and bone marrow, cisplatin has been used in combination with 5-FU in the treatment of anal cancer. Complete response rates of 90% to 95% (Table 16–5) and colostomy-free survival rates of 86% at 3 years have been reported. Hematologic toxicity is significantly less with cisplatin than with mitomycin C. In an ECOG study of radiation therapy plus 5-FU and cisplatin (Martenson et al, 1996), only 1 patient had grade 4 thrombocytopenia, and no patient had a grade 5 hematologic side effect. At M. D. Anderson Cancer Center, no patient has developed a grade 3 or more severe hematologic side effect with infusional cisplatin.

Another study compared radiation alone to radiation and cisplatin (50 mg/m^2) used as a single agent. Local-regional failure rates were 41% in the radiation-alone arm and 23% in the radiation-and-cisplatin arm. A survival benefit was observed with cisplatin used as a single agent: the 2- and 5-year overall survival rates were 46% and 13%, respectively, with radiation alone, and 72% and 36%, respectively, for radiation and cisplatin ($P < .01$). A survival benefit was observed because toxicity was limited with cisplatin.

Other Issues

To summarize, the optimal schedule of chemotherapy and radiation therapy for anal cancer remains undetermined. The total radiation dose necessary to achieve local control is dependent on the bulk of disease. Questions remain regarding the type of chemotherapy that should be administered with radiation. It is clear that 5-FU alone is not as effective as combined chemotherapeutic regimens. However, it is unknown whether an advantage exists for the administration of mitomycin C over cisplatin with 5-FU. The answer to this question will need to be based not only on rates of local control but also on the toxicity profile.

Special Treatment Issues

Posttreatment Biopsy

Patients should have frequent clinical evaluations after chemoradiation for anal cancer. The determination of persistent or progressive disease should be based on clinical evaluation. Biopsies should be avoided unless the information will directly affect clinical decision-making.

Table 16–5. Randomized Phase III Trials of Radiation Therapy plus 5-Fluorouracil and Cisplatin for Anal Cancer

Study	Chemotherapy		Radiation Therapy (Dose/Fractions/Time)	No. of Patients with Primary Tumor Complete Response/Total No. of Patients (%)	Survival Rate
	5-Fluorouracil	Cisplatin			
Concurrent Therapy					
Wagner et al, 1994	1,000 mg/m²/24 h IVI (96 h) days 1–4	25 mg/m² IVB days 2–5	42 Gy/10/days 1–19 plus interstitial boost days 63–64	47/51 (92%)	Approx. 75% 5 years
Martenson et al, 1996	1,000 mg/m²/24 h IVI (96 h) days 43–46	75 mg/m² IVB days 1 and 43	59.4 Gy/33/days 1–59 (split after 36 Gy)	14/17 (82%)	Not stated
Rich et al, 1993	300 mg/m²/24 h IVI 5 days (120 h)/wk days 1–42	4 mg/m² IVB days 1–42, 5 days/wk	45–54 Gy/25–30/days 1–42	20/21 (95%)	91% 2-year actuarial
Induction Therapy					
Brunet et al, 1990	1,000 mg/m²/24 h IVI (120 h) days 2–6; repeat cycles, days 22, 43	100 mg/m² IVB days 1, 22, 43	45 Gy/25/days 64–69 plus boost	17/19 (89%)	No cancer deaths, 10–40 months
Svensson et al, 1993	1,000 mg/m²/24 h IVI (120 h) days 1–5; repeat cycles, days 29, 57	300–350 mg/m² IVB days 1, 29, 57*	66 Gy/33/days 79–125	6/6 (100%)	No recurrences, 8–21 months
Alternating Therapy					
Roca et al, 1990	750 mg/m²/24 h IVI (120 h) days 2–7, 23–28	50 mg/m² IVB days 1–2, 22–23	20 Gy/10/days 8–21, 29–42 plus boost	18/25 (72%)	87% 5-year actuarial

Abbreviations: IVI, continuous intravenous infusion; IVB, intravenous bolus injection.
* Carboplatin rather than cisplatin.
Reprinted with permission from Cummings (1998).

A biopsy was required 6 weeks after radiation therapy in the RTOG/ ECOG study (Flam et al, 1996). Biopsies revealed cancer in 15% of patients treated with 5-FU alone versus 8% who received 5-FU and mitomycin C. If the biopsy revealed disease, an additional 9 Gy in 5 fractions was given with a 4-day infusion of 5-FU ($1,000 \, mg/m^2$) and a single injection of cisplatin ($100 \, mg/m^2$). Half of the 24 patients treated were rendered disease free. However, another study (Miller et al, 1991) found that only half of the patients who had persistently positive biopsy findings after treatment developed progressive disease. It was the authors' conclusion that a positive biopsy after completion of chemoradiation does not always represent a viable tumor and that a positive biopsy alone should not prompt the recommendation of an abdominoperineal resection. Also, administering a delayed boost of radiation, as was done in the RTOG/ECOG study (Flam et al, 1996), may not provide any benefit to a patient whose residual tumor is not viable, and the additional chemoradiation may unnecessarily increase toxicity. Furthermore, repeated biopsies traumatize the irradiated tissues and create a risk for infection, a chronic wound due to delayed healing, and fistula formation.

Treatment of the Elderly and Patients with Comorbid Conditions

Treatment of the elderly and patients with comorbid conditions raises concerns regarding tolerance of chemoradiation. In our experience, full therapy can be administered without significant side effects if close attention is paid to the patient's clinical status during the course of therapy, especially to the fluid and electrolyte status. This involves proactive care, including administration of growth factors to avoid neutropenia, infusion therapy for fluid and electrolyte replacement, nutritional support, and attention to skin care to avoid infection. Using this approach, therapy can be completed in more than 95% of elderly patients, and no differences between elderly patients and younger patients are seen in local control or survival parameters.

Treatment of HIV-Positive Patients

Tolerance of therapy is a significant consideration among HIV-positive patients with invasive anal cancer. Excessive mucosal reactions from radiation and significant cytopenia have been reported during treatment among HIV-positive patients, especially those with a CD4 count less than $200 \, cells/mm^3$. Acceptable toxicity and a 100% complete response rate have been reported among HIV-positive patients with the use of lower doses of radiation (30 Gy in 15 fractions) and mitomycin C ($10 \, mg/m^2$) plus standard doses of 5-FU.

Anal Margin

The anal margin is considered by some to be an anatomically distinct region. The anal margin includes the anal verge and the perianal tissues around the anal canal. Squamous cancers in this region are staged like skin cancers and generally have a good prognosis. Most are well differentiated and keratinized. Visceral metastases are rare, and inguinal metastases are uncommon. Management is dependent on location, tumor extent, and patient factors. Treatment can include local excision or radiation therapy; abdominoperineal resection should be reserved for patients with fecal incontinence at presentation or locally recurrent disease. Local excision is sufficient for T1 lesions, but pelvic and inguinal node irradiation is indicated for T2 lesions. Chemotherapy should be included with radiation for T3 and T4 tumors.

DEFINITIVE CHEMORADIATION

Two basic principles are critical in the treatment of anal cancer. First, a dose-response relationship based on clonogenic burden has been demonstrated. Second, computed tomography–based treatment planning is imperative in patients with inguinal node involvement given the significant range in the depth of the inguinal nodes due to variations in patient anatomy.

A first principle of radiation oncology is that larger tumor volumes require higher total doses of radiation to be controlled. There is evidence of a dose-response relationship based on treatment techniques. In the RTOG/ECOG trial (Flam et al, 1996), the superior border of the radiation field was shifted down from the L5-S1 interspace to the inferior aspect of the sacroiliac joints after 30.6 Gy was given with conventional fractionation (Figure 16–3; no local failures occurred in this area even though only 30.6 Gy was delivered. Uninvolved inguinal nodes, which received a total radiation dose of 36 Gy delivered with reduced radiation fields, also were locally controlled. The M. D. Anderson experience (Janjan et al, 1999; Hung et al, 2001) also provides evidence that 30 Gy with conventional fraction-

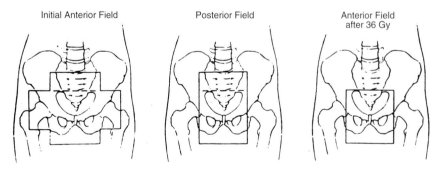

Figure 16–3. The treatment portals used for high-dose radiation therapy in the Radiation Therapy Oncology Group trials. Modified from Martenson et al (1996). Reprinted with permission.

ation may be sufficient to control microscopic disease. The local failure rate was less than 5% among patients with clinically uninvolved inguinal nodes who received 30 Gy.

The M. D. Anderson Technique

On the basis of existing evidence and in an attempt to minimize treatment-related side effects, at M. D. Anderson we administer cisplatin (4 mg/m²/day) and 5-FU (250 mg/m²/day) as a continuous infusion 5 days per week throughout the radiation therapy course.

The radiation course is as follows. First, 30.6 Gy is administered at 1.8 Gy per fraction with anteroposterior-posteroanterior portals that include the inguinal region (Figure 16–4A). An additional 19.8 Gy is then administered to the pelvis using a 3-field technique that includes the use of a belly board (Figure 16–4B) (see also Figure 10–4 for a schematic diagram of the belly board technique). The treatment portals are weighed posteroanterior (2): right lateral (1): left lateral (1), and the radiation dose is prescribed to the 95% isodose curve. As in the RTOG/ECOG trial (Flam et al, 1996), a field reduction is performed, and the superior border of the radiation portal is placed at the inferior aspect of the sacroiliac joints (Figure 16–4B).

A localized boost to the primary tumor is then administered with the 3-field belly board technique, giving an additional dose of 4.6 Gy in 2 fractions. Dosimetry shows that 30 Gy is given to the volume between L5-S1 and the inferior aspect of the sacroiliac joints and to the inguinal region. The lower pelvis receives 50.4 Gy, and the primary tumor receives 55 Gy (Figure 16–5). A supplemental dose of radiation, to a total dose of 55 Gy, is given only to treat clinically involved inguinal nodes. The electron energy is selected from computed tomography–based treatment planning. Since the contribution to the inguinal region from the 3-field belly board technique is negligible, conventional fractionation is used for the electron-beam radiation that is directed to the inguinal region.

A retrospective analysis was performed among 92 patients with M0 squamous cell carcinoma of the anus treated at M. D. Anderson between 1989 and 1998 (Hung et al, 2003). By American Joint Committee on Cancer criteria, 10 patients had T1, 43 had T2, 27 had T3, and 12 had T4 disease.

Figure 16–4. Radiation treatment portals used at M. D. Anderson. (*A*) The anterior/posterior fields used. (*B* and *C*) Field reductions used with the three-field belly board technique. The superior border of the pelvic field now is at the inferior border of the sacroiliac joint. (*C*) Lateral fields used during the belly board technique. The last 4.6 Gy (given in two fractions) is given to a localized boost field using posterior and lateral fields. (*D*) The anterior portal. Modified from Janjan NA, Ballo MT, Delclos ME, Crane CH. The anal region. In: Cox JD, Ang KK, eds. *Radiation Oncology: Rationale, Technique, Results.* 8th ed. St. Louis, MO: Mosby; 2003:537–556. Reprinted with permission.

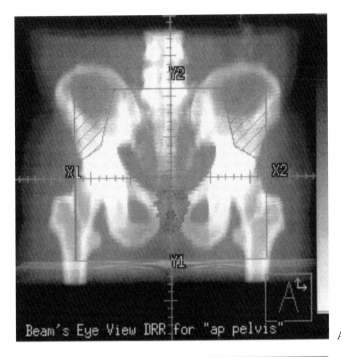

Beam's Eye View DRR for "ap pelvis"   A

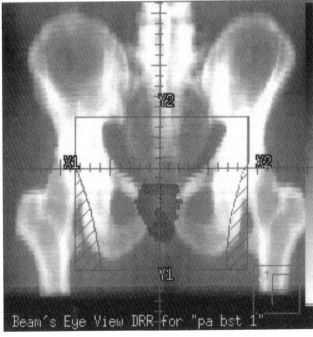

Beam's Eye View DRR for "pa bst 1"   B

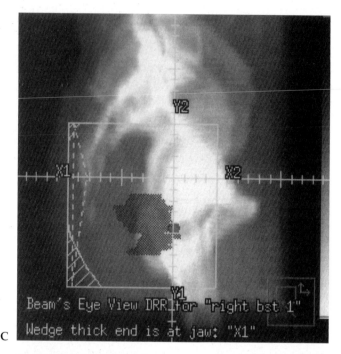

C

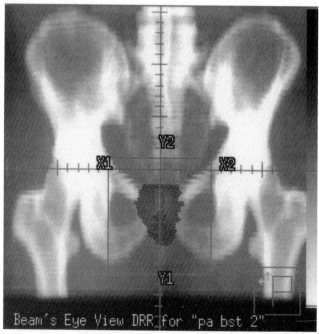

D

Figure 16–4. *Continued*

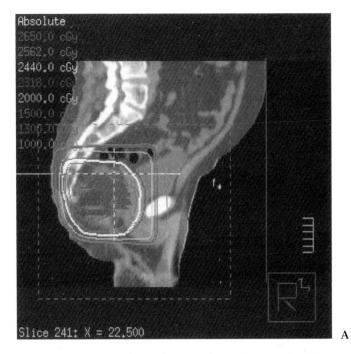

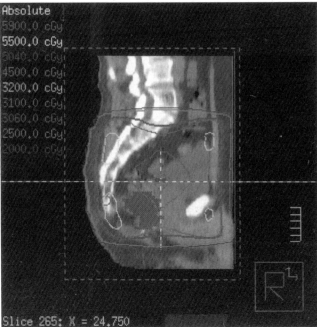

Figure 16–5. Dosimetry of the M. D. Anderson technique. (*A*) Total radiation dose of 24.4 Gy to the primary tumor from the belly board fields (19.8 Gy from the reduced pelvic field and 4.6 Gy from the boost field). When the 30.6 Gy from the initial irradiation and the 24.4 Gy from the belly board fields are combined, the primary tumor receives a total radiation dose of 55 Gy (*B*). Note that the bladder is spared with the 3-field belly board technique.

Seventy-one percent of the patients (n = 65) were node negative; 7 patients had N1 disease, 13 had N2 disease, and 7 had N3 disease. The actuarial 5-year disease-free survival rate was 77%, and the sphincter preservation rate was 83%. Consistent with other reports, local control rates were influenced by T classification and were 100% for T1, 88% for T2, 75% for T3, and 60% for T4 tumors. Local recurrences occurred in 16 patients (17%). Salvage surgery was performed in 13 of these 16 patients, and all of these patients were alive at the time of this writing. Distant metastases occurred in 8 patients (9%); 2 of these patients were rendered free of disease and 1 patient was still alive at the time of this writing. In 90% of cases, local relapses occurred within 13 months and distant relapses occurred within 10 months after completion of therapy. As in other series, the disease-free survival rate was dependent on tumor stage: 100% for T1, 81% for T2, 71% for T3, and 50% for T4 tumors. Of the known prognostic factors, only T classification was predictive of overall survival ($P = .05$).

Treatment Interruptions and Management of Treatment-Related Side Effects

The toxicity of therapy for anal cancer can be significant. However, the consequence of local failure, a colostomy, is also profound. Expert medical management is needed to control the side effects of chemoradiation in anal cancer. Two issues, time-dose considerations and total dose, have been shown to significantly affect the results of treatment in anal cancer.

Time-dose considerations are directly affected by the adequacy of medical management of side effects. In the initial phase of the RTOG/ECOG study (Flam et al, 1996), treatment interruptions were associated with a 23% local failure and colostomy rate. When the planned treatment interruption was eliminated, the local failure and colostomy rate decreased to 11%. However, half of the patients required unplanned toxicity-related interruptions, and the median length of these interruptions was 11 days. Uninterrupted radiation therapy consisting of 50 Gy in 20 fractions with 5-FU and mitomycin C resulted in improved rates of local control, but acute and late side effects were increased. The daily radiation dose was then decreased to 2 Gy per fraction, and an interruption in treatment was planned; these measures decreased treatment-related side effects but also significantly decreased local control rates.

When mitomycin C was omitted from the chemotherapeutic regimen, hematologic side effects were significantly reduced, but local control rates were also compromised. Pretreatment hemoglobin levels of less than 100 g/L were also associated with a worse treatment outcome. Local control rates were improved with radiation doses of greater than 54 Gy and with overall treatment times of less than 40 days. On multivariate analysis, radiation dose and hemoglobin level independently influenced local control, radiation dose influenced disease-free survival, and radiation dose, hemoglobin level, T classification, and HIV status influenced overall survival. Therefore, outcomes are dependent on optimizing radiation dose and chemotherapy and on minimizing treatment-related side effects.

Aggressive medical management is required to prevent and treat the expected side effects of definitive chemoradiation for anal cancer. Supportive care measures can prevent treatment interruption and improve outcomes of therapy. Aggressive supportive care is required both during therapy and after the completion of therapy.

With attentive medical management, fewer than 5% of patients at M. D. Anderson treated with infusional 5-FU and cisplatin have required a treatment interruption. At the first signs of dry desquamation, which generally occur during the end of the second week of radiation therapy, emollients like Aquaphor (Beiersdorf AG) should be used in the inguinal region, and barrier creams like Lantiseptic's Skin Protectant (Marietta, GA) should be used in the perianal region. The barrier cream is especially important to help prevent secondary infection from fecal bacteria. Moist desquamation frequently occurs in the intergluteal region and along the inguinal folds. Sulfadiazine (Silvadene) cream also acts as a barrier cream and can be applied to areas of moist desquamation. Products that act as a skin, like the hydrogel sheet dressing from Vigilon (Bard, Murray Hill, NJ), can be placed over the affected area to prevent secondary infection and trauma and provide a soothing dressing. Secondary infections, especially candidiasis, must be treated. Sitz baths with Domeboro, an aluminum acetate solution (Bayer Corporation, Pittsburgh, PA), help patients maintain good hygiene, improve healing of areas with moist desquamation, and provide comfort during and after therapy. The inguinal region must also be kept clean with warm soaks, and Domeboro may also be used in this area. In addition to the use of barrier creams, warm water can be sprayed over the perineum during urination to avoid pain caused by acidic urine making contact with the skin.

Pain with these skin reactions can be significant. The pain can occur with urination, defecation, and movement because of reactions in the perineal region. The constipating effects of opioid analgesics can also be exploited to control frequent stooling associated with pelvic irradiation and chemotherapy. Frequently stooling and pain can be controlled with a defined 3-step bowel management program (described in detail in chapter 19) that includes the use of antidiarrheal agents—like the combination of diphenoxylate hydrochloride and atropine sulfate (Lomotil) or loperamide (Imodium)—and opioid analgesics. The goal is for the patient to have 3 or fewer stools per day. This is important to avoid fluid and electrolyte imbalances and reduce trauma and possible infection in the perianal region. In this 3-step bowel management program, in response to the initial symptoms, antidiarrheal agents are used as needed. When the patient requires antidiarrheal agents at least 3 times per day, they are then administered on a scheduled basis (1 to 2 tablets 3 to 4 times a day). If symptoms persist, opioid analgesics are given. For patient convenience and to avoid episodic diarrhea, a long-acting analgesic preparation is preferred. Principles used in pain management are applied. Short-acting analgesics should also be available until the dose of long-acting analgesic is established; the analgesics should be titrated to effect. In general, short-acting analgesics that contain acetaminophen should be avoided because of the potential for renal and hepatic side effects, particularly when acetaminophen is administered in conjunction with cisplatin, and the possibility of masking of fever from an infection. For procedural pain or for pain related to defecation or urination, oral fentanyl, which is rapidly absorbed through the mucous membranes, is of particular benefit.

Blood counts need to be closely monitored, and administration of cytokines should be considered, especially if mitomycin C is given, to avoid treatment interruption and side effects. Profound fatigue can occur during chemoradiation. This can affect nutrition and result in fluid and electrolyte imbalances as well. During administration of cisplatin, the magnesium levels must also be closely monitored because of the magnesium wasting that can occur with cisplatin administration.

Follow-Up Evaluations

Close follow-up is necessary after completion of chemoradiation until re-epithelialization is complete. During this time, patients must be evaluated for symptom control, infection, and blood counts, and the fluid and electrolyte status must be closely monitored. Response to therapy can be monitored during this time, but biopsy of a residual abnormality is discouraged when tumor regression continues to be evident. Fatigue may also be present for several months after completion of therapy. Treatable causes of fatigue, like anemia and hypothyroidism, should be excluded. Long-term bowel management strategies should be pursued, especially with the scheduled use of antidiarrheal agents and fluid management to maximize control and improve quality of life (see chapter 19 for additional information).

Excellent long-term functional outcomes are achieved after definitive chemoradiation among patients who are rendered free of disease and who have limited presenting symptoms. Ten-year follow-up of patients who received combined-modality therapy in the RTOG/ECOG study (John et al, 1996) showed low rates of side effects. Only 4 patients (12%) had a grade 3 or 4 side effect (Table 16–6). Twenty-nine percent of patients had no long-term sequelae, and 58% had either a grade 1 or 2 side effect as their most severe side effect. These side effects involved the skin, anus, and bowel. If anorectal dysfunction occurs after chemoradiation, it is related to sensory and motor abnormalities in the external anal sphincter muscle, a reduced rectal reservoir, and impaired sensory function in the anorectal region.

Table 16–6. Incidence of Late Side Effects from Chemoradiation in 34 Patients with Anal Cancer*

Toxicity	No. (%) of Patients with Side Effects				
	Grade 0	Grade 1	Grade 2	Grade 3	Grade 4
Small or large intestine	17 (50)	9 (26)	7 (20)	1 (3)	0
Skin	24 (70)	4 (12)	3 (9)	1 (3)	2 (6)
Anal canal	18 (53)	5 (15)	10 (29)	1 (3)	0
Worst side effect	10 (29)	10 (29)	10 (29)	2 (6)	2 (6)

* In addition to the side effects listed above, 1 patient developed ureteral stenosis, and 1 patient developed uterine prolapse.

Reprinted with permission from John et al (1996).

KEY PRACTICE POINTS

- Definitive chemoradiation permits sphincter preservation with good functional outcomes in most patients with anal cancer.

- The optimal schedule of chemotherapy and radiation therapy for anal cancer remains undetermined. The total radiation dose necessary to achieve local control depends on the bulk of disease. It is clear that 5-FU is not as effective as combined chemotherapeutic regimens.

- Treatment-related side effects that cause treatment interruptions can compromise local control. Aggressive supportive care and clinical strategies are imperative.

- Patients should have frequent clinical evaluations after chemoradiation for anal cancer. The determination of persistent or progressive disease should be based on clinical evaluation. Biopsies should be avoided unless this information will directly affect clinical decision-making.

- Salvage surgery should not be pursued unless there is clinical evidence of disease progression.

SURGICAL SALVAGE

Abdominoperineal resection is essential for surgical salvage therapy in patients with anal cancer. About 50% of patients with isolated disease recurrence can be rendered disease free. In a study by Allal et al (1999a), 42 patients with local failure were treated with supportive care (n = 16) or curative resection (n = 26). The overall 5-year survival rate was 28%, but the 5-year survival rate among the patients who underwent abdominoperineal resection was almost 45%. Salvage surgery should not be pursued unless there is clinical evidence of disease progression.

Suggested Readings

Allal AS, Laurencet FM, Reymond MA, et al. Effectiveness of surgical salvage therapy for patients with locally uncontrolled anal carcinoma after sphincter-conserving treatment. *Cancer* 1999a;86:405–409.

Allal AS, Obradovic M, Laurencet F, et al. Treatment of anal carcinoma in the elderly: feasibility and outcome of radical radiotherapy with or without concomitant chemotherapy. *Cancer* 1999b;85:26–31.

Allal AS, Sprangers MA, Laurencet F, Reymond MA, Kurtz JM. Assessment of long-term quality of life in patients with anal carcinomas treated by radiotherapy with or without chemotherapy. *Br J Cancer* 1999c;80:1588–1594.

Bartelink H, Roelofsen F, Eschwege F, et al. Concomitant radiotherapy and chemotherapy is superior to radiotherapy alone in the treatment of locally advanced anal cancer: results of a phase III randomized trial of the European Organization for Research and Treatment of Cancer Radiotherapy and Gastrointestinal Cooperative Groups. *J Clin Oncol* 1997;15:2040–2049.

Brunet R, Becouarn Y, Pigneux J, et al. Cisplatine et fluorouracile en chimiotherapie neoadjuvante des carcinomas epidemoides du canal anal. *Lyon Chirurgical* 1990;87:77.

Chawla AK, Willett CH. Squamous cell carcinoma of the anal canal and anal margin. *Hematol Oncol Clin North Am* 2001;15:321–344.

Cleator S, Fife K, Nelson M, Gazzard B, Phillips R, Bower M. Treatment of HIV-associated invasive anal cancer with combined chemoradiation. *Eur J Cancer* 2000;36:754–758.

Constantinou EC, Daly W, Fung CY, Willett CG, Kaufman DS, DeLaney TF. Time-dose considerations in the treatment of anal cancer. *Int J Radiat Oncol Biol Phys* 1997;39:651–657.

Cummings BJ. Anal canal. In: Perez CW, Brady LW, eds. *Principles and Practice of Radiation Oncology.* 3rd ed. Philadelphia, Pa: Lippincott-Raven; 1998:1511–1524.

Cummings BJ, Keane TJ, O'Sullivan B, Wong CS, Catton CN. Epidermoid anal cancer: treatment by radiation alone or by radiation and 5-fluorouracil with and without mitomycin C. *Int J Radiat Oncol Biol Phys* 1991;21:1115–1125.

Cummings BJ, Keane TJ, Thomas GM, et al. Results and toxicity of the treatment of anal canal carcinoma by radiation therapy or radiation therapy and chemotherapy. *Cancer* 1984;54:2062–2068.

Doci R, Zucoli R, LaMonica G, et al. Primary chemoradiation therapy with fluorouracil and cisplatin for cancer of the anus: results in 35 consecutive patients. *J Clin Oncol* 1996;14:3121–3125.

Flam MS, John M, Pajak TF, et al. Role of mitomycin in combination with fluorouracil and radiotherapy and of salvage chemoradiation in the definitive non-surgical treatment of epidermoid carcinoma of the anal canal: results of a phase III randomized intergroup study. *J Clin Oncol* 1996;14:2527–2539.

Frost DB, Richards PC, Montague ED, et al. Epidermoid cancer of the anorectum. *Cancer* 1984;53:1285–1293.

Gerard JP, Ayzac L, Hun D, et al. Treatment of anal canal carcinoma with high dose radiation therapy and concomitant fluorouracil-cisplatinum. Long term results in 95 patients. *Radiother Oncol* 1998;46:249–256.

Grabenbauer GG, Matzel KE, Schneider IH, et al. Sphincter preservation with chemoradiation in anal canal carcinoma: abdominoperineal resection in selected cases? *Dis Colon Rectum* 1998;41:441–450.

Greene FL, Page DL, Fleming ED, Fritz AG, Balch CM, Haller DG, Morrow M, eds. *AJCC Cancer Staging Manual*. 6th ed. New York, NY: Springer-Verlag New York, Inc.; 2002:129–130.

Hoffman R, Welton ML, Klencke B, et al. The significance of pretreatment CD4 count on the outcome and treatment tolerance of HIV-positive patients with anal cancer. *Int J Radiat Oncol Biol Phys* 1999;44:127–131.

Hu K, Minsky BD, Cohen AM, et al. 30 Gy may be an adequate dose in patients with anal cancer treated with excisional biopsy followed by combined-modality therapy. *J Surg Oncol* 1999;70:71–77.

Hung AV, Ballo MT, Crane C, et al. Platinum-based combined modality therapy for anal carcinoma [abstract]. *Proceedings of the American Society of Clinical Oncology* 2001;19:A679.

Hung A, Crane C, Delclos M, et al. Cisplatin-based combined modality therapy for anal carcinoma—a wider therapeutic index. *Cancer* 2003;97:1195–1202.

Janjan NA, Crane CH, Ajani J, et al. 30 Gy is a sufficient dose to control micrometastases from anal cancer—dosimetric evaluation of N0 patients undergoing chemoradiation. *Cancer J* 1999;5:117. Abstract 11.

John M, Flam M, Palma N. Ten-year results of chemoradiation for anal cancer: focus on late morbidity. *Int J Radiat Oncol Biol Phys* 1996;34:65–69.

John MJ, Pajak TJ, Flam MS, et al. Dose escalation in chemoradiation for anal cancer: preliminary results of RTOG 92–08. *Cancer J* 1996;2:205–211.

Joon DL, Chao MWT, Ngan SYK, Joon ML, Guiney MJ. Primary adenocarcinoma of the anus: a retrospective analysis. *Int J Radiat Oncol Biol Phys* 1999;45:1199–1205.

Leichman L, Nigro N, Vaitkevicius VK, et al. Cancer of the anal canal. Model for preoperative adjuvant combined modality therapy. *Am J Med* 1985;78:211–215.

Martenson JA Jr, Gunderson LL. External radiation therapy without chemotherapy in the management of anal cancer. *Cancer* 1993;71:1736–1740.

Martenson JA, Lipsitz SR, Wagner H, et al. Initial results of a phase II trial of high dose radiation therapy, 5-fluorouracil and cisplatin for patients with anal cancer (E4292): an Eastern Cooperative Oncology Group study. *Int J Radiat Oncol Biol Phys* 1996;35:745–749.

Mendenhall WM, Zlotecki RA, Vauthey JN, Copeland EM. Squamous cell carcinoma of the anal margin. *Oncology* 1996;10:1843–1854.

Miller EJ, Quan SH, Thaler T. Treatment of squamous cell carcinoma of the anal canal. *Cancer* 1991;67:2038–2041.

Myerson RJ, Karnell LH, Menck HR. The National Cancer Data Base report on carcinoma of the anus. *Cancer* 1997;80:805–815.

Nigro N, Vaitkevicius V, Considine B. Combined therapy for cancer of the anal canal: a preliminary report. *Dis Colon Rectum* 1974;15:354–356.

Papillon J, Montbarbon JF. Epidermoid carcinoma of the anal canal. A series of 276 cases. *Dis Colon Rectum* 1987;30:324–333.

Peddada AV, Smith DE, Rao AR, et al. Chemotherapy and low-dose radiotherapy in the treatment of HIV-infected patients with carcinoma of the anal canal. *Int J Radiat Oncol Biol Phys* 1997;37:1101–1105.

Rich T, Ajani JA, Morrison WH, et al. Chemoradiation therapy for anal cancer. Radiation plus continuous infusion of 5-fluorouracil with or without cisplatin. *Radiother Oncol* 1993;27:209–215.

Roca E, De Simone G, Barugel M, et al. A phase II study of alternating chemoradiotherapy including cisplatin in anal canal carcinoma [abstract]. *Proceedings of the American Society of Clinical Oncology* 1990;9:128.

Roelofsen F, Bosset JF, Eschwege F, et al. Concomitant radiotherapy and chemotherapy are superior to radiotherapy alone in the treatment of locally advanced anal cancer: results of a phase III randomized trial of the EORTC Radiotherapy and Gastrointestinal Cooperative Group [abstract]. *Proc Am Soc Clin Oncol* 1995;14:194.

Schneider IHF, Grabenbauer GG, Reck T, et al. Combined radiation and chemotherapy for epidermoid carcinoma of the anal canal. *Int J Colorectal Dis* 1992;7:192–196.

Sischy B, Doggett RLS, Krall JM, et al. Definitive irradiation and chemotherapy for radiosensitization in management of anal carcinoma: interim report on Radiation Therapy Oncology Group study no. 8314. *J Natl Cancer Inst* 1989;81:850–856.

Svensson C, Goldman S, Friberg B. Radiation treatment of epidermoid cancer of the anus. *Int J Radiat Oncol Biol Phys* 1993;27:67–73.

Tanum G, Tveit K, Karlsen KO, et al. Chemoradiotherapy and radiation therapy for anal carcinoma. Survival and late morbidity. *Cancer* 1991;67:2462–2466.

UKCCCR Anal Cancer Trial Working Party. Epidermoid anal cancer: results from the UKCCCR randomized trial of radiotherapy alone versus radiotherapy, 5-fluorouracil, and mitomycin. *Lancet* 1996;348:1049–1054.

Wagner JP, Mahe MA, Romestaing P, et al. Radiation therapy in the conservative treatment of carcinoma of the anal canal. *Int J Radiat Oncol Biol Phys* 1994;29:17–23.

17 GASTROINTESTINAL STROMAL TUMORS

Dejka M. Steinert and Jonathan Trent

CHAPTER OVERVIEW

Over the past 60 years, basic scientists, pathologists, and clinical investigators have studied gastrointestinal stromal tumors (GISTs), with no major advances in patient care. Recent discoveries have led to an understanding of the biological role of Kit in GISTs and the development of one of the most exciting examples of targeted therapy to date. The success of the Kit tyrosine kinase inhibitor imatinib mesylate (Gleevec) has caught the attention of the medical community. Understanding the mechanisms of response and resistance to imatinib will broaden our understanding of cancer biology and lead to strategic approaches in the treatment of other malignancies. This understanding will take place more rapidly with faster patient accrual to clinical trials, such as those designed at M. D. Anderson Cancer Center. Thus, all oncologists should do their best to place their patients with GISTs on clinical trials.

INTRODUCTION

Gastrointestinal (GI) stromal tumors (GISTs) are typically spindle-shaped neoplasms of the GI tract that may also be described as epithelioid or pleomorphic. In the 1940s, GISTs were designated as smooth muscle tumors of the GI tract (GI leiomyosarcoma, leiomyoblastoma, leiomyosarcoma, and leiomyoma). Electron microscopy later provided ultrastructural evidence that GISTs were not of smooth muscle origin. Gottlieb et al (1974) at M. D. Anderson Cancer Center observed that leiomyosarcomas originating from the GI tract do not respond to conventional chemotherapy, whereas those arising from other organ systems are more likely to respond to doxorubicin-based therapies. Our understanding of the responses of GISTs was refined by others, and it became clear that patients with GISTs had poor response rates not only to standard therapy but also to a number of investigational agents.

Most mesenchymal tumors of the GI tract are GISTs and express the Kit receptor (stem cell factor receptor, CD117) as shown by immunohistochemical analysis. Since most GI smooth muscle tumors are GISTs, the published data from older clinical trials of smooth muscle tumors are largely representative of GISTs. GISTs account for approximately 2% of all stomach cancers, 14% of all small-intestine tumors, and 0.1% of colon cancers. A recent increase in the number of GISTs diagnosed is the result of increased recognition of this entity and use of immunohistochemical analysis to detect the Kit receptor in tumors from patients with intra-abdominal sarcomas.

The incidence of GIST in the United States, previously thought to be 300 to 500 cases per year, is now believed to be 5,000 to 6,000 cases annually (Fletcher et al, 2002). GIST is equally prevalent in men and women, and its incidence peaks in the fourth through sixth decades of life. Most patients with GIST are white; fewer than 10% are black or Hispanic. GISTs arise most commonly in the stomach (60% to 70% of GISTs), small intestine (20% to 30%), colon and rectum (5%), and esophagus (<5%), although they can arise anywhere along the GI tract. Omental or mesenteric GISTs have been reported as primary but may represent a metastatic tumor arising from an occult primary tumor; it is not unusual for the primary site of an extensively metastatic GIST to remain occult. About a third of patients with GISTs present with metastases or unresectable disease. The most common sites of metastases are the liver, peritoneum, and abdominal wall. Metastases involving the central nervous system, lymph nodes, lung, and bone have been reported but are exceedingly rare in our experience. In 191 patients with GIST at M. D. Anderson, as many as 47% had invasion of adjacent organs, peritoneal sarcomatosis, or metastasis at presentation (Ng et al, 1992a,b). There are no known environmental risk factors for GIST.

FAMILIAL SYNDROMES ASSOCIATED WITH GIST

GIST has been defined as a component of several familial syndromes. The Carney triad is an association of GIST, functioning extra-adrenal paraganglioma, and pulmonary chondroma. This triad is thought to be hereditary because affected patients are often young and the tumors are multifocal, although the precise germline abnormality remains elusive. It was first described in 7 unrelated young females (Carney et al, 1977). A later report (Carney, 1999) described 79 patients (12 male and 67 female) with the Carney triad. Twenty percent of the patients had all 3 of the tumor types, and the remainder had 2 of the 3. Only 2 of the 79 patients, however, had family members with any of these tumors, suggesting that the Carney triad does not follow a simple mode of inheritance. A yet later report (Carney and Stratakis, 2002) suggested that a heritable syndrome of paraganglioma and GIST distinct from the Carney triad may exist. In that study, 12 patients (7 males and 5 females; mean age, 23 years) from 5 unrelated families manifested paraganglioma, GIST, or both. The tumors were inherited in an apparently autosomal dominant manner, with incomplete penetrance. Seven patients had paraganglioma, 4 had paraganglioma and GIST, and 1 had GIST. The paragangliomas were multicentric, and the GISTs were multifocal.

A familial syndrome of dysphagia with multiple GISTs was recently reported (Hirota et al, 2000). Family members with the germline *kit* mutation reported dysphagia, with uncoordinated contractions of the esophagus without normal peristalsis, but those without the mutation did not. A mutation at Asp-820 in the tyrosine kinase II domain of the *kit* oncogene was found in both tumors and normal tissue. Mutations in the tyrosine kinase II domain had not previously been found in GISTs, and this was the first report of GISTs with tyrosine kinase II domain mutations.

Commonality of specific mutations among patients with GISTs and their family members has been reported. One report described 2 siblings with cutaneous hyperpigmentation since their late teens who developed multiple GISTs by 45 years of age. These tumors were Kit and CD34 positive and encoded a mutation at codon 559 of exon 11. The same point mutation was found in peripheral leukocytes obtained from the patients' older sister, younger sister, and younger sister's 2 children (Maeyama et al, 2001).

In a separate family, a mother and daughter had hyperplasia of the interstitial cells of Cajal and had multiple GISTs that encoded a point mutation at codon 557, which was also found in peripheral leukocytes isolated from both relatives (Hirota et al, 2000).

In a mother and son with multiple GISTs and diffuse hyperplasia of the myenteric plexus layer, a single base mutation resulted in the substitution of Glu for Lys at codon 642 in the kinase I domain (Isozaki et al, 2000).

Nishida et al (1998) studied 3 family members (a woman, her niece, and her nephew) with multiple GISTs. Tumors from each of the 3 overexpressed Kit protein by immunohistochemical analysis and had an activating deletion of the valine at codon 559. The same deletion was detected in peripheral leukocytes from the 3 patients and 2 family members without GIST.

CLINICAL PRESENTATION

The symptoms at presentation often reflect the site of origin of the tumor. Patients with esophageal GISTs most often present with dysphagia, odynophagia, weight loss, dyspepsia, retrosternal chest pain, or hematemesis. Modified barium swallow or endoscopic evaluation is often diagnostic.

Patients with gastric GISTs typically present with vague symptoms, including abdominal pain, anorexia, weight loss, and GI hemorrhage. These GISTs are most commonly diagnosed at esophagogastroduodenoscopic evaluation for unrelated conditions.

Small-bowel tumors are rare, but GISTs account for more than 10% of neoplasms in this location. Patients with GISTs of the small intestine often present with nonspecific abdominal complaints, such as pain or hemorrhage. These tumors may be misdiagnosed as peptic ulcer disease, gastroesophageal reflux, or cholelithiasis. In many cases, they are initially detected by the small-bowel follow-through portion of a barium swallow; larger lesions may be detected by computed tomography (CT) radiography, and bleeding lesions may be detected by angiography.

Colorectal GISTs are rare, accounting for less than 0.1% of all colorectal tumors. Colorectal GISTs arise predominantly in the cecum and the rectum. Patients may present with abdominal discomfort, hemorrhage, a change in pattern or character of bowel movements, obstruction, or perforation. Diagnosis is most often made by a colonoscopic biopsy.

Patients with GISTs arising from the esophagus, stomach, small intestine, or colon may present with a life-threatening hemorrhage. If discovered by palpation, these tumors are generally large or metastatic to the liver. Patients with liver metastases may have lower-extremity edema, ascites, and even jaundice in the later stages of disease.

Some GISTs are discovered incidentally during evaluation for other medical conditions or as part of a screening program. These incidental GISTs may be found during physical examination, laparoscopic procedures, surgery, radiographic testing, or endoscopy and are generally smaller.

DIAGNOSTIC TESTS

Prior to initiation of therapy, the disease is carefully staged to rule out metastatic disease and provide a baseline for the assessment of therapy (Table 17–1). Staging is performed preoperatively to avoid unnecessary surgery in patients with advanced disease. Staging procedures should include routine laboratory evaluation of renal, liver, and hematopoietic function. Laboratory testing should also be performed as a baseline before systemic therapy is begun. In view of the neutropenia and elevated transaminase levels reported with imatinib mesylate (Gleevec; see the section on imatinib later in this chapter), careful attention should be paid to liver function and absolute neutrophil counts for patients receiving this drug.

Radiographic modalities routinely used to visualize GISTs include barium swallow, CT, magnetic resonance imaging (MRI), and ultrasonography.

Table 17–1.   Recommended Staging Tests for Patients with GIST

Laboratory tests
  Complete blood count with differential and platelet counts
  Electrolyte levels
  Creatinine level
  AST, ALT, LDH, total bilirubin, and alkaline phosphatase levels
Radiographic tests
  Computed tomography radiography of abdomen and pelvis
  Plain chest radiography
  Positron emission tomography scan*
Pathologic tests
  Hematoxylin-eosin stain
  Kit (CD117)
  CD34
  Smooth muscle actin
  Desmin†
  S-100†

* We recommend positron emission tomography scan before initiation of imatinib therapy, as part of a clinical trial if possible.
† Desmin and S-100 are usually not expressed by GISTs on immunohistochemical analysis.

Because GISTs are intra-abdominal, CT is generally more useful than MRI in the diagnosis and monitoring of this type of sarcoma. Of clinical importance, CT radiography provides 3-dimensional information about tumor size, tumor density (tumor necrosis), and intratumoral hemorrhage and about whether there has been sufficient downstaging to allow resection. Abdominal CT is necessary for adequate diagnosis, staging, and monitoring for response, relapse, or recurrence. Liver metastasis occurs in up to 65% of patients with metastatic GISTs, making CT radiography of the abdomen and rectum a critical component of diagnosis and monitoring.

The standard measurements of response, bidimensional or unidimensional diameters by CT scan, may not accurately reflect tumor cell death. We have seen patients with large GISTs that contained minimal viable tumor cells at resection. Clinical response to imatinib may include a decrease in tumor size, a decrease in tumor radiodensity, or both by CT radiography (Figure 17–1). We have also seen tumors enlarge after 2 months of therapy with imatinib, only to later regress (Figure 17–2).

MRI is occasionally useful in diagnosing GISTs because of the level of soft-tissue contrast, tissue specificity, and the modality's multiplanar nature. MRI often helps to narrow a differential diagnosis owing to differences in tissue characteristics. Preoperative MRI allows optimal staging, delineation of tissue planes, and evaluation of neurologic or vascular involvement.

Ultrasonography is used to guide diagnostic biopsy but may also be used to evaluate response to therapy or possible recurrent disease. Ultrasonography is often a useful adjunct to inconclusive MRI or CT and is particularly useful in the evaluation for nodal metastases. However, nodal metastases have been reported in only 6% of patients with metastatic GISTs. In cases that require a tissue diagnosis, ultrasonography provides a useful and relatively inexpensive method for directing a biopsy.

Positron emission tomography (PET) is useful in evaluating tumors of many histologic subtypes and may be useful in evaluating GISTs. We have found that response to imatinib is detected by PET scanning earlier than by conventional unidimensional or bidimensional CT radiographic measurements (Figure 17–3). In fact, PET has detected changes even after a single dose of imatinib, laying the groundwork for additional clinical trials designed to determine whether PET can rapidly assess and predict clinical response in the first few days of therapy. Van den Abbeele and colleagues (2002) reported that patients with advanced GIST who had a PET response (standardized uptake value ≤2.0) as early as day 1 after the start of therapy maintained a long-term response. However, patients who had no PET response (standardized uptake value >2.0) had progressive disease. In many cases, PET predicted response before significant changes were seen on CT radiography (Van den Abbeele et al, 2002). However, the clinical implications of and role for PET scanning in the management of GISTs remain investigational. At M. D. Anderson, we are developing a

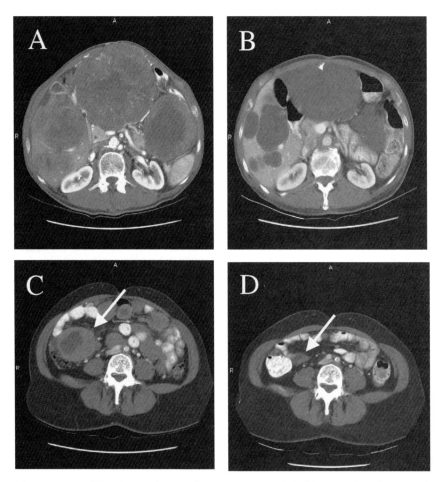

Figure 17–1. CT radiographic results in patients with GISTs treated with imatinib mesylate. (*A*) CT radiograph of a large intra-abdominal GIST that is heterogeneous with central necrosis. (*B*) CT radiograph of the patient shown in *A* after 3 months of imatinib therapy. The tumor has shrunk and appears homogeneously cystic with a decrease in radiodensity. (*C*) CT radiograph of a GIST with central necrosis. (*D*) CT radiograph of the patient shown in *C* after 2 months of therapy with imatinib. There has been a significant decrease in tumor size. Arrow denotes the site of the tumor.

novel clinical trial designed to study the early biological effects of preoperative imatinib in patients with resectable GISTs who have early PET responses. This will provide insight into the direct molecular and radiographic effects of imatinib in GIST. The Radiation Therapy Oncology Group in conjunction with the American College of Radiology Imaging Network is also evaluating the utility of early PET scanning (1 to 7 days after initiation of therapy with imatinib) in patients with operable malignant GISTs who receive preoperative imatinib. In our experience, the decision to discontinue therapy should not be based solely on imaging but instead should be made on the basis of the patient's overall clinical condition.

The diagnosis of GIST has been a subject of debate for many years. Many pathologists believe that, with very few exceptions, Kit expression should be a requirement for the diagnosis of GIST. Most GISTs show Kit positivity in 90% of tumor cells, but a small minority show more focal staining in as few as 5% to 20% of tumor cells. The clinical relevance of this more limited expression is not known, but it may give rise to sampling error in small biopsy samples (Fletcher et al, 2002). Despite the use of anti-Kit antibodies as well as refined immunohistochemical analyses, including antigen retrieval, to identify GISTs, a small proportion of GISTs show either faint expression of Kit or negative staining (Fletcher et al, 2002; de Silva and Reid, 2003). Tumors that have the undeniable clinicopathologic features of GIST but are Kit negative may be classified as GIST, but controversy surrounds this issue. One author suggests that the diagnosis of a Kit-negative GIST should only be rendered by an expert (Greenson, 2003). The assumption of Kit negativity based on very small needle biopsy samples or fine-needle aspirates should be discouraged.

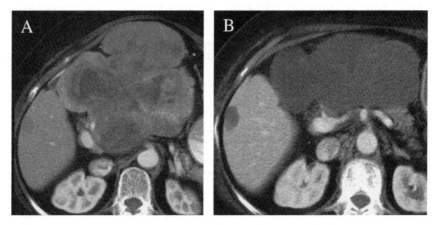

Figure 17–2. Paradoxical response to therapy with imatinib mesylate. (*A*) CT radiograph of the primary tumor and a liver metastasis in a patient with a GIST prior to initiation of imatinib therapy. (*B*) Repeat CT radiograph 2 months after initiation of imatinib therapy reveals that the tumor has increased in unidimensional diameter but has become cystic and homogeneous, with decreased radiodensity. Although the tumor appears larger in 1 dimension, the patient continued receiving imatinib, and the tumor subsequently shrank.

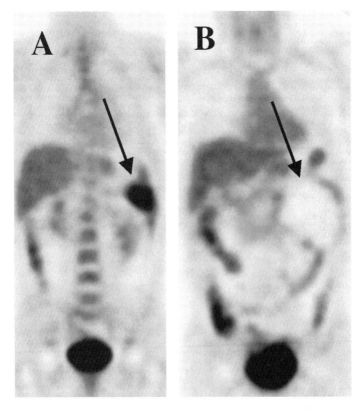

Figure 17–3. 18-fluorodeoxyglucose (FDG)-PET radiographic effects of imatinib mesylate therapy on tumor uptake in a patient with a GIST. (*A*) 18-FDG-PET scan prior to initiation of imatinib therapy. The 18-FDG-avid tumor is black and indicated by the arrow. (*B*) 18-FDG-PET scan after 2 months of therapy with imatinib. The tumor is no longer 18-FDG-avid.

The immunohistochemical approach to intra-abdominal sarcomas is to stain for Kit (CD117), CD34, smooth muscle actin, desmin, and S-100. Unlike leiomyosarcoma and other intra-abdominal sarcomas, GISTs are generally Kit positive, CD34 positive, desmin negative, and S-100 negative (Table 17–1).

DIFFERENTIAL DIAGNOSIS

GISTs constitute the largest group of mesenchymal tumors of the stomach and small intestine (Miettinen et al, 2000b). Other mesenchymal tumors that need to be differentiated from GISTs include inflammatory fibroid polyps, fibromatoses, inflammatory myofibroblastic tumors, solitary fibrous tumors, schwannomas, leiomyomas, and leiomyosarcomas.

Inflammatory fibroid polyps are benign lesions most often found in the stomach and small intestine. These lesions typically are submucosal and consist of a mixture of small granulation tissue–like vessels, spindle cells, and inflammatory cells, including eosinophils. The majority of these lesions are CD34 positive, and therefore, confusion with GISTs is possible. Although the stromal component of these tumors is Kit negative, mast cells within the tumor are Kit positive, providing yet another possible source of confusion with GISTs (Greenson, 2003).

Fibromatoses, also called desmoid tumors, are spindle cell tumors that can occur in the mesentery or retroperitoneum and grow into the lumen of the gut, mimicking a GIST (Greenson, 2003). Depending on the specific antibody used, fibromatoses may express Kit (Miettinen et al, 2001). Unlike GISTs, however, the tumor cells of fibromatoses do not stain for CD34 (Yantiss, 2000). Although fibromatoses can be locally aggressive and recur, they do not metastasize, and therefore, they should be differentiated from GISTs (Greenson, 2003).

Inflammatory myofibroblastic tumors are uncommon mesenchymal lesions characterized by a proliferation of spindle cells mixed with lymphocytes and plasma cells. While GISTs are usually found in patients older than 50 years of age, inflammatory myofibroblastic tumors are often seen in children. Histologically, these lesions are composed of elongated spindle cells (myofibroblasts) that can mimic GISTs. However, these lesions are typically CD34 and Kit negative (Greenson, 2003).

Solitary fibrous tumors occasionally occur in the peritoneal cavity and adhere to the bowel. Histologically, they have a random pattern of spindle cells and collagen. These lesions are CD34 positive and therefore may be confused with GISTs (Greenson, 2003). However, solitary fibrous tumors do not express Kit (Shidham et al, 2002).

Gastrointestinal schwannomas usually occur in the stomach, although they can also be found in the colon and esophagus. These lesions have a characteristic cuff of lymphoid aggregates around their periphery. Immunohistochemically, schwannomas are positive for S-100 but negative for Kit. Some have focal CD34 positivity. It is important to distinguish these lesions from GISTs since schwannomas of the gut are generally benign (Greenson, 2003).

Although much less common than GISTs, true leiomyomas and leiomyosarcomas do occur in the gut. Most arise in the esophagus, although they can occur in the colon, rectum, and anus. Leiomyomas, like GISTs, usually express actin but do not express desmin. In contrast, however, leiomyomas are negative for Kit and CD34. Leiomyosarcomas stain negatively for Kit and positively for actin, but these lesions are usually also positive for desmin (Greenson, 2003).

STAGING AND GRADING

Data concerning prognostic features were obtained in large part before imatinib was used to treat patients with Kit-expressing GISTs. As the clinical experience with imatinib grows, the prognostic features will be reevaluated since imatinib appears to alter the natural history of GIST in patients with advanced disease. The current prognostic factors are presented in Table 17–2.

Although several staging systems are available for sarcomas, none are clinically useful for GISTs. The American Joint Committee on Cancer (AJCC) staging system, the most commonly used for sarcoma, was developed from studies of localized soft-tissue sarcomas of the extremities (Greene et al, 2002). However, the AJCC system does not address histologic heterogeneity of sarcomas, and none of the studies used to develop the AJCC system incorporated GISTs. Sarcomas as divergent as rhabdomyosarcoma and GIST are as divergent as breast cancer and lung cancer. Unfortunately, the rarity of sarcomas has prevented the development of a meaningful staging system for each sarcoma histologic subtype. Although this makes application of the AJCC staging system and prognostic factors less appealing, the general principles seem to apply.

The exact criteria for estimating the risk for metastasis remain controversial. It is apparent that the most important features that estimate the malignant behavior of a tumor are mitotic rate and tumor size. Evaluation of these features is reproducible, inexpensive, and clinically relevant.

The AJCC staging system incorporates histologic grade and tumor size as the primary determinants of clinical stage. This staging system classifies tumors as T1 (<5 cm) and T2 (≥5 cm). Although this cutoff point is somewhat arbitrary, it is clear that as primary tumor size increases, time to recurrence and overall survival duration decrease.

Table 17–2.   Prognostic Factors in Patients with GISTs

Poor Prognosis	Good Prognosis
Tumor >10 cm	Tumor <5 cm
High mitotic rate (>5 per 10 HPF)	Low mitotic rate (<2 per 10 HPF)
High proliferation index	Low proliferation index
Necrosis	Absence of necrosis
Metastatic or extragastrointestinal primary tumor	Esophageal or gastric primary tumor
Male sex	Female sex
Age ≥40 years	Age <40 years

Abbreviation: HPF, high-power field.

The malignant potential of GIST is subject to disagreement, but clearly, the risk of recurrence increases with increasing tumor size and mitotic rate. In studies at M. D. Anderson involving primarily gastric and small-intestine GISTs, the median disease-free survival durations were 19 and 17 months for patients with tumors 5 to 10 cm and larger than 10 cm, respectively, and 36 months for patients with tumors smaller than 5 cm (Ng et al, 1992a). Thus, tumors larger than 5 cm should be considered malignant. However, it should be noted that tumors smaller than 5 cm are not necessarily benign. Some pathologists believe GISTs are so unpredictable that "benign" GISTs may not exist. We have seen very small lesions (<3 cm) with metastasis to the peritoneum or liver.

The prognostic significance of *kit* mutations is controversial. In a series of 124 patients described by Taniguchi and colleagues (1999), exon 11 mutations were identified in 57% of the GISTs and seemed to correlate with a poor prognosis. Several other authors have also shown a correlation between exon 11 *kit* mutations and poor prognosis (Ernst et al, 1998; Lasota et al, 1999). Contrary to these reports, however, some authors have reported that *kit* mutations are not restricted preferentially to higher-grade tumors, and that in fact, they are frequently found in pathologically low-risk GISTs (Sakurai et al, 1999; Rubin et al, 2001; Corless et al, 2002). Determining whether the *kit* mutation will prove to be an independent prognostic factor awaits the completion of larger studies.

In a study by Evans (1985), high mitotic rate (>10 mitoses per high-powered field [HPF]) was associated with shorter survival, although the exact number of mitoses per HPF used to predict malignant versus benign behavior is controversial. Some GISTs with low mitotic activity display an aggressive clinical pattern; we have seen tumors with very low mitotic rates (even <1 per 10 HPFs) metastasize. This unpredictability has led some pathologists to designate small (<5 cm), mitotically inactive GISTs (<1 mitosis per HPF) as having "uncertain malignant potential." It is actually now thought that categorizing GISTs into low-risk, intermediate-risk, and high-risk tumors on the basis of an estimation of their potential for recurrence and metastasis is more appropriate than dividing them into benign and malignant categories (de Silva and Reid, 2003).

In general, small tumors (<5 cm) with a low mitotic number (<1 per HPF) usually have a very low risk of metastasis. GISTs with more than 1 mitosis per HPF are designated malignant, and those with more than 10 mitoses per HPF are designated high grade. With prolonged follow-up, it appears that almost any GIST that causes clinical symptoms or signs leading to treatment has malignant potential. Moreover, studies at M. D. Anderson have clearly advanced the concept that most if not all GISTs will recur if the patient is evaluated for a sufficient period of time.

Several other large studies have identified prognostic factors in patients with GI leiomyosarcomas. In a multivariate analysis (DeMatteo et al, 2000), the most important negative prognostic factors were male sex, tumor size greater than 5 cm, and incomplete resection or unresectable tumor. Another study (Ng et al, 1992b) identified several factors significantly associated with improved survival after relapse. These were initial disease-free interval of 18 months or more, recurrences either isolated to the peritoneal cavity or within the liver, or complete resection of peritoneal recurrences or liver metastases. In contrast, recurrences at multiple sites, extra-abdominal metastases, and unresectable disease were associated with significantly shorter survival (Ng et al, 1992b).

Adverse prognostic features for GISTs include tumor size greater than 5 cm, presence of coagulative tumor necrosis, local recurrence, peritoneal seeding at time of surgery, high Ki-67 score, aneuploidy, and high-grade tumor.

MOLECULAR BIOLOGY

Proliferation, angiogenesis, and apoptosis of mesenchyme-derived cells are coordinated by peptide growth factor ligands that bind the corresponding cell surface receptor, resulting in protein tyrosine kinase activity (Ruddon, 1995; Remmelink et al, 1998). Receptor tyrosine kinases subsequently undergo autophosphorylation and dimerization, with transduction of the signal through the cell membrane to downstream molecules. Growth factors can be produced by the tumor cell; stromal cells, such as fibroblasts and endothelial cells; or circulating cells, such as platelets and leukocytes. Growth factor receptors are expressed on the surface of sarcoma cells as well as the surrounding normal cells, creating a complex network of autocrine and paracrine growth stimulation.

Group III membrane receptor tyrosine kinases include Kit and are important signaling molecules in sarcoma. These receptor tyrosine kinases contain immunoglobulin-like extracellular domains, a transmembrane domain, and 2 intracellular tyrosine kinase domains that contain phosphorylation sites (Figure 17–4). As is the case with many other receptor tyrosine kinases, the binding of ligand to receptor results in autophosphorylation, homodimerization, and activation of downstream molecules, such as mitogen-activated protein kinase, Stat, and Akt (Figure 17–5A) (Schlessinger, 2000). This activation is blocked by imatinib (Figure 17–5B).

The natural ligand of Kit is known as stem cell factor, steel factor, or Kit ligand. Kit is expressed on hematopoietic precursors, mast cells, germ cells, melanocytes, and the interstitial cells of Cajal (ICC) (Nocka et al, 1989). c-kit mutations are common in GISTs but not in leiomyomas or uterine leiomyosarcomas (Lasota et al, 1999). Mutation results in constitutive activation and ligand-independent proliferation (Hirota et al, 1998).

Activation of Kit by stem cell factor prevents apoptosis-in Ewing's sarcoma and other neuroectodermal tumors by an unclear mechanism

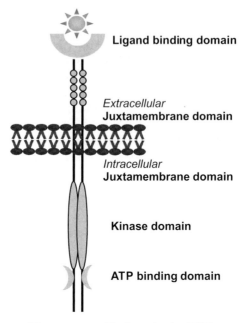

Figure 17–4.   Kit domains in GISTs.

(Ricotti et al, 1998). Kit overexpression has been observed in more than 50% of angiosarcomas (Miettinen et al, 2000a). Preclinical data have shown that intratumoral mast cell release of stem cell factor modulates tumor growth and angiogenesis (Zhang et al, 2000).

The ICC, autonomic pacemaker cells of the GI tract, also express Kit by immunohistochemical analysis. Because of the immunohistochemical and morphologic similarity between GIST cells and ICC, the ICC are thought to be the precursor cells for GISTs. This is supported by the finding that Kit-defective mice have GI motility dysfunction. Moreover, ICC and GIST cells also both express the CD34 antigen. Alternatively, GISTs may arise from a precursor cell that morphologically resembles the ICC upon activating mutation of the *kit* gene. Investigators have shown that ICC have a common precursor with smooth muscle cells and can differentiate into cells with a smooth muscle morphology, similar to some GISTs.

Kit receptor is expressed on mast cells, melanocytes, germ cells, mammary ductal epithelia, and certain cutaneous epithelial cells. It is expressed in angiosarcomas, Ewing's sarcoma, melanoma, seminoma, and mast cell neoplasms.

Approximately 80% of GISTs express the Kit receptor tyrosine kinase by immunohistochemistry. Most tumors that express the Kit receptor encode an activating mutation in the c-*kit* proto-oncogene. Most mutations occur within exon 11 (codons 550 through 552), which encodes the

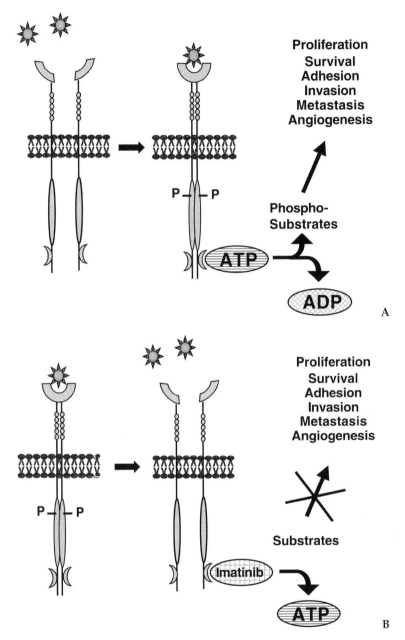

Figure 17–5. Effects of imatinib mesylate on Kit kinase domain. (*A*) In wild-type Kit, stem cell factor binds to the Kit receptor, resulting in homodimerization, autophosphorylation, and activation of the kinase domain. ATP then donates a phosphate to downstream substrates that induce phenotypic alterations. (*B*) Imatinib mesylate is thought to displace ATP from the ATP binding site of the Kit kinase domain. This results in abrogation of downstream signaling and reversal of the tumor phenotype.

Table 17–3.   Kit Mutation Status and Response Rate in Patients with GIST in
the USA-Finland Phase II Study of Imatinib*

Mutation	Frequency	Response Rate	Median Time to Progression	P
Exon 11	65%	79%	Not reached	
Exon 9	18%	46%	213 days	.003
Exon 13	2%			
Exon 17	2%			
Wild-type (no mutation)	13%	19%	90 days	.0001

* Heinrich et al (2002).

intracellular juxtamembrane regulatory domain. These mutations are most frequently missense mutations or frameshift deletions. Less commonly, there is a mutation in exon 9, 13, 14, 15, or 17 (Corless et al, 2002; Sjogren et al, 2002) (Table 17–3). These mutations result in ligand-independent activation of Kit tyrosine kinase activity. Stable transfection of the activated *kit* gene into murine tumor cells results in transformation in vitro.

kit-activating mutations were originally reported in the juxtamembrane domain (exon 11) of the gene (Hirota et al, 1998). However, mutations in extracellular (exon 9) and intracellular (exons 13 and 17) *kit* domains have also been described. The genetic location of specific *kit* mutations appears to be important in predicting response to targeted therapy with imatinib. Recent evidence suggests that most *kit* mutations occur in the juxtamembrane domain and predict a greater likelihood of response to imatinib. The response rates were 79% for patients whose tumors had an exon 11 juxtamembrane domain, 46% for patients with an exon 9 mutation, and 19% for patients with wild-type *kit*, suggesting that juxtamembrane mutations alter the structure of Kit such that the receptor is constitutively activated but can be inactivated by imatinib. On the other hand, imatinib does not appear to inactivate Kit molecules with a mutation in exon 9. The wild-type Kit molecule is sensitive to the inhibitory effects of imatinib. Tumors with wild-type Kit do not respond to imatinib, suggesting that inhibition of Kit is insufficient to result in antitumor activity. This may result from activation of parallel or downstream molecules by a mechanism not involving Kit. For instance, a subset of GISTs could harbor an activated proliferation pathway, such as mitogen-activated protein kinase, or may have activation of an antiapoptotic pathway, such as AKT. This provides the rationale for combining imatinib with other targeted therapies directed at downstream or parallel signaling pathways.

A recent evaluation has demonstrated activation (phosphorylation) of Kit in GISTs that lack detectable *kit* mutations (Rubin et al, 2001;

Heinrich et al, 2002). Mechanisms that might account for Kit activation in mutation-negative GISTs are undetected mutations, inactivation of Kit-inhibitory phosphatases, up-regulation of the Kit ligand, and Kit homo-dimerization with other activated receptor tyrosine kinase proteins (Heinrich et al, 2002). *kit* mutations in tumors that are small (10 mm or less), clinically incidental, or morphologically benign are identical to those identified in larger GISTs. In addition, the overall frequency of mutations (85%) in the incidental tumors is not significantly different from that seen in advanced and metastatic GISTs (86%). These observations suggest that activating mutations in *kit* are acquired very early in the pathogenesis of GISTs (Corless et al, 2002).

Therapeutic Options

Resection of Primary Tumors

GISTs are generally not responsive to chemotherapy or radiation therapy, and complete surgical resection remains the mainstay of treatment of primary tumors. Unlike carcinomas, GISTs rarely metastasize to lymph nodes; thus, lymph node dissection or biopsy is not routinely employed. Wedge resection of the stomach or segmental resection of the intestine provides adequate therapy and has been shown at M. D. Anderson to be associated with improved overall survival (Ng et al, 1992a). DeMatteo and colleagues (2000) at Memorial Sloan-Kettering Cancer Center reported that in a series of 200 patients with GISTs, the median survival was 66 months for patients with primary disease who underwent complete resection, compared with 22 months for patients who underwent incomplete resection or whose tumor was unresectable. In the DeMatteo study, 80 patients had primary tumor without metastasis and underwent complete surgical resection. The overall survival rate was 55% at a median follow-up of 24 months. On multivariate analysis, tumor size was an independent prognostic factor for survival: patients with tumors larger than 10 cm had a disease-specific 5-year survival rate of only 20% after resection.

Studies at M. D. Anderson have shown that tumor rupture before or during resection is a predictor of poor outcome. Surgical dissection by a skilled sarcoma surgeon is imperative to avoid tumor rupture and intraperitoneal dissemination during resection.

GISTs of the esophagus are rare, and few data exist regarding the efficacy of surgical resection. However, extrapolating from data on sarcomas of other histologic subtypes, 75% of esophageal sarcomas are amenable to complete resection. Nonetheless, the 5-year overall survival rate is only 30%.

Long-term follow-up shows that most GISTs recur locally. In an M. D. Anderson series (Ng et al, 1992b), 119 (90%) of 132 patients who underwent an initial complete resection had either local or metastatic recurrence after a median follow-up of 68 months. The median time to relapse was 18 months, and most recurrences occurred within 2 years of initial resection. Prognostic factors associated with recurrence were tumor size greater than 5 cm, high grade, tumor rupture, and small-bowel primary tumor site.

Resection of Metastases

The liver is the most common site of GIST metastasis. Most liver metastases from GIST are unresectable owing to multiple, bilobar intrahepatic metastases, very large metastases, or intraperitoneal sarcomatosis. However, select patients appear to derive benefit from resection of hepatic metastases. In a recent study (DeMatteo et al, 2000), the 1-year and 3-year survival rates for patients with GIST or intra-abdominal leiomyosarcoma who underwent hepatic resection of all visible disease were 90% and 58%, respectively.

Hepatic Artery Embolization of Liver Metastases

Hepatic artery embolization or chemoembolization seems to be an effective palliative option for patients with liver metastases from GIST and is thought to be effective because these tumors are often hypervascular. Chemoembolization mechanically occludes the arterial blood supply to the tumor, increases intratumoral concentration of drug, and minimizes systemic toxicity because of systemic dilution and metabolism. We often repeat embolization, for the same or alternate lesions. Mavligit et al (1995) performed intra-arterial chemoembolization of liver metastases in 14 patients with GI leiomyosarcomas using polyvinyl alcohol sponge particles mixed with cisplatin powder (150 mg) followed by intrahepatic arterial vinblastine administration (10 mg/m^2); 70% of patients had a partial or complete response lasting from 8 to 31 months (median, 12 months) after an average of 2 embolizations. Toxicity was limited to mild myelosuppression, right upper quadrant pain, minimally elevated hepatic enzyme levels, and transient ileus. Although this was a small series, these results are better than those obtained with systemic chemotherapy. Other investigators (Rajan et al, 2001) studied chemoembolization to treat liver metastases in patients with intra-abdominal sarcomas (11 GISTs and 5 leiomyosarcomas). Partial responses were observed in 13%, and stable disease was achieved in an additional 69% of patients, lasting a median of 8 months. Side effects were mild and not unexpected. Patients with ascites or hyperbilirubinemia are considered to be at high risk for complications and should not undergo this therapy.

It is interesting that we have seen disease stabilization in patients receiving bland embolization (i.e., polyvinyl alcohol sponge particles without chemotherapy). It is not completely clear whether the results of chemoembolization are due to increased exposure of the tumor to chemotherapy or blockage of the blood supply to the tumor. Hepatic arterial embolization or chemoembolization therapy should be considered for patients whose hepatic tumors are resistant to or relapse after therapy with imatinib.

Radiation Therapy

Radiation therapy has a limited role in the treatment of patients with GIST. These tumors are relatively radioresistant. It is difficult to deliver adequate cytotoxic doses of radiation to GISTs owing to the proximity of vital organs, such as the kidney, spleen, liver, and bowel. These same organs make delivery of meaningful adjuvant radiation therapy impossible. Radiation therapy has an occasional role in the management of metastatic GIST; it can be used to palliate pain from a tumor fixed in the pelvis or to the abdominal wall. Otherwise, the pattern of metastasis in the liver and peritoneum involves too large a field to be amenable to radiation therapy.

Intraperitoneal Chemotherapy

Some patients present with intra-abdominal sarcomatosis and minimal other organ involvement. A review of the M. D. Anderson experience (Bilimoria et al, 2002) found that tumor volume was a prognostic factor. The 2-year overall survival rate was 75% for patients with tumors less than 5 cm in diameter or with less than 10 peritoneal nodules but only 14% for patients with tumors greater than 5 cm in diameter or with more than 50 peritoneal nodules.

Eilber et al (1999) used intraperitoneal mitoxantrone after surgical debulking to treat 54 patients with intra-abdominal sarcomatosis, 33 of whom had GISTs. Mitoxantrone was chosen because it is an anthracycline that binds to intraperitoneal tissues and produces high local drug concentrations with minimal systemic absorption. The 5-year overall survival rate was 46% for patients with peritoneal-only disease, but only 5% for those with liver metastases. In the 27 patients with peritoneal-only disease, the median time to recurrence was increased from 8 to 21 months by the addition of postoperative intraperitoneal mitoxantrone, although 83% of patients had recurrent disease after a median time of 11 months. Therefore, intraperitoneal chemotherapy may provide benefit for patients with peritoneal-only disease. Additional studies of intraperitoneal chemotherapy for recurrent GIST are ongoing at M. D. Anderson for patients with imatinib-resistant tumors.

Systemic Chemotherapy

Only since the availability of Kit immunohistochemical analysis and discovery of the unprecedented activity of imatinib has GIST been routinely distinguished from intra-abdominal leiomyosarcoma. It is therefore difficult to interpret the results of most trials of chemotherapy for intra-abdominal soft-tissue sarcoma. Many, if not most, tumors previously classified as GI leiomyosarcoma were actually GISTs.

Until the development of imatinib, there was no effective therapy for metastatic GIST. Doxorubicin and ifosfamide are the 2 most active agents against sarcoma and are the centerpiece of most regimens used to treat soft-tissue sarcomas. However, these 2 agents have very limited activity against GIST. We reviewed our experience at M. D. Anderson with patients treated for GI leiomyosarcomas (stomach and small bowel, presumably GISTs) between 1948 and 1989. Of 120 patients with measurable disease who were treated with a doxorubicin-based regimen, 4 (3%) had objective responses (1 complete and 3 partial). Three partial responses were seen with the combination of cyclophosphamide, doxorubicin, and dacarbazine, and 1 partial response and 1 complete response were seen with cyclophosphamide, vincristine, doxorubicin, and dacarbazine (Plager et al, 1991). We also reviewed our experience with ifosfamide in patients treated for GI leiomyosarcoma between 1985 and 1989. Of 30 patients with evaluable disease, 4 (13%) had objective responses (Patel et al, 1991). This observation has been confirmed by investigators at Mayo Clinic: only 1 (5%) of 21 patients with GISTs who were treated with the combination of doxorubicin, dacarbazine, mitomycin, and cisplatin had an objective response (Edmonson et al, 1999). We recently completed several phase II trials evaluating new agents for activity against GIST. We found only an occasional partial response until our recent trials with imatinib. These data reflect the refractory nature of GISTs to systemic treatment with standard cytotoxic chemotherapy drugs.

Because conventional agents have yielded disappointing results, it has been difficult to recommend any particular agent or combination of drugs as standard therapy for metastatic GIST. The mechanism of resistance of GIST to chemotherapy is currently unknown but may relate to elevated levels of multidrug resistance protein compared to those found in leiomyosarcoma. It is interesting to speculate that oncogenic activation of Kit in GISTs may contribute to chemoresistance through upregulation of antiapoptotic signaling or activation of other drug-resistance mechanisms.

Imatinib Mesylate for Metastatic or Unresectable GIST

One patient with refractory, metastatic GIST at the University Hospital of Helsinki, Finland, was treated with once-daily doses of 400 mg of imatinib. This patient's tumor had previously been documented to express the Kit protein (CD117) and was subsequently found to encode a mutation in exon 11 of the *kit* gene. An objective response was revealed by 18-fluorodeoxyglucose-PET and CT radiography. The patient's tumor remained stable after a year of therapy. The patient had only mild GI side effects. Serial tumor biopsies revealed myxoid degeneration.

These encouraging results led to rapid deployment of large-scale studies of imatinib in GIST. A multicenter phase II clinical trial of imatinib in patients with unresectable or metastatic GIST began in July 2000.

Table 17–4. Toxicity Associated with Imatinib Mesylate Therapy in the USA-Finland Trial* of 147 Patients with Advanced GIST (N = 147)

Side Effect	All Grades	Grade 3/4
Fluid retention	72.8	4.1
Superficial edema	72.1	2.0
Other fluid retention	6.1	2.0
Nausea	55.1	2.7
Diarrhea	51.0	3.4
Abdominal pain	36.7	4.8
Muscle cramps	35.4	0
Fatigue	35.4	0.7
Rash	32.0	2.7
Headache	29.9	0
Vomiting	22.4	2.0
Flatulence	19.7	0
Hemorrhage	17.0	6.1
Intratumoral hemorrhage	2.7	2.7
Cerebral hemorrhage or subdural hematoma	0.7	0.7
Upper GI tract	5.4	2.7
Musculoskeletal pain	15.0	1.4
Nasopharyngitis	12.9	0
Anemia	11.6	4.1
Insomnia	10.9	0

* von Mehren et al (2002).

Imatinib was shown to be effective and to have minimal toxicity (Table 17–4).

This trial was subsequently expanded to include an additional 145 patients, and the preliminary results were presented at the plenary session of the American Society of Clinical Oncology (ASCO) meeting in 2001 (Blanke, 2001). Patients with unresectable or metastatic GIST were randomized between 2 different dose levels of imatinib therapy (400 mg vs 600 mg daily oral dose) for up to 24 months. Patients were required to have a *kit*-expressing GIST. This study had a crossover design. Of 147 patients randomized to treatment with imatinib at a dose of 400 or 600 mg per day, 59% had partial responses, and only 13% had progressive disease.

Updated results from this trial were presented at the 2002 ASCO meeting. At a median follow-up of 24 months, 63% of patients had objective responses (all partial responses), 19% of patients had stable disease, and 12% of patients had confirmed tumor progression. At the median follow-up of 15 months, 18% of the responders had progressive disease, and 73% remained in the study. The median time to progression was 72 weeks, but the median survival had yet to be reached. The response rates did not differ significantly between the 2 doses, although there was a trend toward a higher response rate at the 600-mg dose (62% vs 65%) (von Mehren et al, 2002).

The preliminary trials of imatinib in GIST were so successful that sarcoma investigators met at the National Cancer Institute in November 2000 to discuss the results and to design a study to expand access to this agent for GIST patients who might benefit from it. With more than 100 patients enrolled in 8 months, M. D. Anderson became the lead institution in the North American Sarcoma Intergroup study S0033. This study was designed to test whether imatinib 800 mg/day provides better clinical outcomes than does imatinib 400 mg/day. The optimal dose of imatinib in GIST patients remains unknown, and investigators await the final results of these large, randomized clinical trials.

In a phase II study by the European Organization for Research and Treatment of Cancer, 27 patients with Kit-expressing, metastatic or unresectable GISTs were treated with 400 mg of imatinib daily. The objective response rate was 71%, with 1 complete response and 18 partial responses. Interestingly, the median time to response was 4 months, and the time to progression had not been reached (Judson et al, 2002). Early toxicity results of a phase III international trial of 946 patients with advanced, Kit-expressing GIST were reported by the European Organization for Research and Treatment of Cancer, Italian Sarcoma Group, and Australasian Gastro-Intestinal Trials Group. This trial randomized patients to receive either 400 mg or 800 mg of oral imatinib daily. Most side effects were mild to moderate, although 88% of patients developed anemia, 67% had edema, 60% developed fatigue, and 32% were neutropenic. One patient died of drug-related neutropenic sepsis.

Recently, Bauer and colleagues (2003) reported a patient whose metastatic GIST responded well to imatinib treatment despite the tumor's near absence of Kit expression. The tumor was morphologically typical for a GIST, stained positively for CD34, and had an in-frame deletion in *kit* exon 11. These findings suggest that even GISTs with very low levels of Kit expression may respond to imatinib (Bauer et al, 2003).

On the basis of the preliminary data presented at the 2002 ASCO meeting, imatinib is clearly safe and effective at doses of 400 to 800 mg per day orally. The toxicity profile of imatinib in patients with GIST is also very favorable. The major side effects include mild fatigue, periorbital edema, diarrhea, and intermittent muscle cramping. The most medically severe side effects could actually come from excessive anticancer activity of the drug. A few patients have had significant GI bleeding episodes, postulated to be associated with massive tumor necrosis induced by this active agent.

The appropriate management of metastatic GIST that has not responded or has become resistant to imatinib is not currently known. Investigators at M. D. Anderson and other institutions are currently developing new clinical trials to evaluate imatinib in combination with other agents as first-line therapy and upon relapse. Current clinical trials for imatinib-resistant or -refractory GIST include trials of G3139 (antisense Bcl-2, Genta Pharmaceuticals) and irinotecan. Physicians should be encouraged to refer patients with GIST to centers that have access to these clinical trials.

Preoperative and Postoperative Adjuvant Imatinib for Primary GIST

The role of adjuvant imatinib is being evaluated because of the drug's marked efficacy and safety in patients with metastatic disease. The hypothesis is that imatinib may prevent or delay recurrence and prolong survival in patients with completely resected GISTs. The American College of Surgeons Oncology Group (ACOSOG) developed a phase II trial to test the benefit of adjuvant imatinib (400 mg/day for 1 year) in patients after complete resection of high-risk primary GIST (tumor >10 cm, tumor rupture, or multifocal tumors) as compared with historical controls. A phase III trial led by ACOSOG is ongoing that will include patients with both high-risk and moderate-risk tumors (i.e., >3 cm). Patients will be randomized to receive either placebo or imatinib (400 mg/day for 1 year). A patient assigned to placebo will receive imatinib therapy in the event of tumor recurrence. An M. D. Anderson study has been designed to determine the mechanism of antitumor activity of imatinib in patients with GIST. As noted above, patients with GIST may have PET scan responses after as little as 24 hours of therapy with imatinib. Additionally, GIST patients treated for 4 weeks have minimal viable tumor after resection. In the M. D. Anderson preoperative-plus-postoperative imatinib study, patients with Kit-expressing GIST undergo baseline PET scan, perfusion CT, and tumor biopsy. Patients are then treated with imatinib 600 mg by mouth each day for 3, 5, or 7 days. Subsequently, patients undergo repeat PET scan and perfusion CT. Patients undergo resection followed by adjuvant therapy with imatinib 600 mg each day for 2 years. The pre- and post-imatinib tumor samples will be subjected to molecular analysis for imatinib-induced alterations in gene expression, tumor vascularity, and tumor cell apoptosis. This information will lead to an understanding of the mechanisms by which imatinib is efficacious in GISTs.

The role of imatinib in the preoperative and postoperative setting has not been clearly defined. Trials such as these will help determine the proper role, dose, and duration of therapy with this drug. Nonetheless, it is likely that adjuvant therapy with imatinib will improve outcomes if applied early in the course of GIST therapy.

Patients whose disease responds to imatinib may become candidates for surgical resection. After prolonged therapy with imatinib, resected

GISTs are found to have undergone myxoid degeneration. Patients with stable disease may continue imatinib treatment until disease progression becomes evident. Patients whose disease becomes refractory to imatinib are eligible for palliative therapy, such as hepatic artery embolization, radiation therapy, surgical debulking, and intraperitoneal chemotherapy. Surgery remains the principal treatment for primary disease, but its outcome may be improved by neoadjuvant or adjuvant imatinib.

CONCLUSION

Imatinib has quickly become the most active targeted, small-molecule therapy in patients with solid tumors. Imatinib is the first-line agent for metastatic GIST and is currently being evaluated against other tumor types. Also, several ongoing studies of imatinib in GIST at M. D. Anderson address the important issues of efficacy of adjuvant therapy, efficacy of neoadjuvant therapy, duration of therapy, safety in the perioperative period, and the pathologic and molecular meaning of a response by PET imaging. The use of imatinib for treating patients with GIST will be tailored by the final results of neoadjuvant, adjuvant, and metastatic clinical trials and their associated correlative studies.

The identification of imatinib as an agent to specifically target the critical pathogenetic mechanisms of GIST represents a major advance in the treatment of this disease. The information gained from the success of imatinib in GIST will enhance drug development for oncology in general. Many challenges lie ahead in the applications of these strategies to other human cancers.

On the basis of studies published in abstract form, it appears that very few patients with metastatic GIST exhibit complete responses to imatinib therapy, perhaps owing to relatively slow responses or imatinib's failure to induce cell death. The exact cause may be determined by studies in which GIST patients receive imatinib preoperatively. If indeed imatinib arrests cell growth but does not induce apoptosis, combination therapy with a proapoptotic agent would be intriguing. If imatinib has no effect on tumor vasculature, perhaps combination with an antiangiogenic agent would enhance efficacy.

The mechanisms of primary and acquired resistance to imatinib are not known and are being actively investigated. It is possible that the site of the mutation on the *kit* gene determines the kinetics of Kit inhibition by imatinib. Tumors from patients whose disease relapses after an initial response to imatinib therapy may be undergoing clonal selection for tumor cells encoding a *kit* mutation in an imatinib-resistant domain, such as the ATP binding site. Alternatively, resistance may develop by activation of pathways located downstream or in parallel to Kit and therefore not sensitive to inhibition by imatinib.

KEY PRACTICE POINTS

- Patients with metastatic GIST should be treated initially with 400 mg to 600 mg orally each day of imatinib.

- Response of patients with GIST to imatinib should be carefully evaluated by CT radiography with emphasis on changes in tumor density.

- Neoadjuvant and adjuvant therapy for GIST should be administered in the setting of a clinical trial.

- Patients with imatinib-resistant or -refractory GIST should be evaluated for enrollment in a clinical trial.

Whatever the outcome, this is an amazing opportunity to understand the biological basis of resistance to one of the most successful therapeutic advances in oncology.

It appears that the wild-type expression of Kit is not sufficient to confer antitumor activity of imatinib. Thus, inhibiting a normal target may not have antitumor activity if the target does not provide an essential function to the tumor cell. Therefore, identification of molecular abnormalities that are essential for tumorigenesis will lead to the development of new anticancer therapies.

Diseases such as GIST appear to be pathogenetically simpler than other common human malignancies, such as carcinomas of the breast, lung, colon, and prostate, which are the result of complex multistep tumorigenesis. Understanding diseases such as GIST may lay the foundation for understanding the more complex types of human cancer.

SUGGESTED READINGS

Bauer S, Corless CL, Heinrich MC, et al. Response to imatinib mesylate of a gastrointestinal stromal tumor with very low expression of KIT. *Cancer Chemother Pharmacol* 2003;51:261–265.

Bilimoria MM, Holtz DJ, Mirza NQ, et al. Tumor volume as a prognostic factor for sarcomatosis. *Cancer* 2002;94:2441–2446.

Blanke C. Evaluation of the molecularly targeted therapy STI571 in patients with unresectable or metastatic gastrointestinal stromal tumors expressing KIT [abstract]. *Proc Am Soc Clin Oncol* 2001;20. Abstract 1.

Carney JA. Gastric stromal sarcoma, pulmonary chondroma, and extra-adrenal paraganglioma (Carney triad): natural history, adrenocortical component, and possible familial occurrence. *Mayo Clin Proc* 1999;74:543–552.

Carney JA, Sheps SG, Go VL, et al. The triad of gastric leiomyosarcoma, functioning extra-adrenal paraganglioma and pulmonary chondroma. *N Engl J Med* 1977;296:1517–1518.

Carney JA, Stratakis CA. Familial paraganglioma and gastric stromal sarcoma: a new syndrome distinct from the Carney triad. *Am J Med Genet* 2002;108:132–139.

Corless CL, McGreevey L, Haley A, et al. KIT mutations are common in incidental gastrointestinal stromal tumors one centimeter or less in size. *Am J Pathol* 2002;160:1567–1572.

DeMatteo RP, Lewis JJ, Leung D, et al. Two hundred gastrointestinal stromal tumors: recurrence patterns and prognostic factors for survival. *Ann Surg* 2000; 231:51–58.

de Silva MV, Reid R. Gastrointestinal stromal tumors (GIST): C-kit mutations, CD117 expression, differential diagnosis and targeted cancer therapy with imatinib. *Pathol Oncol Res* 2003;9:13–19.

Edmonson J, Marks R, Buckner J, et al. Contrast of response to D-MAP + sargramostatin between patients with advanced malignant gastrointestinal stromal tumors and patients with other advanced leiomyosarcomas. *Proc Am Soc Clin Oncol* 1999;18:541a.

Eilber FC, Rosen G, Forscher C, Nelson SD, Dorey FJ, Eilber FR. Surgical resection and intraperitoneal chemotherapy for recurrent abdominal sarcomas. *Ann Surg Oncol* 1999;6:645–650.

Ernst SI, Hubbs AE, Przygodzki RM, et al. KIT mutation portends poor prognosis in gastrointestinal stromal/smooth muscle tumors. *Lab Invest* 1998;78:1633–1636.

Evans HL. Smooth muscle tumors of the gastrointestinal tract. A study of 56 cases followed for a minimum of 10 years. *Cancer* 1985;56:2242–2250.

Fletcher CD, Berman JJ, Corless C, et al. Diagnosis of gastrointestinal stromal tumors: a consensus approach. *Int J Surg Pathol* 2002;10:81–89.

Gottlieb J, Baker L, O'Bryan R, et al. Adriamycin (NSC-123-127) used alone and in combination for soft tissue and bony sarcomas. *Cancer Chemotherapy Reports* 1974;6:271–282.

Greene FL, American Joint Committee on Cancer, American Cancer Society. *AJCC Cancer Staging Manual*. 6th ed. New York, NY: Springer-Verlag; 2002.

Greenson JK. Gastrointestinal stromal tumors and other mesenchymal lesions of the gut. *Mod Pathol* 2003;16:366–375.

Heinrich MC, Rubin BP, Longley BJ, et al. Biology and genetic aspects of gastrointestinal stromal tumors: KIT activation and cytogenetic alterations. *Hum Pathol* 2002;33:484–495.

Hirota S, Isozaki K, Moriyama Y, et al. Gain-of-function mutations of c-kit in human gastrointestinal stromal tumors. *Science* 1998;279:577–580.

Hirota S, Nishida T, Isozaki K, et al. Familial gastrointestinal stromal tumors associated with dysphagia and novel type germline mutation of KIT gene. *Gastroenterology* 2002;122:1493–1499.

Hirota S, Okazaki T, Kitamura Y, et al. Cause of familial and multiple gastrointestinal autonomic nerve tumors with hyperplasia of interstitial cells of Cajal is germline mutation of the c-kit gene. *Am J Surg Pathol* 2000;24:326–327.

Isozaki K, Terris B, Belghiti J, et al. Germline-activating mutation in the kinase domain of KIT gene in familial gastrointestinal stromal tumors. *Am J Pathol* 2000;157:1581–1585.

Judson I, Verweij J, van Oosterom A, et al. Imatinib (Gleevec) an active agent for gastrointestinal stromal tumors (GIST), but not for other soft tissue sarcoma (STS) subtypes not characterized for KIT and PDGF-R expression. Results of

EORTC phase II studies [abstract]. *Proc Am Soc Clin Oncol* 2002. Abstract 1609.

Lasota J, Jasinski M, Sarlomo-Rikala M, et al. Mutations in exon 11 of c-Kit occur preferentially in malignant versus benign gastrointestinal stromal tumors and do not occur in leiomyomas or leiomyosarcomas. *Am J Pathol* 1999;154:53–60.

Maeyama H, Hidaka E, Ota H, et al. Familial gastrointestinal stromal tumor with hyperpigmentation: association with a germline mutation of the c-kit gene. *Gastroenterology* 2001;120:210–215.

Mavligit GM, Zukwiski AA, Ellis LM, Chuang VP, Wallace S. Gastrointestinal leiomyosarcoma metastatic to the liver. Durable tumor regression by hepatic chemoembolization infusion with cisplatin and vinblastine. *Cancer* 1995;75: 2083–2088.

Miettinen M, Sarlomo-Rikala M, Lasota J. KIT expression in angiosarcomas and fetal endothelial cells: lack of mutations of exon 11 and exon 17 of C-kit. *Mod Pathol* 2000b;13:536–541.

Miettinen M, Sobin LH, Sarlomo-Rikala M. Immunohistochemical spectrum of GISTs at different sites and their differential diagnosis with a reference to CD117 (KIT). *Mod Pathol* 2000a;13:1134–1142.

Miettinen R, Pitkanen A, Miettinen M. Are desmoid tumors kit positive? [comment]. *J Comp Neurol* 2001;432:440–465.

Ng EH, Pollock RE, Munsell MF, et al. Prognostic factors influencing survival in gastrointestinal leiomyosarcomas. Implications for surgical management and staging. *Ann Surg* 1992a;215:68–77.

Ng EH, Pollock RE, Romsdahl MM. Prognostic implications of patterns of failure for gastrointestinal leiomyosarcomas. *Cancer* 1992b;69:1334–1341.

Nishida T, Hirota S, Taniguchi M, et al. Familial gastrointestinal stromal tumours with germline mutation of the KIT gene. *Nat Genet* 1998;19:323–324.

Nocka K, Majumder S, Chabot B, et al. Expression of c-kit gene products in known cellular targets of W mutations in normal and W mutant mice— evidence for an impaired c-kit kinase in mutant mice. *Genes Dev* 1989;3:816–826.

Patel S, Legha S, Salem P, et al. Evaluation of ifosfamide in metastatic leiomyosarcomas of gastrointestinal origin. *Proc Am Soc Clin Oncol* 1991;31:352.

Plager C, Papadopolous N, Salem P, et al. Adriamycin based chemotherapy for leiomyosarcoma of the stomach and small bowel [abstract]. *Proc Am Soc Clin Oncol* 1991;10:352.

Rajan DK, Soulen MC, Clark TW, et al. Sarcomas metastatic to the liver: response and survival after cisplatin, doxorubicin, mitomycin-C, Ethiodol, and polyvinyl alcohol chemoembolization. *J Vasc Intervent Radiol* 2001;12:187–193.

Remmelink M, Decaestecker C, Darro F, et al. The in vitro influence of eight hormones and growth factors on the proliferation of eight sarcoma cell lines. *J Cancer Res Clin Oncol* 1998;124:155–164.

Ricotti E, Fagioli F, Garelli E, et al. c-kit is expressed in soft tissue sarcoma of neuroectodermic origin and its ligand prevents apoptosis of neoplastic cells. *Blood* 1998;91:2397–2405.

Rubin BP, Singer S, Tsao C, et al. KIT activation is a ubiquitous feature of gastrointestinal stromal tumors. *Cancer Res* 2001;61:8118–8121.

Ruddon R. *Cancer Biology.* New York, NY: Oxford University Press; 1995.

Sakurai S, Fukasawa T, Chong JM, et al. C-kit gene abnormalities in gastrointestinal stromal tumors (tumors of interstitial cells of Cajal). *Jpn J Cancer Res* 1999;
90:1321–1328.

Schlessinger J. Cell signaling by receptor tyrosine kinases. *Cell* 2000;103:211–225.

Shidham VB, Chivukula M, Gupta D, et al. Immunohistochemical comparison of
gastrointestinal stromal tumor and solitary fibrous tumor. *Arch Pathol Lab Med*
2002;126:1189–1192.

Sjogren H, Meis-Kindblom JM, Stenman G, et al. The complexity of KIT gene mutations and chromosome rearrangements and their clinical correlation in gastrointestinal stromal (pacemaker cell) tumors. *Am J Pathol* 2002;160:15–22.

Taniguchi M, Nishida T, Hirota S, et al. Effect of c-kit mutation on prognosis of
gastrointestinal stromal tumors. *Cancer Res* 1999;59:4297–4300.

Van den Abbeele A, Badawi R, Cliche J-P, et al. 18F-FDG PET predicts response to
imatinib mesylate (Gleevec) in patients with advanced gastrointestinal stromal
tumors (GIST) [abstract]. *Proc Am Soc Clin Oncol* 2002. Abstract 1610.

Van Oosterom A, Judson I, Verweij J. STI57, an active drug in metastatic gastrointestinal stromal tumors (GIST), an EORTC phase I study [abstract]. *Proc Am Soc
Clin Oncol* 2001;20:1a. Abstract 2.

von Mehren M, Blanke C, Joensuu H, et al. High incidence of durable responses
induced by imatinib mesylate (Gleevec) in patients with unresectable and
metastatic gastrointestinal stromal tumors (GISTs) [abstract]. *Proc Am Soc Clin
Oncol* 2002. Abstract 1608.

Yantiss RK. Gastrointestinal stromal tumor versus intra-abdominal fibromatosis of
the bowel wall: a clinically important differential diagnosis. *Am J Surg Pathol*
2000;24:947–957.

Zhang W, Stoica G, Tasca SI, et al. Modulation of tumor angiogenesis by stem cell
factor. *Cancer Res* 2000;60:6757–6762.

18   PALLIATIVE THERAPY

Nora A. Janjan, Edward H. Lin,
Marc E. Delclos, Christopher Crane,
Miguel A. Rodriguez-Bigas, John M. Skibber,
and Charles Cleeland

CHAPTER OVERVIEW

More than 70% of all cancer patients develop symptoms from either their primary tumor or metastatic disease. Approximately half of patients diagnosed with cancer will develop metastatic disease. Controlling symptoms due to cancer or its treatment is an important obligation in cancer care. When cancer is not curable, it should be treated like a chronic disease with interventions aimed to prevent or control newly developed symptoms. Treatment needs to be indexed to the site and volume of disease and the prognosis. The time required for palliative care and the toxicity of palliative care must be minimized. Patients should not spend a disproportionate percentage of their remaining life receiving palliative treatment. Ineffective therapies that involve morbidity and cost and provide little or no palliative benefit should not be administered. The burden of palliative care should not exceed the burden of disease.

INTRODUCTION

Palliative care is defined as care that prevents or relieves symptoms of disease, and it can be broad in its application. It is important to remember that palliative care is not restricted to terminally ill patients and that palliative care is an important aspect of overall cancer management. Patients may live with cancer for many years. Although the clinical presentations for which palliative care is appropriate are broad, the principle of palliative care remains focused on relieving symptoms and improving functional outcome for the remainder of the patient's life. The goal of palliative care is to relieve symptoms effectively and efficiently with the fewest treatment-related symptoms and to maintain the maximum quality of life for the duration of the patient's life. Acknowledging the importance of quality of life, the Joint Commission on Accreditation of Healthcare Organizations has instituted standards for the appropriate assessment and management of pain and other symptoms. Unlike the case in other realms of cancer therapy, tumor control and survival are not the end points of therapeutic success in palliative care.

Vigano et al (2000) studied predictors of survival in a cohort of patients diagnosed with terminal disease. Among 208 patients with metastatic cancer, the overall median survival was 15 weeks. Shorter survival times were independently associated with the following factors: primary tumor site in the lung as opposed to the breast or gastrointestinal tract, liver metastases, comorbid conditions, weight loss of greater than 8 kg in the previous 6 months, and clinical estimate by the treating physician of a survival time of less than 2 months. Laboratory assessments associated with a poor prognosis included serum albumin levels of less than 35 g/L, a lymphocyte count of less than 1×10^9/L, and a lactate dehydrogenase level of more than 618 U/L. These independent prognostic factors are important in palliative-care decisions.

The type and severity of symptoms predict survival and add to the prognostic information derived from the Karnofsky performance status and extent of disease. The symptoms among 350 hospice inpatients with cancer correlated with patient characteristics, general condition, tumor location, and medications. The mean number of symptoms correlated directly with Karnofsky performance status; performance status was 10 to 20 in patients with 7 symptoms, 30 to 50 in patients with 6 symptoms, and 60 or greater in patients with 4 symptoms. Pain, dry mouth, constipation, change in taste, lack of appetite and energy, feeling bloated, nausea, vomiting, weight loss, feeling drowsy, and feeling dizzy portend a poorer prognosis.

Cancer symptoms are controlled through direct treatment of the symptoms (e.g., administration of opioids to control pain) and through treatment of the site where cancer is causing symptoms. Palliation constitutes a large part of oncology practice. For example, about 25% of all radiation treatments administered at M. D. Anderson Cancer Center are with palliative intent, and this pattern of practice has been stable for more than 40 years. At M. D. Anderson, multimodality treatment is used in palliative as well as curative approaches to therapy.

PRINCIPLES OF PALLIATIVE THERAPY

The goal of palliative therapy is the prompt and cost-effective relief of symptoms with little treatment-related morbidity.

Control of cancer-related pain with the use of analgesics is imperative to allow patient comfort during therapeutic interventions and while the patient awaits response to such interventions. Pain represents a sensitive measure of disease activity. Symptoms that recur or worsen most commonly result from localized regrowth of tumor. Patients should be followed up closely after any palliative therapeutic intervention, and diagnostic studies should be performed as indicated to identify progressive disease. It is important to realize that pain may not completely resolve after palliative therapy, which generally shrinks but does not eradicate a tumor. Residual symptoms must still be controlled using established principles of pain management.

Effective palliation of symptoms from cancers involving the gastrointestinal tract requires a clear evaluation of the prognosis. Among the considerations are the resectability of the disease and the presence and volume of metastatic disease. As in other realms of cancer care, a multidisciplinary approach is generally needed for effective palliative care.

CLINICAL PRESENTATIONS REQUIRING PALLIATIVE MANAGEMENT

There are many types of clinical presentation that necessitate palliative management for tumors involving the gastrointestinal region. Among the most common are symptoms caused by recurrent rectal cancer and biliary obstruction caused by pancreatic cancer. Nausea and vomiting due to gastrointestinal obstruction may require surgical decompression. Metastases from gastrointestinal malignancies can occur in any location, become symptomatic, and necessitate palliative care.

Pelvic Tumors

Pelvic tumors that cause symptoms are generally primary colorectal, cervical, or urinary tract tumors, although metastases from any primary tumor site can occur in the pelvis. Obstructive symptoms can result from a primary rectal cancer or from extrinsic tumor compression of the rectum by cervical or urinary-tract tumors. Urinary symptoms can result from ureteral or bladder obstruction or hematuria. Edema of the genitalia and lower extremities can result from lymphatic obstruction. Pain and other symptoms can result from metastatic involvement of the pelvic bones and lumbosacral plexus.

Anemia or Bleeding

In patients with unexplained anemia or bleeding, colorectal cancers are often the cause. Radiation therapy is an effective treatment, stopping active bleeding within 1 to 2 days of the first radiation fraction. Endoscopic laser ablation or surgical intervention may also be necessary to emergently stop active bleeding.

Obstructive Symptoms

Colorectal cancers may also result in intestinal obstruction necessitating stent placement to maintain the integrity of the visceral lumen. Occasionally a diverting colostomy will be required to bypass intestinal obstruction or fistula formation. If these procedures are not performed, intestinal colic can be palliated quickly with opioids. Opioids must be used carefully because they may worsen a partial bowel obstruction owing to their constipating effect. Anticholinergics—like scopolamine, atropine, and loperamide—also decrease peristalsis in the smooth muscle of the intestinal tract.

Intestinal obstruction resulting in nausea and vomiting can be palliated with nasogastric decompression and administration of pharmacologic agents. Octreotide, an analogue of somatostatin, reduces gastrointestinal secretions, motility, and splanchnic blood flow. Octreotide has a proabsorptive effect on water and ions and may inhibit the secretion of vasoactive intestinal peptide. Nasogastric decompression and administration of pharmacologic agents also helps to disrupt the cycle of abdominal distention that results in further intestinal secretion followed by peristalsis and bleeding.

The pelvic lymph nodes and major blood vessels may become obstructed by tumor. Lymphovascular obstruction results in painful edema that is refractory to diuretic and other therapies. When obstruction is severe, fluid and electrolyte imbalances can occur. Pelvic irradiation can relieve lymphovascular obstruction through tumor regression.

Pain

Pelvic tumors can also invade the sacral plexus and cause intractable pain. Tumor can spread along nerve roots and can be associated with bony invasion of the sacrum. Pain due to visceral or lymphovascular obstruction often responds more rapidly to palliative irradiation than does the neuropathic pain seen with sacral plexus involvement. Analgesic management of neuropathic pain can include use of adjuvant analgesics, like steroids and neuroleptic agents. Interventional pain management techniques, like intrathecal administration of analgesics, are frequently required to control pain associated with sacral plexus involvement.

Treatment Plan

The presence, volume, and location of metastatic disease influence the palliative treatment plan. Palliative chemoradiation can relieve symptoms of pain and bleeding in about 70% of cases. High-grade obstructive symptoms may require a diverting colostomy; urinary diversion may also be necessary. The following represent clinical approaches considered in a palliative treatment plan:

- If the disease is operable, surgery may be undertaken first to stop bleeding or decompress intestinal obstruction. Depending on the prognosis, postoperative chemoradiation may be recommended to prevent symptoms resulting from local recurrence.
- Patients with inoperable disease may benefit from chemoradiation to relieve symptoms, and if there is significant regression after radiation therapy, the tumor may become resectable. The schedule of chemoradiation used depends on the extent of local disease and whether metastases are present.
- If metastases are present and resectable or limited in volume, a more aggressive therapeutic approach consisting of preoperative chemoradiation to the pelvis followed by surgery may be appropriate. The course of the disease can be evaluated during the 6 weeks between completion of chemoradiation and surgery.
- If the local and metastatic disease is stable in the 6-week interval, local tumor resection can be undertaken for control of pelvic disease.
- If disease progresses during the 6-week interval, the chemoradiation administered to the pelvis should induce sufficient local tumor regression to relieve symptoms for the duration of the patient's life.
- If metastases are present and unresectable, palliative care should focus on relief of tumor-related symptoms.

These strategies focus on prompt relief of pelvic-related symptoms that is indexed to prognosis.

Symptoms of bleeding and obstruction due to inoperable pelvic tumors can be palliated with chemoradiation. Like the approach used in rectal cancer, 5-fluorouracil (5-FU) is administered during radiation therapy. Palliative radiation schedules used at M. D. Anderson have included 35 Gy in 14 fractions, 30 Gy in 10 fractions, and 30 Gy in 6 fractions given twice weekly for 3 weeks. In a series of 80 patients with metastatic rectal cancer treated at our institution (Crane et al, 2001), 16% of patients required a diverting colostomy before radiation therapy. No significant treatment-related side effects were observed, and symptoms from the primary tumor resolved in 94% of cases. Durable control of pelvic symptoms, defined as symptom control 3 or more months after treatment, did not differ significantly between the groups—rates were 81% for palliative chemoradiation and 91% for preoperative chemoradiation. The endoscopic complete response rate was 36%. Twenty-five patients underwent primary tumor resection. Although the 2-year survival rate was greater in the group that underwent resection (46% vs 11%), the colostomy-free survival rate was greater in the group that did not undergo resection (79% vs 51%). Predictors of a worse prognosis included pelvic pain at presentation, biologically equivalent dose at 2 Gy per fraction of less than 35 Gy, and poor tumor differentiation. Among patients with locally advanced rectal cancer who also had liver metastases at presentation, the median survival was 17 months among patients treated with palliative chemoradiation.

These results are similar to those with palliative radiation at the Princess Margaret Hospital. In that series, the most frequent palliative radiation schedule for locally advanced rectal cancer was 50 Gy in 20 fractions in 4 weeks. Five-year survival rates were directly dependent on the extent of the tumor: rates were 48% for patients with mobile tumor, 27% for patients with partially fixed tumors, and only 4% for patients with fixed tumors. Tumor extent also predicted response to radiation therapy: 50% of patients with mobile, 30% of patients with partially fixed, and only 9% of patients with fixed tumors had a complete clinical response to radiation. The rate of tumor regression was slow; only 60% of the complete responses occurred by 4 months, and not until 9 months had 90% of the complete responses occurred. Of the complete responders, approximately half of those with mobile or partially fixed tumors and more than 70% of those with fixed tumors developed progressive disease. Salvage surgery to relieve symptoms was accomplished without significant complications in more than 90% of patients who developed progressive or recurrent disease.

The decision to proceed with surgical resection depends on the volume of primary and metastatic disease, the patient's underlying medical condition, the possibility of complete tumor resection, and the ability to relieve symptoms, such as bowel obstruction. In a study by Videtic et al (1998), preoperative radiation therapy to a total dose of 54 Gy and continuous-infusion 5-FU was administered to 29 patients with inoperable rectal cancer. Resection was then undertaken in 23 patients, and in 18 of these patients, resection was performed with curative intent. Thirteen patients had an abdominoperineal resection, 3 underwent a low anterior resection, and 2 had a local excision. Pathologic findings included a complete response in 13% and pathologic evidence of tumor regression in 90%. With a median follow-up of 28 months, 15 patients were free of disease. Multivisceral resection resulted in a survival rate of approximately 50% at 5 years among patients with initially inoperable, locally advanced rectal cancer.

The risk of recurrence after pelvic exenteration exceeds 80% if radiation therapy is not administered. This is substantially higher than the risk of local recurrence after treatment of locally advanced but operable rectal cancer. Local control rates are also improved when intraoperative radiation therapy (IORT) is used to treat patients initially presenting with inoperable rectal cancer. In one series, the local control rate without IORT was only 33%, whereas the local control rate when IORT was added to external-beam therapy was 92% (Kim et al, 1997).

Techniques that localize the radiation dose to the recurrent tumor and limit the dose to the surrounding normal tissues allow reirradiation of recurrent tumors. Such techniques include conformal external-beam radiation therapy, intensity-modulated radiation therapy (IMRT), IORT, and brachytherapy. Conformal radiation therapy techniques precisely localize the radiation dose and give very low doses of radiation through a number of beams, such that no one area of normal tissues receives a significant dose of radiation. The tumor receives the sum of the radiation from all of the beams and receives a high dose of radiation. This technique has allowed high doses of radiation to be administered and has allowed for reirradiation of normal tissues. IMRT is a form of conformal external-beam radiation therapy that even more precisely administers radiation. For example, with IMRT, the center of the tumor may receive 2.20 Gy with each radiation treatment to a total dose of 66 Gy over 30 fractions in 6 weeks. The periphery of the tumor may receive 2.0 Gy with each radiation treatment to a total dose of 60 Gy. The normal tissues within 2 cm of the tumor (clinical tumor volume to account for possible microscopic tumor extension) may receive 1.8 Gy with each radiation treatment to a total dose of 54 Gy. Any shape or configuration of radiation dose, like an hourglass, can be designed with IMRT. Because of these factors, this radiotherapeutic tool is extremely helpful for unresectable tumors and tumors that recur in a previously irradiated field.

Gastroesophageal Tumors

The most common presenting symptoms of gastric and esophageal cancers are upper abdominal discomfort, weakness from anemia, weight loss, and hematemesis. Exophytic tumors can cause significant bleeding. Infiltrative tumors can invade the celiac plexus and cause severe back pain like that observed with pancreatic cancer. Tumor infiltration resulting in linitis plastica is associated with an extremely poor prognosis. Epigastric pain from gastric cancer can also result from acid secretion. Early satiety, hematemesis, and melena occur less commonly. Obstructing lesions in the antrum can cause vomiting, and obstructing lesions in the cardia can cause dysphagia. Several series indicate that 50% to 75% of patients experience improvement of bleeding, gastric outlet obstruction, and pain.

Gastric cancer can spread via direct extension, lymphatic or hematologic invasion, and transperitoneal dissemination. Critical organs such as the pancreas, diaphragm, transverse colon, duodenum, spleen, jejunum, liver, left kidney, left adrenal gland, and celiac axis are in close proximity to the stomach and are frequently involved. Lymphatic spread initially occurs to the mediastinal nodes and the perigastric nodes along the lesser and greater curvatures, and then occurs to lymphatics that accompany all 3 branches of the celiac axis. Remote lymphatic spread can occur to the hepatoduodenal, peripancreatic, superior mesenteric, and para-aortic nodal chains. Similar to the case with tumors of the esophagus and duodenum, clinically occult spread beyond the gross lesion can occur through the abundant subserosal and submucosal lymphatics. Sixteen to thirty-five percent of patients have positive peritoneal cytology findings at the time of tumor resection, but not all patients with positive cytology findings are destined to develop peritoneal carcinomatosis. However, transperitoneal spread occurs in 23% to 43% of patients after gastrectomy. Distant metastasis occurs most commonly via the portal venous drainage to the liver. Lung involvement is less common, but tumors involving the gastroesophageal junction have a stronger tendency to spread to the lungs.

All treatment modalities are involved in the palliative treatment of gastroesophageal cancer. The modality used depends on the patient's condition and the extent of disease. Localized therapies include surgery and radiation therapy. Among operable patients with extensive bleeding, surgery is often the first palliative approach. Radiation therapy can also palliate localized bleeding and tumor obstruction. Symptoms caused by disease infiltration of retroperitoneal structures also can respond to localized radiation therapy. Systemic chemotherapy is administered concurrently with radiation therapy and when disease is extensive or no longer localized. The most active single chemotherapeutic agents in gastric cancer are 5-FU, mitomycin, and doxorubicin. Although randomized studies have shown an advantage in median survival for multiagent chemotherapy compared to best supportive care, no corresponding advantage in long-term survival has been seen, and the median survival with chemotherapy is relatively short (5 to 7 months) in most studies.

Aggressive supportive care provided by a multidisciplinary care team is vital in the treatment of the abdominal region. This is illustrated by the Gastrointestinal Tumor Study Group experience. Even though patients treated with chemoradiation eventually had a better outcome, 6 of 45 patients in that group died because of sepsis or nutritional inadequacy. Prior to initiation of chemoradiation for gastric cancer, laparoscopic placement of a jejunostomy feeding tube may be necessary to support the extended need for nutrition and hydration. Prophylactic antiemetic therapy, like that given to patients treated with systemic therapy, should be administered prior to and during the course of chemoradiation as needed. A proton-pump inhibitor or H2 blocker is also recommended during the course of chemoradiation. Common antiemetics, like prochlorperazine, may be sufficient to control symptoms, but frequently patients will require other agents.

The critical structures in a typical radiation field for gastric cancer include the stomach itself, the small intestine, and the liver, kidneys, and spinal cord. The radiation sensitivity of these structures, though, limits the role of radiation therapy as a regional treatment modality. When 50% of a single kidney receives a radiation dose of more than 26 Gy, the creatinine clearance decreases by 10%. When the entire kidney receives more than 26 Gy, a 24% decrease in creatinine clearance has been observed. The development of clinically relevant compromise of kidney function is rare when 1 kidney is spared from the radiation field, especially in patients with limited life expectancy. Radiation-induced liver disease, often called radiation hepatitis, is characterized by the development of anicteric ascites approximately 2 weeks to 4 months after hepatic irradiation. The whole liver has been treated safely to doses greater than 20 Gy, but a significant risk of radiation hepatitis exists when doses of more than 35 Gy are given. The risk of radiation hepatitis is dependent on both the radiation dose and the volume of liver treated. Small volumes of the liver can tolerate high doses of irradiation.

Although treatment plans can limit the radiation dose to fixed structures like the liver and kidneys, it is not possible to exclude the small bowel from radiation fields in the upper abdomen. Unlike the case in treatment of rectal cancer, where much of the small bowel can be displaced from the radiation field using techniques like use of a belly board, in treatment of the upper abdomen, the radiation tolerance of the small bowel is a more important issue. Localized segments of the small bowel can tolerate doses of 45 to 50 Gy with conventional fractionation of 1.8 to 2.0 Gy per fraction, but tolerance of radiation is significantly less if significant volumes of small bowel are in the radiation field or if high radiation doses are used for each treatment fraction. These are critical factors for radiation therapy or if reirradiation of the abdomen is considered for progressive disease, especially when surgery and chemotherapy are not possible.

Brachytherapy involves placement of radioactive sources within a tumor bed and represents another means of administering well-localized radiation therapy to limit the dose to adjacent uninvolved structures. With brachytherapy, uninterrupted radiation therapy is delivered precisely to the tumor bed over a determined number of minutes or hours. Brachytherapy has been used for definitive treatment of localized disease, for a boost in conjunction with external-beam irradiation, and for treatment of disease recurring in a previously irradiated area.

High-dose-rate brachytherapy is often used to treat tumors involving the biliary tract, esophagus, cervix, or bronchus. The percentage of patients experiencing relief of dysphagia ranges from 70% to 85% in a number of published reports of brachytherapy used in the treatment of esophageal cancer. A combination of a short course of external-beam irradiation (30 Gy in 10 fractions) plus high-dose-rate brachytherapy used as a localized radiation boost relieves dysphagia from esophageal cancer for 3 to 6 months. Relative contraindications include a tumor length of 10 cm or more, extension to the gastroesophageal junction or cardia, skip lesions,

extensive extraesophageal spread of disease, macroscopic regional ade-
nopathy, tracheoesophageal fistula, cervical esophageal involvement, and
stenosis that cannot be bypassed.

Therapeutic options for patients who have extensive disease depend on
the clinical presentation and include supportive care, interventional or
surgical procedures to treat bleeding or obstruction, chemotherapy alone
or in combination with radiation therapy, and participation in clinical
trials evaluating new agents or treatment combinations.

Small Bowel Tumors

Small bowel tumors are rare, and the symptoms of such tumors are difficult to palliate given the propensity for widespread peritoneal involvement. When the cause of symptoms like obstruction or bleeding can be
localized, surgery or radiation therapy may provide palliative benefit.
Systemic chemotherapy, as in the case of gastroesophageal cancers, does
not significantly affect survival but can be considered for treatment of
widespread disease if the toxicity of the chemotherapy is limited.

Most cancers of the small bowel are treated with surgical resection.
Since the small bowel and surrounding mesenteric lymphatics are mobile,
regional treatment for malignancies of the jejunum and ileum would have
to include very large radiation fields that would be associated with significant toxicity. However, it is possible to use radiation to palliate the
symptoms of a tumor at the fixed region of the duodenum (the C-loop)
around the pancreas, especially if there is local infiltration into adjacent
visceral structures and the celiac plexus that would prohibit surgical
resection.

Pancreatic Tumors

The initial goals in the evaluation and treatment of symptomatic patients
with pancreatic cancer are to determine resectability and to re-establish
biliary tract outflow if necessary. The most common presenting symptoms
of pancreatic cancer are jaundice, weight loss due to anorexia and exocrine
insufficiency, and abdominal pain. Jaundice is usually a presenting
symptom in lesions of the pancreatic head. Lesions arising in the body or
tail of the pancreas more often present with pain. Pain is a symptom of
locally advanced disease. It is typically described as sharp and knife-like
and located in the midepigastric region, with the pain radiating to the
back, and is often a clinical indicator of unresectable disease. After treatment with surgery alone, 50% to 80% of patients with pancreatic cancer
develop local recurrence of disease. The most common distant sites of
failure are the liver and peritoneum. The lungs and bone are involved less
commonly by distant disease.

The pancreas is drained by an abundant supply of lymphatics. Primary
drainage occurs to the pancreaticoduodenal, suprapancreatic, pyloric
lymph, and pancreaticosplenic nodal regions, which all drain to the celiac
lymph nodes and to the superior mesenteric nodes. The porta hepatis

nodal region can also be involved, especially in advanced disease. The pancreatic duct and common bile duct are closely related as they travel through the head of the pancreas on their way to the ampulla of Vater. Invasion or compression of the common bile duct and main pancreatic duct is responsible for the presenting symptoms of jaundice and pancreatic exocrine insufficiency. The divisions of the vagus and splanchnic nerves form the celiac and superior mesenteric plexuses. Nerve fibers reach the pancreas and other abdominal organs by traveling along the celiac and superior mesenteric artery and their branches. Direct extension of tumor to the first and second celiac ganglia posteriorly leads to characteristic sharp pain, which is perceived as back pain.

Despite the generally poor overall prognosis for patients with pancreatic cancer, most treatment programs for pancreatic cancer will administer chemotherapy and radiation therapy over 4 to 6 weeks to deliver 45 to 60 Gy. However, at M. D. Anderson, we found no survival advantage with the use of higher doses of radiation in the definitive treatment of pancreatic cancer. Routinely, we administer 30 Gy in 10 fractions. This treatment is well tolerated for both definitive and palliative therapy. Furthermore, this fractionation schedule limits treatment time, which is of particular importance in the palliative setting. A study that compared preoperative chemoradiation (50.4 Gy and rapid-fractionation chemoradiation totaling 30 Gy over 2 weeks) plus pancreaticoduodenectomy with pancreaticoduodenectomy plus postoperative adjuvant chemoradiation (50.4 Gy over 5.5 weeks with 5-FU) found that no patient who received preoperative chemoradiation experienced a delay in surgery because of chemoradiation toxicity. In contrast, one third of patients in the postoperative-chemoradiation group required hospitalization because of acute gastrointestinal side effects. Also, 24% of patients in the postoperative-chemoradiation group did not receive the intended postoperative chemoradiation because of delayed recovery following pancreaticoduodenectomy.

Computed tomography–based treatment planning allows precise definition of the symptoms caused by disease and permits reduction of the radiation fields and thus reduction in the side effects of treatment. Supportive-care recommendations for patients with pancreatic tumors are similar to those for patients with gastroesophageal cancers, but less nausea and diarrhea generally occur in the treatment of pancreatic tumors because less of the stomach is included in the radiation field and the radiation field is generally smaller. When pancreatic cancer is found to be unresectable at laparotomy, improvements in local and symptomatic control have been shown when IORT is used.

Because the risk of intra-abdominal and systemic failure is so high, paclitaxel and gemcitabine chemotherapies have been administered. A randomized trial of gemcitabine versus 5-FU as first-line therapy among patients with advanced pancreatic adenocarcinoma demonstrated a modest median survival benefit (4.41 months vs 5.65 months, $P = .0025$) for patients who received gemcitabine. Gemcitabine was approved for use among patients with inoperable or metastatic pancreatic cancer on the basis of improvement in quality-of-life parameters compared to outcomes with supportive care, although no survival advantage was seen with gemcitabine.

Because gemcitabine is a potent radiation sensitizer, a significant increase in toxicity without long-term impact on survival or quality of life was initially observed when gemcitabine was combined with palliative radiation therapy. Because the gemcitabine dose limitation is predominantly attributable to gastrointestinal toxicity within the radiation field, the size of the radiation field is a critical variable. Weekly doses of gemcitabine in the range of 200 to 400 mg/m² are tolerated when the radiation fields encompass the primary tumor and regional lymphatics. Doses in the range of 700 to 1,000 mg/m² have been given with smaller fields. These prospective clinical data appear to indicate that the tolerated dose of gemcitabine with radiation is inversely related to the radiation dose and the radiation field size.

Because surgical resection of the primary tumor remains the only potentially curative treatment for pancreatic cancer, preoperative chemoradiation has been studied for its ability to convert locally unresectable pancreatic cancer to resectable disease. Only 10% of patients with clinically unresectable disease treated with 5-FU- or paclitaxel-based chemoradiation are able to eventually undergo margin-negative resection. Preliminary reports indicate that the margin-negative resectability rate

---

KEY PRACTICE POINTS

- The goals of palliative therapy are palliation of symptoms with limited treatment-related toxicity.

- Multimodality recommendations for care must be individualized on the basis of clinical presentation.

- Although the gastrointestinal tract can be the site of metastatic disease, locally advanced disease from a gastrointestinal malignancy is the most common cause of gastrointestinal-tract symptoms.

- In patients with incurable disease, surgical resection of the primary tumor often allows durable control of symptoms from the primary tumor. Surgery can also quickly palliate obstruction and bleeding. Localized symptoms can effectively be managed with endoscopic techniques and radiation therapy. Chemotherapy, used in the palliative setting for cytoreduction, can also provide relief of symptoms.

- In all cases, aggressive supportive care is required to limit treatment-related side effects and manage persistent symptoms of disease.

could be as high as 40% to 50% among selected patients with unresectable disease treated with gemcitabine-based chemoradiation.

Ulceration of Skin and Subcutaneous Tissues

Tumors can cause ulceration of the skin and subcutaneous tissues, which is often painful and distressing because of constant drainage. Such ulceration increases the risk of sepsis in immunocompromised patients. Localized radiation therapy can be applied to destroy tumor and allow re-epithelialization of the skin. Radiation is generally used to treat only the skin and subcutaneous tissues (electron-beam therapy) to avoid radiation side effects to underlying uninvolved normal structures. Surgical resection and flap placement can also be considered for selected cases.

SUGGESTED READINGS

Blinkert CA, Ledermann H, Jost R, Saurenmann P, Decurtins M, Zollikofer CL. Acute colonic obstruction: clinical aspects and cost-effectiveness of preoperative and palliative treatment with self-expanding metallic stents—a preliminary report. *Radiology* 1998;206:199–204.

Brierly JD, Cummings BJ, Wong CS, et al. Adenocarcinoma of the rectum treated by radical external radiation therapy. *Int J Radiat Oncol Biol Phys* 1995;31:255–259.

Camunez F, Echenagusia A, Simo G, Turegano F, Vazquez J, Barreiro-Meiro I. Malignant colorectal obstruction treated by means of self-expanding metallic stents: effectiveness before surgery and in palliation. *Radiology* 2000;216:492–497.

Chang VT, Thaler HT, Polyak TA, Kornblith AB, Lepore JM, Portenoy RK. Quality of life and survival: the role of multidimensional symptom assessment. *Cancer* 1998;83:173–179.

Coia LR, Myerson RJ, Tepper JE. Late effects of radiation therapy on the gastrointestinal tract. *Int J Radiat Oncol Biol Phys* 1995;31:1213–1236.

Crane CH, Janjan NA, Abbruzzese JL, et al. Effective pelvic symptom control using initial chemoradiation without colostomy in metastatic rectal cancer. *Int J Radiat Oncol Biol Phys* 2001;49:107–116.

Dawson LA, McGinn CJ, Normolle D, et al. Escalated focal liver radiation and concurrent hepatic artery fluorodeoxyuridine for unresectable intrahepatic malignancies. *J Clin Oncol* 2000;18:2210–2218.

Evans DB, Abbruzzese JL, Cleary KR, et al. Preoperative chemoradiation for adenocarcinoma of the pancreas: excessive toxicity of prophylactic hepatic irradiation. *Int J Radiat Oncol Biol Phys* 1995;33:913–918.

Glimelius B, Ekstrom K, Hoffman K, et al. Randomized comparison between chemotherapy plus best supportive care with best supportive care in advanced gastric cancer. *Ann Oncol* 1997;8:163–168.

Goldberg RM, Fleming TR, Tangen CM, et al. Surgery for recurrent colon cancer: strategies for identifying resectable recurrence and success rates after resection. *Ann Intern Med* 1998;129:27–35.

Grabowski CM, Unger JA, Potish RA. Factors predictive of completion of treatment and survival after palliative radiation therapy. *Radiology* 1992;184:329–332.

Hayes N, Wayman J, Wadehra V, Scott DJ, Raimes SA, Griffin SM. Peritoneal cytology in the surgical evaluation of gastric carcinoma. *Br J Cancer* 1999;79:520–524.

Janjan NA, Breslin T, Lenzi R, Rich TA, Skibber JM. Avoidance of colostomy placement in advanced colorectal cancer with twice weekly hypofractionated radiation plus continuous infusion 5-fluorouracil. *J Pain Symptom Manage* 2000;20: 266–272.

Janjan NA, Waugh KA, Skibber JM, et al. Control of unresectable recurrent anorectal cancer with Au198 seed implantation. *J Brachytherapy Int* 1999;15:115–129.

Kim HK, Jessup JM, Beard CJ, et al. Locally advanced rectal carcinoma: pelvic control and morbidity following preoperative radiation therapy, resection, and intraoperative radiation therapy. *Int J Radiat Oncol Biol Phys* 1997;38:777–783.

Lamont EB, Christakis NA. Some elements of prognosis in terminal cancer. *Oncology* 1999;13:1165–1170.

Luna-Perez P, Delgado S, Labastida S, Ortiz N, Rodriguez D, Herrera L. Patterns of recurrence following pelvic exenteration and external radiotherapy for locally advanced primary rectal adenocarcinoma. *Ann Surg Oncol* 1996;3: 526–533.

Mancini I, Bruera E. Constipation in advanced cancer patients. *Support Care Cancer* 1998;6:356–364.

Mohiuddin M, Marks GM, Lingareddy V, Marks J. Curative surgical resection following reirradiation for recurrent rectal cancer. *Int J Radiat Oncol Biol Phys* 1997;39:643–649.

Morris DE. Clinical experience with retreatment for palliation. *Semin Radiat Oncol* 2000;10:210–221.

Pyrhonen S, Kuitunen T, Nyandoto P, Kouri M. Randomised comparison of fluorouracil, epidoxorubicin, and methotrexate (FEMTX) plus supportive care versus supportive care alone in patients with non-resectable gastric cancer. *Br J Cancer* 1995;71:587–591.

Rousseau P. Management of malignant bowel obstruction in advanced cancer: a brief review. *J Palliat Med* 1998;1:65–72.

Salo JC, Paty PB, Guillem J, Minsky BD, Harrison LB, Cohen AM. Surgical salvage of recurrent rectal carcinoma after curative resection: a 10-year experience. *Ann Surg Oncol* 1999;6:171–177.

Videtic GM, Fisher BJ, Perera FE, et al. Preoperative radiation with concurrent 5-fluorouracil continuous infusion for locally advanced unresectable rectal cancer. *Int J Radiat Oncol Biol Phys* 1998;42:319–324.

Vigano A, Bruera E, Jhangri GS, Newman SC, Fields AL, Suarez-Almazor ME. Clinical survival predictors in patients with advanced cancer. *Arch Intern Med* 2000;160:861–868.

Wesselmann U, Burnett AL, Heinberg LJ. The urogenital and rectal pain syndromes. *Pain* 1997;73:269–294.

Willett CG, Tepper JE, Orlow EL, Shipley WU. Renal complications secondary to radiation treatment of upper abdominal malignancies. *Int J Radiat Oncol Biol Phys* 1986;12:1601–1604.

19 BOWEL MANAGEMENT IN PATIENTS WITH CANCER

Annette K. Bisanz

Chapter Overview

This chapter addresses concepts used as a foundation for bowel management in patients with cancer. Because cancer treatment can be very noxious and disrupt bowel function, a preventive approach is an important part of bowel management for patients with cancer. The 6 steps to good bowel management are assessment and diagnosis of bowel dysfunction, normalization of the bowel, establishment of expectations for bowel-movement frequency, development of a bowel management program, assessment of outcomes, and adjustment of the bowel management program through problem-solving. New and innovative approaches to management of bowel dysfunction covered in this chapter are (1) differentiation between low and high impactions in the treatment of impactions; (2) administration of milk-and-molasses enemas; (3) use of a bowel training program for patients with constipation or diarrhea or frequent stooling; and (4) use of a proven, nontraditional fiber regimen for patients with frequent stooling after colorectal surgery. Opiate-induced constipation may be effectively prevented using senna and docusate sodium. Gastrointestinal gas may be decreased through controlling the intake of certain foods. Diarrhea in patients with cancer may have various noncancer causes, including impaction, lactose intolerance, food allergies, and medication. The cause of diarrhea, not the symptom, must be treated for optimal relief. New and innovative approaches, including strengthening the anal sphincter, slowing the gastrointestinal tract, and training the bowel, help patients achieve better outcomes. Involving the patient as a partner in bowel management is crucial because many problems are encountered outside the immediate supervision of the health care team.

Introduction

Alteration in bowel function is a common source of distress for patients with cancer, not only causing discomfort but also affecting daily activities, nutritional intake, and socialization. Fifty percent of people with cancer experience constipation, and that percentage increases to 78% for terminally ill patients with cancer (Levy, 1991). An estimated 10% of patients in the United States who have advanced cancer (more than 20,000 people) will experience diarrhea (Levy, 1991). In addition, about 43% of patients undergoing bone marrow transplantation develop diarrhea as a result of radiation therapy or graft versus host disease (Cox et al, 1994). Diarrhea mandates equal vigilance because of the potential complications and discomfort.

There is no common medical definition of constipation or diarrhea. For the purposes of this chapter, constipation is defined as the condition in which stool is hard and difficult to eliminate; the term does not refer to the frequency of stooling. Diarrhea is defined as more than 3 loose stools per day. The normal number of stools varies from 3 per day to 3 per week (Cimprich, 1985; Lembo and Camilleri, 2003).

Some patients never experience alterations in bowel function before they are diagnosed with cancer. Many cancer treatments cause either constipation or diarrhea, however, and it is very important to take a preventive approach and teach patients how to manage bowel function before symptoms begin. To illustrate, it is much more difficult to treat a myelosuppressed patient for an impaction, owing to limited treatment options, than it is to prevent the impaction initially. Prevention of symptoms, not just temporary relief of symptoms, should be a primary focus in bowel management.

In many cases, patients with cancer also have health problems unrelated to cancer that need to be explored. Often, bowel problems are erroneously thought to be related to the cancer and cancer treatment. Properly diagnosing these problems will lead to the best outcome for the patient and save time in providing relief.

Because each patient's gastrointestinal (GI) tract reacts differently to the amount and type of food, solutions to bowel dysfunction may vary by patient. To help meet individual needs, patients should be enrolled in a basic program and then guided toward effective bowel management by learning to problem-solve using basic principles, which will be presented in this chapter.

Admittedly, the bowel is not easy to manage. Effective management involves a problem-solving approach and may take some time to accomplish. Patients who are not compliant with a bowel management program typically will not show a good outcome. Patients need to be active partners in managing the bowel, keeping the health care team informed so that any necessary changes can be made.

This chapter presents some principles that have been helpful in bowel management in patients with GI cancer. It is not meant to provide comprehensive coverage of all possibilities but to share new, innovative treatment regimens that have proven to be successful in guiding patients with GI cancer to good bowel management. This chapter is presented in a simplified manner, reflecting the approach and education that patients need to understand how to help themselves.

It is important to impress upon the reader that input from members of an interdisciplinary health care team is invaluable in the arena of bowel management. Many of the successful elements of the regimens presented in this chapter were discovered over the years through collaboration among pharmacists, clinical dietitians, physicians, and nurses. Frequently, patients who do not initially have a favorable outcome find a solution when a member of the interdisciplinary team involves the entire team of experts in problem-solving together for an individual patient.

Quality-of-life issues for patients with bowel management problems involve many facets. From a quality-of-life perspective, issues such as having no more than 3 bowel movements per day, being able to leave the house without fear of not finding a bathroom, having the perianal skin intact without irritation and pain, and having regular bowel movements to prevent pain, bloating, and cramping are extremely important.

Because bowel management can be a very delicate topic, it is helpful to inform patients that bowel management needs to be discussed so that the appropriate guidance can be provided to lead patients to the quality of life most people desire. Maintaining a sense of humor is essential. Frequently, it is not hard to smile at the way patients describe their predicament; smiling may help patients understand that making light of their burden may actually help to lessen it. It is nice to know that someone understands, that patients are not alone, and that someone wants to guide them to better outcomes. Patients who have accidents do better if they can make light of the problem, carry with them a change of clothing, and be thankful that they can rectify the situation. Additionally, it is helpful for patients to realize that they can learn to manage their bowel function.

Patients are inevitably affected by bowel changes during cancer treatment or disease progression. Too often, clinicians wait until a serious symptom arises to address this potential problem. Oncology care would be enhanced if a more proactive, aggressive approach to bowel management were taken.

STEPS TO EFFECTIVE BOWEL MANAGEMENT

There are 6 steps to good bowel management: assessment and diagnosis of bowel dysfunction, normalization of the bowel, establishment of expectations for bowel-movement frequency, development of a bowel management program, assessment of outcomes, and adjustment of the bowel management program through problem-solving.

Assessment and Diagnosis of Bowel Dysfunction

Thoroughly assessing bowel function and obtaining a bowel history together constitute the most important step in bowel management. Unless the cause of the dysfunction or problem is diagnosed, the wrong treatment may be prescribed, leading to an unfavorable outcome. The assessment should include the following: vital signs; hydration status; abdominal status; perianal or peristomal skin integrity; frequency of bowel movements in the previous 2 weeks; consistency of stool (liquid, soft formed, or hard and hard to eliminate); number of impactions since cancer diagnosis; appetite (ranging from 3 big meals per day to only sips of liquid); daily fluid intake; daily fiber intake; medications currently being taken, particularly those that affect bowel elimination; presence of abdominal pain or cramping; concomitant diseases that affect bowel function (e.g., diabetes, Crohn's disease, and irritable bowel syndrome); presence of abdominal distention; frequency of bowel movements before cancer diagnosis; usual time of day that bowel movements occur; effective corrective measures previously used for bowel problems; extent of cancer; current treatments for cancer; laboratory results; and diagnostic imaging results. This information provides a comprehensive picture, allowing the problem to be correctly diagnosed and its causes to be identified.

Comorbid conditions unrelated to cancer need to be assessed, along with consumption of over-the-counter drugs; changes in the patient's physiologic make-up secondary to surgery, disease process, or treatment; and dietary habits. All of these factors must to be weighed when advising patients about a bowel management program.

Normalization of the Bowel

Normalization means bringing the bowel back to a normal state without constipation or impaction and with no more than 3 bowel movements per day. When a patient is constipated or has a fecal impaction, the buildup of stool or the impaction must be removed. If a patient has diarrhea, the motility of the GI tract must be slowed to decrease the frequency of bowel movements to 3 or fewer per day. A bowel management program will be ineffective if it is begun before the bowel is returned to a normal state.

Establishment of Expectations for Bowel-Movement Frequency

The amount of stool output is directly related to the amount of food consumed; this idea is central to expectations about the frequency of bowel movements. Such expectations help patients with cancer intervene at the first sign of bowel irregularity. At M. D. Anderson Cancer Center, patient-education materials clearly outline normal expectations. For instance, patients who eat 3 full meals per day can expect to have a bowel movement daily; patients who eat half of their normal amount can expect to have a bowel movement every other day; and patients who eat one third of their normal amount can expect to have a bowel movement every third day. Under the guidelines, the failure to have a bowel movement at the expected time signals the patient to induce a bowel movement. Patients with no expectations to have bowel movements at set intervals tend to ignore irregularity, which leads to complications, such as impaction from constipation or dehydration from diarrhea. Patient education is crucial in helping patients prevent bowel problems.

Development of a Bowel Management Program

A bowel management program for long-term use should not be initiated until therapy that has side effects on the GI tract is completed. During treatment, however, bowels can be managed using a symptom management approach. After the patient finishes all chemotherapy, radiation therapy, and biotherapy, the patient's present pattern of elimination is assessed, and a long-term bowel management program can be initiated.

All bowel programs must consider the titration of food, fluids, fiber, and medication. This is the fundamental, founding principle of bowel management.

All patients need to be on a bowel management program; few need to be placed in a bowel training program, which will be addressed later in this chapter.

Assessment of Outcomes

Patients must understand the importance of informing the health care team if defecation does not occur as expected. The bowel management program can then be altered.

Adjustment of Bowel Management Program to Achieve the Desired Outcome

The bowel management program may need to be altered multiple times to obtain the optimal outcome for an individual patient. Patients should adhere to each change in the regimen for 3 days to allow the bowel to adjust and to permit determination of the consistent response to that change.

Patients need to be taught how to problem-solve, adjusting the regimen regularly every 3 days until the desired response is obtained. They should be encouraged to understand their own bodies so that once they learn the principles of a bowel management program, they can alter the regimen of food, fluid, fiber, and bowel medication independently of the health care team. Again, prevention is the key, and patient education is a requirement.

REQUIREMENTS FOR ADEQUATE BOWEL FUNCTION

Adequate bowel function requires GI motility, mucosal transport, defecation reflexes, and intact anal sphincter muscles.

GI motility requires muscle contraction; secretions supplied by the salivary glands, stomach, biliary system, pancreas, and small intestine; an adequate central nervous system; and adequate nutrition and hydration.

Mucosal transport promotes the absorption of nutrients, water, and electrolytes in the small bowel, leaving water resorption to take place in the large bowel. If the stool moves through the large bowel too quickly, less water is reabsorbed and the stool remains liquid. The longer the stool remains in the large bowel, the more fluid is removed and the harder the stool becomes.

Spontaneous mass movements occur three or four times a day when the colon becomes filled and distended (Society of Gastroenterology Nurses and Associates Core Curriculum Committee, 1993). This usually occurs after a big meal, and thus a substantial decrease in oral intake alters the normal function of the GI tract. Defecation reflexes are initiated by rectal distention. The primary function of the colon is to store and concentrate fecal material before defecation. As the involuntary internal anal sphincter muscle relaxes, the longitudinal muscle of the rectum contracts to expel the stool (Portenoy, 1987; Levy, 1992).

Patients with GI cancer have a great risk for alterations in 1 or more of these mechanisms required for good GI function, depending on the anatomic location of the cancer and the treatments prescribed. The GI changes induced by the disease and treatment must be factored into any bowel management program. For example, the flow of stool may be altered by an intraluminal tumor in the GI tract. Likewise, extraluminal pressure on the gut or neural innervation change may affect flow through the GI tract.

A common culprit causing fecal impaction is recent diagnostic procedures using barium. This type of impaction can be prevented by routinely prescribing a laxative to be taken until evidence of barium excretion abates. Although laxatives are prescribed in many cases, the dose may be too small to fully eliminate the barium. Patients need to be instructed about the desired outcome from laxatives after barium ingestion so that they can inform their health care professional if the laxative does not work. If patients are assessed as having a high risk for constipation, a request to use Gastrografin (mixture of meglumine diatrizoate with sodium diatrizoate) in place of barium is appropriate.

Advanced disease or carcinomatosis commonly obstructs the flow through the GI tract. Thus, a plan should be made and implemented to ensure that patients have regular soft to semiliquid elimination, even if only with a medicinal supportive-care regimen.

COMPONENTS OF AN EFFECTIVE BOWEL MANAGEMENT PROGRAM

Any bowel management program should include fluid, fiber, food, and medication (Figure 19–1). This is verified in recent literature by Rao (2003) and Lembo and Camilleri (2003). Additionally, patients must understand

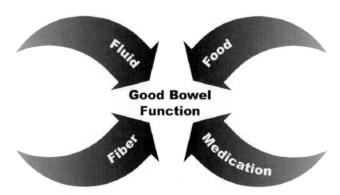

Figure 19–1.   Four essential elements of any bowel management program.

the need to balance these 4 components—this is the most fundamental concept in managing their bowels. A balanced scale, with 2 components in each basket that must be balanced for the bowel to function properly, is a good image to bring to patients' attention. When patients understand this concept and experiment using the problem-solving approach, this indicates that patients are convinced of the importance of each of the components affecting good bowel function. This can represent a real change for many patients because they have never had to comply with a bowel management program to have good bowel health.

Fluid

The average fluid intake required is 2 quarts per day. Many patients describe their fluid intake as much less than the prescribed amount, although occasional patients report consuming more than the average daily requirement. Excessive volumes of fluid increase the frequency of defecation because the fluid increases distention and therefore motility.

For the purpose of measuring fluid intake, fluids include liquids and food items that break down into fluid at room temperature (e.g., gelatin dessert and ice cream). For good bowel management, it is very beneficial for patients to consume at least 50% by volume of their daily intake in the form of water. Americans consume large amounts of beverages that contain caffeine. Caffeinated beverages have a diuretic effect and consequently are eliminated largely through the kidneys. The ratio of a patient's dietary liquids that contain caffeine to those that do not is important in the evaluation of constipation. Optimally, the intake of liquids that contain caffeine should not exceed the intake of liquids that do not contain caffeine.

Environmental factors affect the body's need for fluid, and patients need to be aware of this effect. For example, profuse sweating due to heat or sun exposure causes loss of a considerable amount of fluid through the skin. Elevated body temperature necessitates the replacement of lost fluids. If lost fluid is not replaced, the stool may become firmer. Stool softeners also help to retain fluid in the GI tract and may be titrated as needed.

Medications can affect fluid levels in the body. For example, diuretics decrease the amount of fluid in the GI tract by increasing excretion of fluid through the kidneys.

Specific diseases can affect the fluid balance. For instance, diabetes precipitates a tendency toward constipation if the patient maintains a high glucose level because the unmetabolized sugar cannot be excreted through the kidneys without a solvent, and this situation deprives the GI tract of the normal fluid level. A sudden complaint of constipation by a diabetic patient with cancer alerts the clinician that the patient's blood sugar level may be out of control.

Hot fluids tend to increase peristalsis. This is a very effective concept to incorporate into any bowel management education.

Also influencing fluid balance in the GI tract is fiber intake, discussed in the next section.

In summary, methods to maintain adequate fluid in the GI tract include increasing oral fluid intake, decreasing intake of drinks that contain caffeine, lowering elevated body temperature, avoiding being outside in extreme heat, taking stool softeners, and consuming an adequate amount of fiber and the correct amount of fluid to hold the fluid in the stool and keep it soft.

Fiber

Fiber, which is one of the most important components of good bowel function, acts in several ways. It increases water content in the stool, increases fecal bulk, promotes softer consistency of the stool, replenishes bacteria in the colon, can be used to increase or decrease fecal transit time, decreases intraluminary pressure, and keeps the intestinal villi healthy. People need both the water-soluble and bulk-forming types of fiber in their diet. Water-soluble fiber is found in oat products, legumes, fruits, and pectin. Insoluble bulk-forming fiber (celluloses and hemicelluloses) is present in wheat, vegetables, all-bran cereals, and apple skin.

The daily requirement for fiber ranges from 30 to 40 grams per day. The average American eats 10 to 20 grams per day. However, a sudden increase in daily fiber consumption from 20 grams per day to the optimal daily allowance overnight would cause the GI tract to overreact, resulting in gas, bloating, cramping, and diarrhea. This demonstrates the importance of the concept of titration and why patients need to understand it. For patients experiencing bowel difficulties, medicinal fiber is typically provided instead of nutritional fiber for bowel management. Patients need to be aware of the need to gradually increase fiber intake to avoid becoming disenchanted by an overreaction of the bowel resulting from rapid increases.

Medicinal fiber—i.e., psyllium (Metamucil) and methylcellulose (Citrucel)—has distinct benefits. Patients may have less gas with one or the other of the 2 types of medicinal fiber, and they can be used interchangeably. Medicinal fiber can be given in the right quantity and titrated to meet the patient's individual need more easily than dietary fiber can, and because most people do not consume enough fiber (30 to 40 grams per day), medicinal fiber helps them reach their daily requirement for good bowel function. Locke (2000) described nutritional and medicinal fiber as frontline therapy for constipation. However, it is not for patients who cannot meet fluid requirements for proper action or patients at risk for obstruction.

Fiber can be used to either speed up or slow down GI motility (Wyman et al, 1976; Iseminegr and Hardy, 1982; Bisanz, 1997; Lembo and Camilleri, 2003). This basic concept has given patients more options to normalize their bowels. Unfortunately, the label directions for taking supplemental medicinal fiber apply only to the treatment of constipation. The label directions do not provide instructions on how or when to introduce medicinal fiber for frequent stooling or diarrhea.

Ingesting medicinal fiber in very little fluid allows excess fluid to be reabsorbed by the fiber, which slows GI motility. This concept, described in the literature by Iseminegr and Hardy (1982) and Wyman (1976), was translated into a clinical protocol at M. D. Anderson to help patients with frequent soft-formed stools after colorectal cancer treatment and has been very successful in helping patients regain more normal bowel function (Bisanz, 1997) (see the section Bowel Management Program for Frequent Stooling after Colorectal Surgery later in this chapter).

Contrasting regimens of medicinal fiber to treat patients with constipation or diarrhea are outlined in Table 19–1 (see also Figure 19–2).

Patients taking medicinal fiber to decrease bowel motility frequently ask about commercially packaged fiber (e.g., fiber packaged in pill form or individual doses). In such situations, patients should be advised that commercially packaged fiber is for people with constipation and is more difficult to titrate than the nonpackaged powder form. Only when patients reach a maintenance dose can the equivalent packets or pill form be utilized.

The starting dose of medicinal fiber for patients with constipation is 1 tablespoon in 8 ounces of water followed by 8 additional ounces of water. The starting dose for patients with diarrhea is 1 teaspoon in 2 ounces of water after a meal with no additional fluid for 1 hour after. The dose is then increased gradually as needed to slow the frequent stooling.

It is important to note that fiber is contraindicated in patients who may have an obstruction in either the large or small bowel. Adding bulk may increase the intraluminal content and could worsen the obstruction (Portenoy, 1987).

Food

Food patterns vary greatly from person to person, and it is wise to consider these patterns in advising patients about nutrition. A clinical dietitian can help patients understand how to maintain adequate nutrition

Table 19–1.   Use of Medicinal Fiber to Treat Patients with Constipation or Diarrhea or Frequent Stooling

Symptom	Regimen	Reminders
Constipation	Once a day, take 1 tablespoon of psyllium in 8 ounces of fluid, and then immediately drink 8 additional ounces of fluid. If constipation persists for 3 days, then twice a day, take 1 tablespoon of psyllium in 8 ounces of fluid and then immediately drink 8 additional ounces of fluid. If constipation persists for 3 more days, then three times a day, take 1 tablespoon of psyllium in 8 ounces of fluid and then immediately drink 8 additional ounces of fluid.	Maintain a daily dose of psyllium that produces soft, formed stools. CAUTION: Taking medicinal fiber without adequate fluid can promote constipation.
Diarrhea or frequent stooling	Once a day, take 1 teaspoon of psyllium in 2 ounces of fluid. DO NOT drink extra fluid with this dose. If diarrhea persists for 5 to 7 days, then twice a day, take 1 teaspoon of psyllium in 2 ounces of fluid. Maintain this dose for 5 to 7 days. If diarrhea is still unrelieved, then three times a day, take 1 teaspoon of psyllium in 2 ounces of fluid. Every 5 to 7 days thereafter, until stool is formed, add 1 additional teaspoon of psyllium to each 1-teaspoon dose. Some people need as much as 2 teaspoons of psyllium 3 to 4 times a day (see Table 4–4). Then add a tablespoon at bedtime.	Taking small amounts of psyllium with meals may help to form a food bolus. This small round mass will slow down the passage of stool through the intestine. DO NOT take fluids at mealtime. Instead, drink fluids between meals. Avoid drinking warm liquids. They can initiate diarrhea.

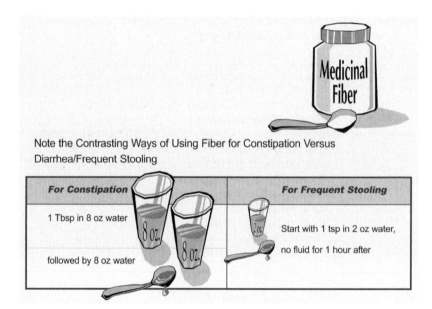

Figure 19–2. Contrasting ways of using fiber for constipation versus diarrhea or frequent stooling.

in a manner that is consistent with their food preferences as they progress through cancer treatment.

Whenever possible, patients are encouraged to eat a regular diet so that they can consume foods that appeal to them. A bowel management program can then be based on the patient's normal diet and avoid dietary restrictions except as required by the patient's individual condition and ongoing treatment.

The foods that most commonly increase GI motility are fried and highly spiced foods and hot liquids. A large meal increases peristalsis, whereas a small meal or snack does not promote a massive peristaltic push. Six small meals per day instead of 3 big meals are recommended for patients with frequent stooling.

Each person's GI tract reacts differently to the same food. For example, 4 ounces of prune juice may cause diarrhea in 1 person and not affect another. Each patient should become aware, by keeping a diet history, of his or her own reactions to specific foods. Patients can tentatively connect certain foods with particular symptoms and then ingest the foods again to see if the response is consistent. Patients can then decide which foods to avoid and which foods will help normalize bowel function.

Medications to Offset Bowel Side Effects of Other Drugs

Many medications can induce either constipation or diarrhea (Table 19–2), and it is important to know what effect a patient's current medications have on bowel function.

When trying to determine the potential side effects of a patient's medication regimen, the clinical pharmacist may provide information about specific drug side effects and drug interactions that contribute to bowel dysfunction. In some cases, the effects can be counteracted; in others, the drug may need to be changed to prevent the unwanted side effect. The pharmacist is the resource needed to guide medication changes based on side effects or drug interactions.

Many of the drugs categorized in Table 19–2 are commonly administered, and in many cases patients do not know that the effects on bowel function may be offset by altering fluid, food, and fiber intake or by adding another medication to compensate for the effect on the bowel.

Failure to ask patients about their use of nonprescription drugs may result in failure to capture a most important clue to a patient's bowel situation. For example, magnesium-based antacids can contribute to diarrhea, and calcium-based antacids can contribute to constipation. Antacids that have equal amounts of calcium and magnesium are now available and best to recommend.

Opiates diminish peristalsis, and because of this, in patients taking opiates, more than the usual amount of fluid is removed from the stool.

Table 19–2. Examples of Types of Drugs that Induce Constipation and Diarrhea

Constipation	Diarrhea
Opioids	Laxatives
Anticholinergic drugs	Antibiotics
Antihistamines	Specific biological drugs
Anti-inflammatory drugs	Magnesium-based antacids
Tricyclic antidepressants	Metoclopramide
Antispasmodics	Specific chemotherapeutic drugs
Anticonvulsant	
Muscle relaxants	
Aluminum antacids	
Bismuth	
Iron	
Neuroleptics	
Anti-Parkinsonism agents	
Specific chemotherapeutic drugs	
Calcium channel blockers	
Angiotensin-converting enzyme (ACE) inhibitors	
Diuretics	
Barbiturates	
Antipsychotics	
Antiarrhythmics	

Source: Levy (1991) and Locke et al. (2003).

This necessitates use of a stimulant laxative and a stool softener, both of which must be titrated up as needed to offset the side effects of the opiates (see the section Prevention of Opioid-Induced Constipation later in this chapter). Opiate-induced ileus is not uncommon in patients with advanced disease, underscoring the need for very aggressive bowel management in patients receiving palliative care.

CONSTIPATION

Definitions of constipation vary from one reference to another. At M. D. Anderson, we define constipation as the condition in which stool is hard and difficult to eliminate. Even if the frequency of bowel movements decreases, as long as the stool remains soft and formed, the patient is not constipated.

Never Underestimate How Much Stool the Intestines Can Hold

The average length of the colon is 4 to 5 feet, and the colon is 2 inches in diameter, which makes possible a large fecal-mass accumulation. Two cases will be presented here to illustrate the need for a very aggressive approach to cleaning out the colon to normalize the GI tract in patients who are eating well and have not had a bowel movement for 5 or more days.

- Case 1: A 110-pound man with a colostomy had not had a bowel movement for 8 days. His colostomy was irrigated, and he eliminated a whole bucket of stool.
- Case 2: A patient from the emergency room was admitted in a crawling position on a stretcher. He had intense pain that was exacerbated by lying on his back. The patient had been eating normally; he had been taking large doses of opioids and had not had a bowel movement for 10 days. An abdominal x-ray series performed in the emergency room showed that the large bowel was full of stool with no signs of obstruction. The patient was given 2 milk-and-molasses enemas (Table 19–3) and then started on 30 mL lactulose (Cephulac) by mouth. Then enemas and lactulose were given 4 times a day until no more formed stool was eliminated. The large bowel was finally cleared of stool after 3 days of this regimen. The patient was then able to lie on his back without pain.

Most healthy people know simple ways to help alleviate simple constipation (e.g., consuming prunes or prune juice). Patients, however—even those who are very intelligent and highly educated (i.e., college professors and physicians)—often do not know how to prevent bowel dysfunction secondary to cancer treatment. Few health care professionals correctly estimate the noxious effects of the treatments patients receive, and many tend to undertreat constipation in patients with cancer, approaching it as they

Table 19–3.   Milk-and-Molasses Enema

Components
    8 ounces hot water (it will cool down before use)
    3 ounces powdered milk (may be purchased at a grocery store)
    4.5 ounces molasses (may be purchased at a grocery store)

Directions for Use
    Put the water and powdered milk in a jar, and shake it until the water and
    milk look fully mixed. Add molasses. Shake the jar again until the mixture
    appears to have an even color throughout. Pour the mixture into an enema
    bag. Gently introduce the tube into your rectum about 12 inches or until the
    tube hits stool. Do not push beyond resistance. When the tube has reached the
    stool, withdraw the tube about half an inch and release the solution.

Modified with permission from Bisanz A. Managing bowel elimination problems in
    patients with cancer. *Oncol Nurs Forum* 1997;24:579–687.

would treat constipation in a healthy individual. It simply does not work
that way. The more serious the cause of a symptom, the more aggressive
the treatment must be.

One common mistake that health care professionals make is to believe
that a positive result from 1 enema solves the problem and restores normal
bowel function. They fail to realize that about 75% of the stool remains in
the colon after a single enema and that if this stool is not removed, the
same problem will resurface in a few days. Thus it is important to normalize the bowel. The goal is to get the bowel back to a normal state so
that the patient can commence a bowel management program that will
prevent the recurrence of severe constipation.

Constipation differs between healthy individuals and patients with
cancer. Many cancer patients go through periods when they eat and drink
less than healthy individuals do and have decreased ambulation or exercise. This decreases peristalsis, leading to impaction in many patients. The
impaction is in many cases in the transverse or descending colon and is
not detected by a digital rectal examination.

Treatment of Low and High Impactions

At M. D. Anderson, health care professionals differentiate low impactions
from high impactions (Figure 19–3). A low impaction is a collection of stool
in the rectum and sigmoid colon. A high impaction is a collection of stool
in the transverse and descending colon with no stool in the sigmoid colon
and rectum.

Patients who present with a low impaction may complain of an inability to sit because they feel like they are sitting on something. They may
feel the need to have a bowel movement, but the stool, which is packed
in the rectum, is too large to expel through the anal opening. They may

High Impaction

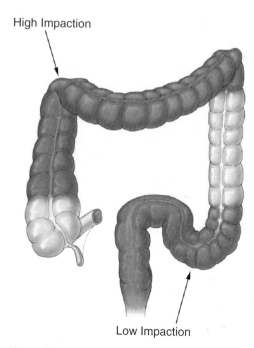

Low Impaction

Figure 19–3. Distinction between high and low impactions.

also complain of bloating, cramping, and gas. In some cases, the patient's abdomen is distended. Liquid stool may be expelled from the small bowel since it leaks around the impacted stool. Patients with a low impaction should be advised to take the following actions:

- Do NOT drink hot liquid or eat a big meal, since this will increase peristalsis and discomfort.
- Lie down and call for professional help.
- Give a Fleet mineral-oil enema very fast to force it high in the colon to help the stool slide out more easily (optional).
- Manually disimpact the stool.
- Administer an enema to help eliminate the stool higher up (e.g., a tap-water, soapsuds, or milk-and-molasses enema).

Patients with a high impaction present with a history of 5 or more days of not having a bowel movement. Patients show no signs of impaction on digital rectal examination and do not have the sensation of stool in the bowel that cannot be eliminated. They have no appetite, eat very little, and feel nauseated after eating or drinking. In many cases, high impactions occur because patients do not eat or drink properly and peristalsis is impaired. Patients do not feel an urge to have a bowel movement until the stool reaches the rectum, and the decreased peristalsis from not eating hinders that process. When these symptoms are present, an abdominal x-ray series is not indicated unless the patient is vomiting and shows signs of obstruction. Patients with a high impaction should be advised by the physician or nurse to take all of the following actions:

- Take 2 tablespoons of mineral oil by mouth if on abdominal palpation the stool is felt to be hard (optional).
- Administer a milk-and-molasses enema every 4 to 6 hours.
- Take 30 mL of lactulose by mouth every 4 to 6 hours once stool begins to be eliminated after the enema is started.
- Continue the prior 2 steps until no more formed stool is eliminated.

In our experience at M. D. Anderson, the milk-and-molasses enema has proven to be relatively easy for patients to take because it has a low volume (1½ cups). It is not a stimulant; instead, it works like an osmotic enema that helps the patient eliminate stool comfortably. In the treatment of patients with high impactions, the enema tube needs to be inserted 12 inches or more until resistance is met or it will not be effective (Figure 19–4). The tube is left in place for 15 minutes after the enema is given to help patients hold the solution.

To self-administer a milk-and-molasses enema for a high impaction, a patient needs an enema bag that will allow the solution to be released close to the impaction. Enema bags sold in drugstores are not made for this type of enema; they usually have about a 3-inch tip, which will deliver the enema solution only about 6 inches into the colon. The correct type of

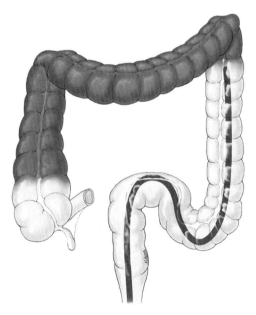

Figure 19–4. Placement of enema tube before release of the solution.

enema bag has 1 continuous length of tubing that is soft and can be inserted higher in the colon; it is usually available at hospital central supply departments or home-care agencies. It may be helpful for physicians to maintain a supply of these enema bags for oncology patients' use.

Milk-and-molasses enemas administered to clean out the colon should be repeated every 4 to 6 hours (every 6 hours at home and every 4 hours in the hospital). Lactulose should be administered simultaneously (30 mL by mouth every 4 to 6 hours) after the patient begins eliminating stool or after 1 or 2 milk-and-molasses enemas. The lactulose draws water into the GI tract, and the increased volume provides pressure to push the stool down through the GI tract. Because lactulose brings more fluid into the bowel, however, patients can become dehydrated and thus must be given sufficient hydration. Patients at home must drink at least 2 quarts of fluid every day.

The goal of the enema and lactulose regimen is to clean out just the large bowel, not the small intestine. Consequently, the enemas and lactulose should be discontinued when the patient stops eliminating formed stool and there is just liquid return.

Effectiveness of Milk-and-Molasses Enemas plus Lactulose

Patients typically tolerate the milk-and-molasses-enema-plus-lactulose regimen well. It involves a very low volume enema (1½ cups) and is not uncomfortable. The patient can usually hold the enema because it is low-volume and administered high in the colon. The caregiver does not mind giving the enema because the solution does not run out of the colon immediately. Any gas pains that the patient has subside as soon as the patient begins eliminating stool because the gas is trapped behind the stool.

Once the patient's GI tract is normalized, the patient should be monitored for 1 week to determine the normal bowel pattern and then placed on a bowel management program. It may be possible to treat the patient with just titration of food, fluid, fiber, and medication. If this does not work, then in addition, the bowel may need to be trained to empty at the same time each day, by using the bowel training program described in the next section.

Bowel Training Program for Constipation

A bowel training program trains the bowel for life to empty at the same time daily with a given stimulus. If patients can eat 3 full meals per day and drink 64 ounces of fluid per day, they are good candidates for bowel training. Patients who cannot eat or drink are not eligible.

Before beginning a bowel-training program, patients must take oral laxatives, enemas, or both to help eliminate the formed stool in the large intestine. Patients start bowel training 3 days later.

Bowel training consists of the following. The patient drinks 4 ounces of prune juice; eats a big meal at the mealtime chosen by the patient; and drinks 1 cup of hot liquid after the meal. Then a bisacodyl suppository is inserted into the rectum and pushed against the mucous membrane of the bowel. These 4 steps are repeated for 14 days. On day 15, a glycerin suppository is substituted for the bisacodyl suppository.

The patient must not take oral stimulant laxatives once the bowel training program has started, although stool softeners may be taken. They will not interfere with the training program because they are not a stimulant cathartic.

If the patient does not respond to the glycerin suppository, the glycerin should be discontinued and the bisacodyl suppository continued for 1 more week before the glycerin is substituted again. If the anal sphincter muscle is tight, the anal opening should be massaged to gently relax the muscle for easy passage of stool. This type of digital stimulation is needed for all patients with spinal cord lesions involving the sacral area. Adjustments to the program should be made 1 at a time and adhered to for 3 days. If there is more than 1 large bowel movement and liquid stool follows, the amount of prune juice should be decreased to 2 ounces, or a half rather than a whole bisacodyl suppository should be inserted into the rectum. If constipation persists, stool softeners should be added to the regimen, and the patient should be directed to eat 5 prunes at bedtime, increase the daily fluid intake, increase the fiber content in the diet, or increase physical activity, of course initiating only 1 change every 3 days.

Bowel Management Program for Constipation

When bowel training is not needed, patients with constipation can be placed on a bowel management program consisting of the following:

- Determine the desired frequency of stooling on the basis of the patient's appetite.
- Prescribe adequate fluid intake, adequate fiber, and at least one good-sized meal for peristaltic pushdown daily, plus medication if needed to counteract side effects of other medicines in the disease process.
- Assess outcome and guide the patient to the program that will be effective, adjusting fluid, fiber, food, and medication.

Patients with advanced disease should be treated using a symptom-management approach. Never allow patients to go more than 3 days without a bowel movement. Do not fear laxative use and abuse. Your goal is to keep patients comfortable. Suppositories or oral laxatives may be used as needed according to circumstances.

Prevention of Opioid-Induced Constipation

When a patient is receiving opioids, a program to prevent constipation should be initiated immediately. The program consists of treatment with senna, a stimulant cathartic, and docusate sodium, a stool softener; the maximum daily dose is eight senna pills and 500 mg of docusate sodium.

Patients start with a lower dose, which is titrated up as the opioid dose is increased. The pill form of senna and docusate sodium may be ordered in bulk at a better price. Patients need to ask their pharmacist about this. Senokot-S (Purdue Frederick Company, Stamford, CT) combines senna and docusate sodium in 1 pill, and up to 8 Senokot-S tablets per day may be taken. Health care professionals often fail to prescribe these medicines in doses sufficient to offset the side effects of opiates and should be more aggressive to prevent the complications that patients frequently experience. Both senna and docusate sodium are available in liquid form and can be given via gastrostomy or jejunostomy tube.

GAS

Because gas is a by-product of food digestion, patients should be advised about which foods create gas. Lamb (1988) explains that many carbohydrates are sources of gas because they nourish the bacteria in the GI tract. These bacteria can break down and digest complex carbohydrates, such as navy beans and soybeans, that the human digestive system cannot. The only carbohydrates that can be absorbed through the intestinal wall are the single sugars—glucose, fructose, and galactose. Enzymes break down starch, table sugar, milk sugar, and most double sugars (disaccharides). Beans, vegetables, and cereal fiber contain complex carbohydrates.

Eliminating milk and milk products from the diet can help to control gaseousness. Lactose intolerance can occur later in life or in many cases after cancer treatment, even if an individual has never had this problem. For example, one patient had very serious frequent stooling (15 to 30 stools per day) after colorectal cancer treatment. His history revealed that he was consuming a gallon of milk each day. After he began abstaining from milk and milk products, the patient made remarkable progress. In other cases, patients may describe their son or daughter as being lactose intolerant, a red flag that needs to be explored since observations in clinical practice indicate that lactose intolerance tends to show up in more than one family member.

The vegetables most likely to cause gas are cucumbers, green peppers, broccoli, cauliflower, onions, asparagus, beans (including soybean products), peas, radishes, carrots, celery, potatoes, and eggplants (Lamb, 1988). The fruits most likely to cause gas are cantaloupe, honeydew melon, watermelon, raisins, bananas, apricots, prunes, prune juice, citrus fruits, and apples.

In the meat group, intestinal gas is caused primarily by fat, so lean meats are better for preventing gas. Carbonated beverages, including beer, produce gas. Chewing gum can also result in gas build-up because air is swallowed during chewing. Highly spiced foods also cause gas.

Interestingly, most patients think it is abnormal to ever expel gas. When they are told that it is normal to expel gas 15 times per day, they are surprised. The misconception may arise from the failure to distinguish between relieving gas in public and relieving gas in private. Patients also need to know that digestion varies between individuals and consequently the same food affects different people differently.

Bowel gas can be treated in many ways, including through dietary adjustments, medication, and exercise. Patients who have problems with gas should be advised to stop or reduce chewing gum and drinking carbonated beverages. Simethicone can provide relief by breaking down large gas bubbles into small ones. Beano is the commercial name of an enzyme that helps digest beans. If milk or milk products create problems, patients can eliminate these from the diet or use lactose-free milk (e.g., Lactaid) or lactose pills whenever consuming dairy products. Patients should review their diet and avoid foods that have tended to cause gas. Anal sphincter exercises will help strengthen the sphincters and thus help patients to avoid expelling gas in public.

As mentioned previously, gaseous distention resulting from constipation is relieved as soon as stool is eliminated.

Diarrhea

Diarrhea is a symptom that can be caused by many things. The cause of the diarrhea, not the symptom, needs to be treated. Assessing the patient for the type of diarrhea and classifying it may help in determining treatment. Types of diarrhea include exudative, secretory, malabsorptive, osmotic, and dysmotility-associated diarrhea. Medications can be specific for each type of diarrhea, but if there are multiple causes, each cause needs to be treated. A good assessment is important in determining the cause and can be very complex. The following case demonstrates the possible complexity.

A patient presented with a history of adenocarcinoma of the cervix and radical resection with positive margins 2 years previously. A portion of her small bowel had been removed, and she had undergone creation of a permanent colostomy with placement of a Hartman's pouch and then radiation therapy. She described a history of diarrhea through the anus, which is abnormal in patients with a Hartman's pouch. She had been taking the combination of diphenoxylate hydrochloride and atropine sulfate (Lomotil) and paregoric to control the diarrhea, without results.

To determine the cause of the patient's symptoms, many factors needed to be considered. Was the diarrhea mucus only (which would be normal in a patient with a Hartman's pouch), colored brown liquid, or clear yellow liquid? Had the patient's urinary output changed? (This would indicate development of a rectal-vesicular fistula.) After review of the pathology report from the patient's prior surgery, it was discovered that she had had a carcinoid tumor of the small bowel resected with free surgical margins several years earlier. It was important to determine if the patient had developed a recurrence of the carcinoid tumor, resulting in secretory diarrhea. Evaluation of serum serotonin levels and 24-hour urine collection for measurement of 5-hydroxyindoleactic acid levels were necessary. These were just some of the multiple possible causes for this patient's diarrhea; others will be described in the rest of this section. The patient could not be successfully treated for diarrhea until the multiple possibilities had been explored.

Specific Noncancer Causes of Diarrhea

Diarrhea can be caused by many factors unrelated to cancer. Impaction can cause diarrhea, with liquid stool from the small bowel seeping around the impaction. Treatment is removal of the impaction. Lactose intolerance may cause diarrhea. Intolerance to milk and milk products is treated by removing these items from the diet or by ingesting the enzyme lactose to help digest dairy products when they are consumed. Another cause of diarrhea is food allergy. Intolerance to specific foods is treated by avoiding foods that cause diarrhea.

Antibiotic therapy can cause diarrhea by killing bacteria that normally live in the intestinal lining. Patients can help to restore the normal flora in the bowel by eating yogurt that contains live cultures (acidophilus), drinking buttermilk, or taking lactobacillus, available over the counter in the pharmacy. Some other causes of diarrhea are nervousness or anxiety; specific medications; opiate withdrawal; rapid increase in fiber intake; some forms of enteral nutrition (a clinical dietitian can help guide the patient); inflammatory bowel diseases; intestinal viral infection—e.g., infection with *Clostridium difficile*, parasitic infections, or gastroenteritis; diabetes (manifested as nocturnal diarrhea with diabetic neuropathy); celiac sprue (gluten malabsorption); fistulas; alcoholism; and excessive use of laxatives.

Bowel Management Program for Treatment of Frequent Stooling after Colorectal Surgery

Diarrhea may also be caused by treatments for cancer, such as surgery. Frequent stooling is a nearly universal symptom after surgery for colorectal cancer that involves a lower anterior resection, coloanal anastomosis, and diverting ileostomy with subsequent reversal of the ileostomy several weeks later. Patients who have undergone this procedure can experience up to 30 stools per day. They describe their stools as being soft-formed, sticky, and very small volume. Patients cannot empty very much at one time. This problem greatly reduces patients' quality of life. On the basis of this author's experience both in the United States and abroad, a new fiber-based approach to this problem was pilot-tested. Eighty-six percent of patients who were compliant with the program had positive results. This specific use of fiber has been developed and researched by this author and adapted as the standard of care for patients with colorectal and anal cancer treated at M. D. Anderson.

The bowel management program described here is a novel approach for helping patients who have undergone surgery for colorectal cancer rehabilitate the bowel after treatment. The program includes 3 steps: strengthening the anal sphincter muscles; slowing and forming the stool; and bowel training, if needed.

Patients need to understand that they are compensating for a shorter or absent colon and, in many instances, the lack of the rectum, which served as a reservoir prior to surgical resection. Patients with rectal tumors are evaluated carefully by the multidisciplinary team, and whenever possible, sphincter-sparing techniques are utilized. After preoperative chemoradiation therapy, a proctectomy and coloanal anastomosis is done with a temporary diverting ileostomy left in place for about 6 weeks to ensure appropriate healing. During the time that the patient has the ileostomy, the anal canal is not used, and those sphincter muscles can become weak. Consequently, the first and a very important process in bowel management for such patients is to keep the anal sphincter muscles strong while they are not being used, to help prevent incontinence when the ileostomy is reversed.

Strengthening the Anal Sphincter Muscles

Specific exercises, which can be started after lower anterior resection when patients no longer experience pain, are used to strengthen the anal sphincter muscles. These so-called Kegel exercises, with specific emphasis on the muscles used to hold back a bowel movement, are as follows:

1. Tighten buttock muscles as if to hold back a bowel movement. Hold this position for 10 seconds, counting "one-one-thousand," "two-one-thousand," "three-one-thousand," etc., up to "ten-one-thousand."
2. Release for 10 seconds, using the same counting method. Notice the difference between tension and relaxation. Repeat this exercise 10 times, four times per day.
3. Practice the exercise while sitting, standing, and walking.

Slowing and Forming the Stool

The primary goal for bowel management in patients who have undergone colorectal surgery is to empty the contents of the colon at the same time every day. However, before that is done, patients need to slow down the bowel by taking the necessary amount of medicinal fiber after a meal and at bedtime so that the stool does not progress down the colon to be eliminated until the trained bowel empties again the next day. (For further detail, see the section Fiber earlier in this chapter.) It is important that patients follow the fiber routine as instructed. Patients must be instructed not to follow any package-insert instructions because they are all written for patients with constipation. If the patient takes fiber the wrong way, increased gut motility—the opposite of the desired outcome—could result. The schedule shown in Table 19–4 is helpful in teaching patients how to gradually titrate the fiber so that the GI tract does not overreact.

Table 19–4. Schedule for Gradually Increasing Medicinal Fiber for Patients Who Have Undergone Colorectal Surgery and Other Patients Who Need to Slow Down Gastrointestinal Motility*

Days	Actual Dates (Fill In)	Fiber Consumption by Time of Day			
		Breakfast	Lunch	Dinner	Bedtime
1–5		1 teaspoon in 2 oz water			
6–10		1 teaspoon in 2 oz water		1 teaspoon in 2 oz water	
11–15		1 teaspoon in 2 oz water	1 teaspoon in 2 oz water	1 teaspoon in 2 oz water	
16–20		1 teaspoon in 2 oz water	1 teaspoon in 2 oz water	1 teaspoon in 2 oz water	1 teaspoon in 2 oz water
21–25		2 teaspoons in 3 oz water	1 teaspoon in 2 oz water	1 teaspoon in 3 oz water	1 teaspoon in 2 oz water
26–30		2 teaspoons in 3 oz water	1 teaspoon in 2 oz water	2 teaspoons in 3 oz water	1 teaspoon in 2 oz water
31–35		2 teaspoons in 3 oz water	2 teaspoons in 3 oz water	2 teaspoons in 3 oz water	1 teaspoon in 2 oz water
36–40		2 teaspoons in 3 oz water	2 teaspoons in 3 oz water	2 teaspoons in 3 oz water	2 teaspoons in 3 oz water
41–45		1 tablespoon in 4 oz water	2 teaspoons in 3 oz water	2 teaspoons in 3 oz water	2 teaspoons in 3 oz water
46–50		1 tablespoon in 4 oz water	2 teaspoons in 3 oz water	1 tablespoon in 4 oz water	2 teaspoons in 3 oz water
51–55		1 tablespoon in 4 oz water	1 tablespoon in 4 oz water	1 tablespoon in 4 oz water	2 teaspoons in 3 oz water
56–60		1 tablespoon in 4 oz water	1 tablespoon in 4 oz water	1 tablespoon in 4 oz water	1 tablespoon in 4 oz water

* As directed in the schedule, take the medicinal fiber dissolved in water right after a meal or at bedtime. DO NOT drink any fluid for 1 hour after drinking this mixture.

Copyright 2002 The University of Texas M. D. Anderson Cancer Center. Reprinted with permission.

While patients gradually titrate up the fiber, antidiarrheal medicines must be used to control symptoms. The goal is to eventually get patients off the antidiarrheals. As the fiber is increased, patients may decrease the antidiarrheal medication. Following are patient instructions for taking antidiarrheal medications:

Table 19–5. Maximum Number of Lomotil (Lom) and Imodium (Imm) Tablets Permitted in Patients Who Have Undergone Colorectal Surgery and Other Patients Who Need to Slow Down Gastrointestinal Motility

6:00 a.m.	9:00 a.m.	Noon	3:00 p.m.	6:00 p.m.	9:00 p.m.	Midnight	3:00 a.m.
2 Lom	2 Imm	2 Lom	2 Imm	2 Lom	2 Imm	2 Lom	2 Imm

Copyright 2002 The University of Texas M. D. Anderson Cancer Center. Reprinted with permission.

- Do not take more than 8 Lomotil or 8 loperamide (Imodium) tablets per day. You may alternate these 2 medicines every 3 hours. The table (Table 19–5) shows the maximum amount of medicine you may take.
- Do not take antidiarrheal medicine unless you need to. If diarrhea stopped after the last dose of medicine, do not take any more until you have more bowel movements. You do not want to revert to constipation. As you gradually increase your intake of fiber, gradually decrease the amount of antidiarrheal medicine you take (Figure 19–5).

Another important part of slowing the motility in the GI tract is to follow the "titration principle" discussed earlier in the chapter (see the section Components of an Effective Bowel Management Program). All 4 components (food, fluid, fiber, and medicine), not the fiber alone, are important, although many patients state that the fiber is really what made the difference. A cautionary note: patients sometimes take too much fiber, which adds so much volume that it produces more stool, causing more frequent bowel movements. If this occurs, the patient should be guided to decrease fiber intake.

Bowel Training for Frequent Stooling

Bowel training for frequent stooling differs slightly from bowel training for constipation. Bowel training for frequent stooling can begin after the stool becomes formed and has slowed down with the use of fiber. Bowel training is done to supply sufficient stimulus to the gut to provide a signal that it is time for a good-sized bowel movement. A consistent, 2 weeks or longer program trains the bowel to eliminate at the same time each day. It is important to remember that each person's gut reacts differently, which

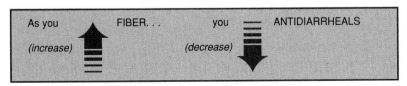

Figure 19–5. In patients with frequent stooling after colorectal surgery, as fiber is increased, antidiarrheals are decreased.

presents a challenge to professionals in guiding patients. Patients should be instructed as follows:

Step 1: Before eating the big meal of your choice, drink the amount of prune juice prescribed (usually not more than 2 ounces). [Sometimes this step is held to see if steps 2 and 3 alone help the patient.]
Step 2: Eat a big meal at the chosen time.
Step 3: Drink 1 cup of hot liquid.
Step 4: Record your progress.

The goal is to empty the contents of just the large bowel each day at the same time. Using the fiber to slow the GI tract in between the daily large bowel movements stops the patient's constant urge to have a bowel movement.

Because each person reacts differently to bowel training, however, the directions above may need to be modified several times to reach the goal. As with bowel training for constipation, only 1 change at a time should be implemented, and this should be continued for 3 days before another change is made. This gives the bowel a chance to adjust to the new program.

If a patient still has diarrhea or extra bowel movements during the day, the bowel training program is too strong. The regimen may be adjusted, 1 option at a time, through the following measures:

- Decrease the amount of fluids taken with a meal. Drink fluids between meals instead.
- Avoid or reduce the intake of hot liquids, which bring on the urge to have a bowel movement.
- Decrease the amount of prune juice by 1 ounce or change the juice to orange juice.
- Stop bowel training. Gradually increase the dose of medicinal fiber. When stools become more formed or decrease in number, restart bowel training.

If the patient becomes constipated, the regimen may be adjusted, 1 option at a time, through the following measures:

- Drink an extra cup of hot liquid.
- Insert a glycerin suppository after the hot liquid.
- Insert half of a bisacodyl suppository instead of a glycerin suppository.
- Increase the amount of prune juice to 3 ounces just before the meal around which you are bowel training.

To help ensure that bowel training is successful, make sure the patient follows the fluid-intake guidelines (i.e., the patient should ingest small amounts of fluids with meals, avoid hot liquids unless the patient wants a bowel movement, and avoid fluids for 1 hour after taking fiber). Bowel training must be planned around a large meal after which a massive peristaltic pushdown occurs. Bowel training must happen at the same time every day. Because bowel training is the formation of a lifelong practice, it is important to maintain the same routine. The only change that may occur is discontinuation of the use of suppositories. Everything else remains the same. Also, the program's success depends on the patient's consistent compliance with directions. Bowel training varies from person to person. These are basic guidelines but need to be adapted according to the patient's response to the program. It is also important to remember that bowel training programs may require changes multiple times before the patient reaches the desired goal.

Bowel Management Program for Copious Output after Ileostomy

Some patients have copious amounts of output in their ileostomy bags following surgery. Once a patient with an ileostomy tolerates liquids and progresses to a soft diet, titration of medicinal fiber helps to slow GI motility. The dose should start at 1 teaspoon (with 3 grams of fiber) in 2 ounces of water after meals and before bedtime and then be increased by 1 teaspoon every 5 days. Medicinal fiber must be started at a low dose and slowly titrated up. Antidiarrheal agents can be utilized once the surgeon has determined that they will not cause an ileus. Patients should be instructed to report a daily output in ostomy bag of greater than 1,500 mL after discharge from the hospital.

Treatment of Diarrhea after Other GI Surgeries

Depending on the kind of GI surgery, patients may need hormonal or enzyme replacements (e.g., pancreatic enzyme replacement) to correct the cause of diarrhea (e.g., after pancreaticoduodenectomy).

Treatment of Diarrhea Caused by Radiation Therapy

Patients who are treated with radiation therapy to the abdomen can develop diarrhea or frequent stooling as a side effect. While receiving radiation therapy and for 2 weeks after treatment, patients should follow a low-fiber diet and take no medicinal fiber. They can initiate or resume a fiber regimen 2 weeks after completion of treatment. Patients are instructed to alternate 2 Imodium tablets with 2 Lomotil tablets every 3 hours. (The optimum dose of each drug is 8 per day.) Patients must not take any more than is needed, however. Once the diarrhea ceases for 3 hours after a dose of either drug, the patient should not take another dose until the symptoms recur. This avoids alternating constipation and diarrhea, which is difficult to treat in any bowel management program and reflects the improper titration of medication to meet the patient's needs. Occasionally, patients do not have an adequate response to the alternating Imodium-Lomotil treatment, even at optimum doses. In such cases, an opiate (e.g., oxycodone) is added because it slows down peristalsis and forms the stool.

Initial studies in the literature have suggested that cholestyramine, a drug that binds bile acids before they pass through to the colon, can be effective in preventing radiation-induced diarrhea when administered in dosages of 4 grams 3 times per day. Other substances being considered for the control of diarrhea are a number of salicylate and other prostaglandin compounds, on the presumption that irradiation increases prostaglandin secretion (Baughan et al, 1993).

It is documented in the literature that in severe cases of radiation-induced diarrhea, oral steroids may be needed. Goldstein and colleagues (1976) note,

Glucocorticoids have an antisecretory action in that they can induce the synthesis of lipomodulin, an intracellular protein that inhibits the action of phospholipase A2, and thus suppress the release of the eicosanoid precursor, arachidonic acid, from the cell membrane. Eicosanoids are a large family of local transmitter substances that include prostaglandins and leukotrienes, both of which are potent secretagogues. Furthermore, chronic radiation-induced enteritis has been shown to be susceptible to a combination of salicylate and sulfonamides, such as salicylazosulfapyridine.

(See Ippoliti [1998] for a classification of antidiarrheal agents [p. 1576]. This reference, however, does not mention the use of steroids or sulfonamides.)

Treatment of Diarrhea Caused by Chemotherapy

Diarrhea is also a significant consequence of chemotherapy for colorectal cancer, with most patients experiencing grade 3 or 4 diarrhea. In Arbuckle and colleagues' study (2000), 56% of patients had to modify their chemotherapy regimen because of diarrhea. It is important that patients with chemotherapy-induced diarrhea be treated appropriately so that patients can maintain their full chemotherapy dose.

When patients are receiving irinotecan, it is important to control diarrhea as soon as the symptom occurs. The longer diarrhea continues, the more difficult it is to stop it. At the first sign of cramping or diarrhea, patients should be started on 2 loperamide tablets and then 1 tablet every 2 hours thereafter. During the night, patients can take 2 pills every 4 hours. Patients may discontinue loperamide after being diarrhea-free for 12 hours. They are encouraged to drink 2 to 3 quarts of fluid per day to replace lost fluids and to avoid dairy products, fruit juice, alcohol, and coffee. They are encouraged to follow the so-called BRAT diet (bananas, rice, applesauce, and toast) and can be placed on a bland diet if they can tolerate it as directed by Pharmacia Upjohn Company, makers of irinotecan (Camptosar).

Patients need to be reminded to eat small meals more frequently, which decreases peristalsis, rather than eating 3 big meals per day. Patients are also taught to avoid hot liquids, another normal physiological precursor to increased GI motility.

Patients need to be instructed to take antidiarrheal medications to keep this symptom under control. Again, an aggressive approach is indicated, with continual guidance of patients based on the outcome of their therapy.

Preliminary studies of glutamine and thalidomide suggest that they may play a role in alleviating the side effects in patients receiving irinotecan (Savarese et al, 2000; Govindarajan et al, 2000). Much is yet to be learned in this area. Ippoliti (1998) outlines the antidiarrheal regimen for patients who have treatment-related diarrhea.

Treatment of Secretory Diarrhea from Neuroendocrine Tumors

Patients with endocrine tumors experience secretory diarrhea. Secretory diarrhea is intestinal hypersecretion stimulated by endogenous mediators that exert a primary effect on intestinal transport of water and electrolytes, resulting in accumulation of intestinal fluids. Causes of secretory diarrhea include vipoma, carcinoid, gastrinoma, insulinoma, glucagonoma, and *Clostridium difficile*. This condition is characterized by large-volume stools (>1,000 mL per day) that persists despite fasting (Rutledge and Engelking, 1998). Secretory diarrhea can be treated with octreotide. Although the exact mechanism of action of octreotide is unknown, a sharp reduction of luminal fluid in the upper jejunum and an inhibition of electrogen chloride secretion with a stimulation of rectal sodium and chloride absorption may be responsible for the observed effect on stool volume (Cascinu et al, 1993). Octreotide also appears to suppress intestinal motility. Because of its effects, octreotide was studied as an antidiarrheal for use after chemotherapy with fluorouracil. Octreotide was more effective than loperamide and probably more cost-effective (Cascinu et al, 1993)

Since medicinal fiber given with very little water has proven to be effective in slowing GI motility after colorectal surgery, studies of the role of fiber given with very little fluid in patients with secretory diarrhea who are no longer undergoing diarrhea-inducing therapy may be beneficial. It is not suggested that low-dose fiber be investigated as a replacement for octreotide; rather, it could be investigated as a supplement to octreotide and other medications.

LAXATIVES

Patients who are undergoing treatment for cancer need particular attention given to the type of laxative used for constipation. It is important to provide immediate relief in the most gentle way, even if an aggressive approach is needed to relieve severe constipation and prevent more severe problems. The patient's total physical condition and the presence of bulky disease in the abdomen must be considered, as addressed in the following paragraphs. Patients undergoing chemotherapy that may cause myelosuppression need preventative laxative therapy because the treatment options for myelosuppressed patients with constipation are limited—manual disimpaction, suppositories, and enemas are contraindicated in patients with low platelet counts or altered prothrombin time or partial thromboplastin time because of the potential for bleeding.

When patients have abdominal pain from a large tumor burden and are constipated, it is best to avoid stimulant cathartics and instead give a hyperosmotic laxative, which pulls fluid into the GI tract and promotes a milder peristalsis and bowel evacuation. Lactulose is commonly used in these circumstances and works very well. When a patient with a large tumor burden and constipation is not myelosuppressed, any impacted stool can be manually disimpacted, a Fleet mineral-oil enema can be given, and a milk-and-molasses enema can be given simultaneously to help the patient eliminate stool from the colorectal area while the lactulose pushes the stool down from the upper GI tract. The combination of lactulose and a milk-and-molasses enema is effective and well tolerated by patients. When a patient has hard stool, an orally administered lubricant cathartic such as mineral oil is indicated, although this treatment should be avoided by patients who might aspirate it. Lubricant cathartics work well in patients who are myelosuppressed and avoid abrasion of the intestinal mucosa as the hard stool moves down the GI tract. A Fleet mineral-oil enema is effective for hard stool in the colorectal area. Bulk laxatives should be avoided in patients who cannot drink enough fluid because they enhance constipation. Stool softeners are needed in many cases to hold the fluid in the GI tract to keep the stool soft and are utilized to offset the side effects of medications that cause constipation.

Many patients who need a stimulant cathartic have used one in the past and can help guide the health care professional about what works best for them. Senna is a generic stimulant cathartic that offsets the side effects of opiates or other medications and may also be available in bulk.

Patients should be advised about contraindications to the use of nonprescription laxatives. This way, if a patient develops the symptoms of an obstruction, he or she will be aware of the contraindications to laxative use. This is especially important for patients who have cancer. The symptoms that indicate a possible obstruction are vomiting, loss of appetite, abdominal pain, and distention when unsure of cause of these symptoms. An abdominal x-ray series can differentiate severe constipation from obstruction.

Prokinetic Drugs

Prokinetic drugs are used to speed up GI motility. Metoclopramide, a cholinergic agonist and dopamine antagonist, is very effective for patients with gastroparesis and nausea whose food does not pass readily into the duodenum. Erythromycin, a motilin agonist, has also been found to accelerate gastric emptying after pancreaticoduodenectomy. It has also been documented for its use to treat symptoms of colonic pseudoobstruction and postoperative ileus.

KEY PRACTICE POINTS

- In patients with cancer, it is very important to take a preventive approach and teach patients how to manage bowel function before symptoms begin.

- It is crucial to involve the patient as a partner in bowel management.

- Thorough assessment of bowel function and a thorough bowel history are the most important steps in bowel management, permitting correct diagnosis of the cause of bowel dysfunction and thus permitting appropriate treatment.

- In any bowel management program, fluid, fiber, food, and medication are the 4 components that must be balanced.

- Fecal impaction is often caused by recent diagnostic procedures using barium. This type of impaction can be prevented by routinely prescribing a laxative to be taken until evidence of barium excretion abates. If a patient is at high risk for barium retention, a request that barium not be used for this patient is appropriate, and gastrographin should be used as a substitute.

- If a patient's colon is packed with stool, 1 enema is not sufficient to normalize the colon. Enemas need to be repeated 4 times a day until no more formed stool is eliminated.

- Medicinal fiber can be used to treat diarrhea or frequent stooling. However, the label directions for taking supplemental medicinal fiber apply only to the treatment of constipation. Patients must be alerted to this fact and given special written instructions for use of fiber to treat frequent stooling.

- During treatment, bowels can be managed using a symptom management approach.

- A formal bowel training program should not be started until (1) treatment with side effects on the GI tract is completed and (2) the bowel has been brought back to a normal state, without constipation or impaction and with no liquid stools.

- After treatment, a long-term bowel management program can be initiated for maintaining regular bowel functions.

Positively Affecting the Patient's Attitude

Positively affecting the patient's attitude is key to the success of any bowel management program. Emphasizing the following points for patients may ease and enhance the process and the outcome of bowel rehabilitation:

- Bowel elimination can be managed.
- There is a bowel management program for everyone.
- Patient compliance is essential to good results.
- Patience and a sense of humor are invaluable.
- Problem-solving increases options.

The challenge to all health care professionals is to give patients hope for bowel management through patient education and ongoing guidance until they reach their goal. Individual guidance is essential for a good outcome.

Suggested Readings

Arbuckle RB, Huber SL, Zacker C. The consequences of diarrhea occurring during chemotherapy for colorectal cancer: a retrospective study. *Oncologist* 2000;5: 250–259.

Baughan CA, Lanney PA, Buchanan RB, et al. A randomized trial to assess the efficacy of 5-aminosalicylic acid for the prevention of radiation enteritis. *Clinical Oncology* 1993;5:19–24.

Bisanz A. Managing bowel elimination problems in patients with cancer. *Oncology Nursing Forum* 1997;24:679–686.

Brocklehurst JC. How to define and treat constipation. *Geriatrics* 1977;32:85–87.

Bruera E, Suarez-Almazor M, Velasco A, et al. The assessment of constipation in terminal cancer patients admitted to a palliative care unit: retrospective review. *J Pain Symptom Manage* 1994;9:515–519.

Cascinu S. Management of diarrhea induced by tumors or cancer therapy. *Curr Opin Oncol* 1995;7:325–329.

Cascinu S, Fedeli A, Fedeli S, et al. Octreotide versus loperamide in the treatment of fluorouracil-induced diarrhea: a randomized trial. *J Clin Oncol* 1993;11:148–151.

Chew SB, Tindal DS. Colonic J-pouch as a neorectum: functional assessment. *Aust N Z J Surg* 1997;67:607–610.

Cimprich B. Symptom management of constipation. *Cancer Nurs Suppl* 1985;8:39–42.

Cox GJ, Matsui SM, Lo RS, et al. Etiology and outcome of diarrhea after marrow transplantation: a prospective study. *Gastroenterology* 1994;107:1398–1407.

Daniele B, Perrone F, Gallo C, et al. Oral glutamine in the prevention of fluorouracil induced intestinal toxicity: a double blind, placebo controlled, randomised trial. *Gut* 2001;48:28–33.

Glare P, Lickiss JN. Unrecognized constipation in patients with advanced cancer: a recipe for therapeutic disaster. *J Pain Symptom Manage* 1992;7:369–371.

Goldstein F, Khoury J, Thornton JJ. Treatment of chronic radiation enteritis and colitis with salicylazosulphapyridine and systemic corticosteroids. A pilot study. *Am J Gastroenterol* 1976;65:201–205.

Govindarajan R, Heaton KM, Broadwater R, et al. Effect of thalidomide on gastrointestinal toxic effects of irinotecan. *Lancet* 2000;356:566–567.

Hensinkveld RS, Mannis MR, Arsistabal SA. Control of radiation induced diarrhea with cholestyramine. *Int J Radiat Oncol Biol Phys* 1978;4:687–691.

Herbst F, Kamm MA, Nicholls RJ. Effects of loperamide on ileoanal pouch function. *Br J Surg* 1988;85:1428–1432.

Hoff P, Ansari R, Batist G, et al. Comparison of oral capecitabine versus intravenous fluorouracil plus leucovorin as first-line treatment in 605 patients with metastatic colorectal cancer: results of a randomized phase III study. *J Clin Oncol* 2001;19:2282–2292.

Ippoliti C. Antidiarrheal agents for the management of treatment-related diarrhea in cancer patients. *Am J Health Syst Pharm* 1998;55:1573–1580.

Iseminegr J, Hardy P. Bran works! *Geriatric Nursing* 1982;3(6):402–404.

Lamb L. Gaseous distention. In: Lawrence E, Lamb P, eds. *The Health Letter* (ISSN 0739–4217). Special Report 95. Irvine, CA: North America Syndicate, Inc. 1988.

Lembo A, Camilleri M. Chronic constipation. *New Engl J Med* 2003;349:1360–1368.

Levy MH. Constipation and diarrhea in cancer patients. *Cancer Bulletin* 1991;43:412–422.

Locke GR III, Pemberton JH, Phillips SF. American Gastroenterological Association medical position statement: guidelines on constipation. *Gastroenterology* 2000;119:1761–1778.

Longo WE, Vernava AM III. Prokinetic agents for lower gastrointestinal motility disorders. *Dis Colon Rectum* 1993;36:696–708.

Mancini I, Bruera E. Constipation in advanced cancer patients. *Support Care Cancer* 1998;6:356–364.

O'Toole D, Ducreux M, Bommelaer G, et al. Treatment of carcinoid syndrome: a prospective crossover evaluation of lanreotide versus octreotide in terms of efficacy, patient acceptability, and tolerance. *Cancer* 2000;88:770–776.

Portenoy RK. Constipation in the cancer patient: causes and management. *Med Clin North Am* 1987;71:303–311.

Pro B, Lozano R, Ajani J. Therapeutic response to octreotide in patients with refractory CPT-11 induced diarrhea. *Invest New Drugs* 2001;19:341–343.

Rao S. Constipation: evaluation and treatment. *Gastroenterol Clin North Am* 2003;32:659–683.

Robinson CB, Fritch M, Hullett L, et al. Development of a protocol to prevent opioid-induced constipation in patients with cancer: a research utilization project. *Clin J Oncol Nurs* 2000;4:79–84.

Rutledge D, Engelking C. Cancer-related diarrhea: selected findings of a national survey of oncology nurse experiences. *Oncol Nurse Forum* 1998;25:861–872.

Savarese D, Al-zoubi A, Boucher J. Glutamine for irinotecan diarrhea. *J Clin Oncol* 2000;18:450–451.

Schang JC, Devroede G. Beneficial effects of naloxone in a patient with intestinal pseudoobstruction. *Am J Gastroenterol* 1985;80:407–411.

Society of Gastroenterology Nurses and Associates Core Curriculum Committee. Large intestine. In: Van Schaik T, ed. *Gastroenterology Nursing a Core Curriculum*. 1st ed. St. Louis, Mo: Mosby Year Book; 1993:146–158.

Wyman JB, Heaton KW, Wicks ACB. The effect on intestinal transit and the feces of raw and cooked bran in different doses. *Am J Clin Nutr* 1976;29:1474–1479.

Yeo CJ, Barry MK, Sauter P, et al. Erythromycin accelerates gastric emptying after pancreaticoduodenectomy. *Ann Surg* 1993;218:229–238.

20 Barrett's Esophagus

Ishaan S. Kalha and Frank A. Sinicrope

Chapter Overview

Barrett's esophagus is an acquired condition in which specialized metaplastic intestinal epithelium with goblet cells replaces the normal stratified squamous epithelium anywhere in the esophagus. The relationship between long-standing gastroesophageal reflux disease (GERD), the development of specialized intestinal metaplasia in the distal esophagus, and subsequent progression to adenocarcinoma has been clearly established. Once Barrett's esophagus is diagnosed, it is critical to extensively biopsy the segment of Barrett's epithelium to exclude dysplasia and cancer. Management of Barrett's esophagus should focus on relieving symptoms of GERD and performing endoscopic surveillance at appropriate intervals. The timing of surveillance endoscopy is governed by the presence of mucosal dsyplasia and its pathologic grade. Recommendations about endoscopic surveillance intervals will undoubtedly be modified as the natural history of Barrett's esophagus becomes better understood. Studies to validate existing biomarkers of cancer risk in patients with Barrett's esophagus have the potential to permit stratification of patients into low-risk and high-risk groups and to eventually guide surveillance intervals. High-grade dysplasia within Barrett's esophagus continues to be managed with esophagectomy; however, the advent of endoscopic ablative techniques has provided alternative management strategies for use in patients who are not optimal candidates for surgery and patients treated in the setting of clinical trials. Endoscopic ablation techniques show promise in the management of high-grade dysplasia but are still unproven in terms of reducing cancer risk. Chemoprevention strategies are being evaluated and have the potential to benefit high-risk patients. Areas for future research include defining appropriate surveillance intervals, improving management of high-grade dysplasia, and finding new and validating existing molecular and cellular biomarkers that can identify patients at low and high risk of developing cancer.

INTRODUCTION

Barrett's esophagus is an acquired condition in which specialized metaplastic intestinal columnar epithelium with goblet cells replaces the normal stratified squamous epithelium anywhere in the esophagus. This intestinal metaplasia occurs in the tubular esophagus and is distinct from intestinal metaplasia of the gastric cardia. At endoscopy, Barrett's-type mucosa appears orange to red compared to the pearly-white appearance of the normal squamous mucosa of the esophagus. Barrett's esophagus is associated with mucosal injury from gastroesophageal reflux and is believed to occur in predisposed individuals. Antireflux strategies including acid-suppressing medications can generally control reflux symptoms and esophagitis; however, once Barrett's esophagus develops, it usually persists. Endoscopic biopsy of the Barrett's-appearing mucosa is required to establish a diagnosis. Once diagnosed with Barrett's esophagus, patients should undergo surveillance endoscopy with biopsies at specified intervals for detection of dysplasia or early cancer.

The intestinal-type cells of Barrett's esophagus are predisposed to develop genetic alterations that can lead to dysplasia and eventually cancer. In recent years, Barrett's esophagus has gained increased attention owing to its established association with adenocarcinoma of the esophagus.

The rate of rise in the incidence of esophageal adenocarcinoma currently exceeds that of all other cancers in the United States (Blot et al, 1991; Pera et al, 1993; Vizcaino et al, 2002). In some patients with Barrett's esophagus, histologic progression to dysplasia is detected. Dysplasia varies from indefinite to low-grade, moderate, or high-grade and can progress to invasive adenocarcinoma. The vast majority of adenocarcinomas of the esophagus are accompanied by intestinal metaplasia (Haggitt et al, 1978; Skinner et al, 1983; Smith et al, 1984; Rosenberg et al, 1985; Paraf et al, 1995). Cytologic and molecular markers indicating which patients with Barrett's esophagus are likely to develop dysplasia or cancer are being actively pursued but are not yet available for use in clinical practice.

This chapter will review Barrett's esophagus, with a focus on diagnosis, pathogenesis, and management.

Definition

Barrett's esophagus is an endoscopically recognizable change in the esophageal mucosa that has been defined in terms of histopathology: Barrett's esophagus is an acquired condition in which specialized metaplastic intestinal columnar epithelium with goblet cells replaces the normal stratified squamous epithelium anywhere in the esophagus (Gadour and Ayoola, 2002). A clinical definition of Barrett's esophagus has been difficult to achieve. The controversy surrounding the clinical definition of Barrett's esophagus stems from the difficulty in identifying the true squamocolumnar junction (z-line) and the gastroesophageal junction, as these 2 locations do not always coincide. Identifying columnar-lined esophagus at endoscopy requires precise criteria by which to delimit the esophagus and the stomach. If the squamocolumnar junction becomes located proximal to the gastroesophageal junction, then the intervening mucosa between the 2 junctions will be lined by a segment of columnar epithelium.

The length of Barrett's esophagus is defined as the extent of columnar epithelium between the anatomic gastroesophageal junction and the most proximal extension of the specialized epithelium. Originally, if the length of Barrett's mucosa was greater than 3 cm, it was termed "long-segment," and if the length was less than 3 cm, it was termed "short-segment." This rather arbitrary classification has undergone changes that may take into account events occurring at the gastroesophageal junction. The American College of Gastroenterology recently redefined Barrett's esophagus as "a change in the esophageal epithelium *of any length* that is recognized as intestinal metaplasia at endoscopy, is in continuity with the gastric epithelium, and is confirmed by biopsy" (Sampliner, 2002). This definition gives greater importance to short-segment Barrett's esophagus and metaplastic changes at the gastroesophageal junction. Of note, many patients with short-segment Barrett's esophagus in the distal esophagus have no symptoms of gastroesophageal reflux disease (GERD), unlike patients with long-segment Barrett's esophagus.

Short-segment Barrett's esophagus needs to be distinguished from intestinal metaplasia of the gastric cardia, which is not recognizable endoscopically and the significance of which remains less well defined (Spechler et al, 1994; Chalasani et al, 1997; Morales et al, 1997). Patches of the gastric mucosa frequently extend up into the distal esophagus as finger-like projections, giving an irregular appearance to the z-line. Such extension may represent changes consistent with Barrett's metaplasia or may represent intestinal metaplasia of the gastric cardia. Previously, this overlap of gastric mucosa in the esophagus was believed to have no clinical consequences. However, recent studies involving biopsies from this region have revealed specialized intestinal epithelium in a significant number of patients. This finding supports the hypothesis that tumors of the gastroesophageal junction arise from specialized intestinal metaplasia—i.e., Barrett's metaplasia—at or near the squamocolumnar junction.

DIAGNOSIS AND HISTOPATHOLOGY

The diagnosis of Barrett's esophagus requires biopsy of the endoscopically abnormal-appearing esophageal mucosa to document intestinal metaplasia. The more biopsies taken and the greater the length of the Barrett's segment, the greater the chance of recognizing intestinal metaplasia. Specialized intestinal metaplasia with goblet cells in biopsy specimens from endoscopically salmon-colored esophageal mucosa is diagnostic of Barrett's esophagus. Biopsy is also essential to exclude dysplasia, the earliest neoplastic change in the mucosa. Both short-segment and long-segment Barrett's esophagus are associated with an increased risk of dysplasia and cancer, and the cancer risk in patients with short-segment Barrett's esophagus is believed to be similar to the risk in patients with long-segment Barrett's esophagus (Spechler, 1997; Falk, 2001).

In patients with Barrett's esophagus, biopsies are not routinely performed from areas of esophagitis because of the difficulty of excluding dysplasia within Barrett's in the setting of active inflammation. In this situation, repeat endoscopy to exclude dysplasia is generally performed after acid-suppression therapy has been administered to control reflux symptoms and resolve the inflammatory changes. Any subtle mucosal abnormalities within the Barrett's segment—such as ulceration, erosion, plaque, nodule, stricture, or other luminal irregularity, no matter how small—

should be biopsied first. Biopsies should then be performed every 2 cm in 4 quadrants. Because of the concern that taking biopsies every 2 cm could miss areas of high-grade dysplasia and adenocarcinoma, investigators at the University of Washington advocate the use of jumbo-biopsy forceps with biopsies every 1 cm in 4 quadrants (Reid et al, 2000a). In a study in which this protocol was employed, the detection rate for adenocarcinoma was 100%, compared to a 50% detection rate if biopsies were performed every 2 cm (Reid et al, 2000a). This biopsy protocol, however, requires passage of a therapeutic endoscope and is labor-intensive and time-consuming. While these factors have limited widespread adoption of this protocol into clinical practice, its use is recommended for patients with high-grade dysplasia within Barrett's esophagus, especially if an esophagectomy is not immediately planned (Reid et al, 2000a; Sampliner et al, 2002).

Endoscopic staining techniques have been employed in an attempt to improve the recognition of Barrett's esophagus. Of the vital stains evaluated to date, methylene blue may be the most promising (Canto et al, 1996, 2000). With chromoendoscopy, there is some evidence to suggest that fewer biopsies may be needed to diagnose Barrett's esophagus and that there is an increased yield in short-segment Barrett's (Sharma et al, 2001). However, these methods are tedious, prolong procedure time, and are associated with issues of reproducibility between practitioners.

As stated in the previous section, short-segment Barrett's esophagus needs to be distinguished from intestinal metaplasia of the gastric cardia. Specialized intestinal metaplasia of the gastric cardia is not recognizable at endoscopy but can be found on biopsy in approximately 20% of Caucasian adults undergoing elective endoscopy, regardless of the indication for the procedure (Spechler et al, 1994; Morales et al, 1997). Furthermore, specialized intestinal metaplasia can be found in 33% to 50% of patients whose squamocolumnar junction appears jagged, irregular, or prominent. Up to 15% of patients with a normal-appearing squamocolumnar junction harbor small foci of intestinal metaplasia at the gastroesophageal junction (Spechler et al, 1994; Morales et al, 1997). However, to date, the significance of these histologic findings remains poorly understood (Spechler et al, 1994; Chalasani et al, 1997; Morales et al, 1997). In Barrett's esophagus, specialized metaplastic intestinal columnar epithelium with goblet cells replaces the normal stratified squamous epithelium anywhere in the esophagus (Gadour and Ayoola, 2002). The recognition of intestinal metaplasia on biopsy—i.e., the presence of goblet cells—can be enhanced using an Alcian blue stain (pH 2.5) (Zwas et al, 1986). Intestinal metaplasia occurs on either side of the gastroesophageal junction. Type I and type II intestinal metaplasia occur on the gastric side. These are associated with *Helicobacter pylori* infection and have a weaker association with cancer (Rugge et al, 2001). Type III intestinal metaplasia occurs on the esophageal side, is believed to be caused by reflux of gastric contents, and is associated with a higher risk of progression to carcinoma than are types I and II (Leung and Sung, 2002).

Most adenocarcinomas of the gastroesophageal junction arise in a background of intestinal metaplasia, which may be in a segment of Barrett's esophagus or in a small area of intestinal metaplasia in the gastric cardia, though in such cases the type of metaplasia is that seen with Barrett's esophagus and not with *H. pylori* (Cameron et al, 2002b). These histologic markers can be useful in distinguishing Barrett's-related esophageal adenocarcinoma from gastric adenocarcinoma. Cytokeratins (CKs) 7 and 20, cytoplasmic structural proteins with restricted expression, can aid the pathologist in determining the origin of many epithelial tumors. A CK7+, CK20– tumor immunophenotype is associated with Barrett's-related esophageal adenocarcinoma (Ormsby et al, 2001).

EPIDEMIOLOGY

Barrett's esophagus is found in 3.5% to 7% of persons with GERD (Cameron and Carpenter, 1997). Although Barrett's esophagus develops in only a minority of patients with GERD, diagnosis of Barrett's esophagus has increased significantly over the past 30 years. Whether the increased recognition of Barrett's esophagus is a real phenomenon or simply parallels the increased use of endoscopy is somewhat controversial (Conio et al, 2001). The prevalence of Barrett's esophagus increases with age and reaches a plateau by the seventh decade. Barrett's esophagus has been shown to develop more than 20 years before the mean age of diagnosis or the subsequent development of esophageal adenocarcinoma (Cameron and Lomboy, 1992). The actual prevalence of Barrett's esophagus may never be known because many patients with the condition are asymptomatic and consequently do not seek medical attention. However, an autopsy study estimated the prevalence of Barrett's esophagus at 376 per 100,000 persons (Cameron et al, 1990).

Risk factors associated with Barrett's esophagus include increased severity and extended duration of reflux symptoms; smoking; obesity; white race; and male sex (Falk, 2002). Persistent GERD is an independent risk factor for esophageal adenocarcinoma (Cossentino and Wong, 2003). Repetitive injury to the esophageal mucosa from exposure to gastric contents appears to predispose individuals to metaplasia. The rate of esophageal adenocarcinoma development in males is 2 to 3 times greater than that in females (Devesa et al, 1998). In patients with long-segment Barrett's esophagus, smoking is believed to be a contributing factor in up to 40% of cases of esophageal adenocarcinoma. Patients in the highest quartile of body mass index have a risk of esophageal adenocarcinoma 2.9 times greater than that of patients in the lowest quartile

(Romero et al, 1997). Most patients with Barrett's esophagus have a hiatal hernia, indicating that hiatal hernia may also be a risk factor (Cameron, 1999). Concordance for GERD symptoms is greater in monozygotic twins than in dizygotic twins, indicating that genetic factors may be involved. It is estimated that heredity may account for up to 30% of GERD cases (Cameron et al, 2002a). GERD symptoms have been shown to be significantly more prevalent among parents and siblings of patients with esophageal adenocarcinoma in the setting of Barrett's esophagus, indicating that this population may have a genetic predisposition to the development of GERD and subsequently adenocarcinoma (Romero et al, 1997).

Over the past 30 years, the incidence of esophageal adenocarcinoma has increased 5- to 6-fold, especially in white males over age 45 years, and during the past 15 years, the rate of increase in the incidence of esophageal adenocarcinoma has exceeded that of all other cancers (Devesa et al, 1998). This has led to greater awareness of Barrett's esophagus. The rate of esophageal adenocarcinoma is 30 to 60 times higher in patients with Barrett's esophagus than in the general population (Cossentino and Wong, 2003). The reported risk of developing cancer in patients with Barrett's esophagus varies, but experts agree that it is lower than was previously reported (Drewitz et al, 1997; Eckardt et al, 2001). Most recent studies put the incidence at 0.5% per year or lower (Falk, 2001). Data from Cameron et al (2002a) indicate that up to 86% of all esophageal adenocarcinomas develop in a background of intestinal metaplasia. Patients with a diagnosis of esophageal adenocarcinoma who are referred for endoscopy may lack evidence of Barrett's epithelium. In these cases, the metaplastic epithelium may have been completely replaced by tumor (Cameron et al, 2002a). While most cases of adenocarcinoma appear to originate from within Barrett's epithelium, some may not.

The prevalence and characteristics of Barrett's esophagus in patients with adenocarcinoma of the gastroesophageal junction are uncertain. In one study, 61 consecutive esophagogastrectomy specimens with adenocarcinoma were examined (Clark et al, 1994; Cameron et al, 1995; Corley et al, 2002). Barrett's esophagus was found in 64% of the cases but had been recognized in only 38% of the patients who had undergone preoperative endoscopy with biopsy. These cases show a striking predominance of male gender and white race, in contrast to the pattern seen with gastric adenocarcinoma but similar to the pattern seen with adenocarcinoma of the gastroesophageal junction without demonstrable Barrett's esophagus (Sharma, 2001b). These results strongly suggest that unlike gastric-cardia carcinoma, adenocarcinoma of the gastroesophageal junction originates within Barrett's esophagus. Data also suggest that most adenocarcinomas of the gastroesophageal junction arise in ultrashort segments of Barrett's esophagus, which may be difficult to detect at endoscopy (Haggitt et al, 1988; Cameron et al, 2002a; Giard et al, 2002).

PATHOGENESIS

Barrett's esophagus appears to develop as a consequence of a complex interaction between molecular, genetic, and environmental factors (Figure 20–1). As mentioned in the preceding section, GERD has been established as a strong risk factor for esophageal adenocarcinoma (Spechler, 2001). Under normal circumstances, the reflux of gastric contents into the esophagus is prevented by a functioning lower esophageal sphincter. Dysfunction of the lower esophageal sphincter, in many cases in combination with the presence of a hiatal hernia, leads to failure of an effective barrier. In such cases, esophageal mucosal damage results from the chronic exposure to gastroduodenal contents (Buttar et al, 2001b).

One hypothesis suggests that Barrett's esophagus develops as a result of an extension of gastric columnar epithelium into the esophagus, a process called "creeping substitution." If this were the case, then older patients would be expected to have longer segments of Barrett's esophagus than younger patients. However, the mean length of Barrett's mucosa appears to be independent of age (Cameron et al, 1995; Benipal et al, 2001). Others have suggested that Barrett's esophagus arises from undifferentiated cells in glands in the esophageal wall and that constant exposure to an acidic environment initiates the process of metaplasia, independent of esophagitis. Regardless of which pathogenesis model is most accurate, there appears to be a strong association between chronic GERD symptoms, the development of specialized intestinal metaplasia in the distal esophagus, and subsequent progression to adenocarcinoma (Chow et al, 1995; Lagergren et al, 1999). These findings serve to establish Barrett's esophagus as a precursor lesion for esophageal adenocarcinoma.

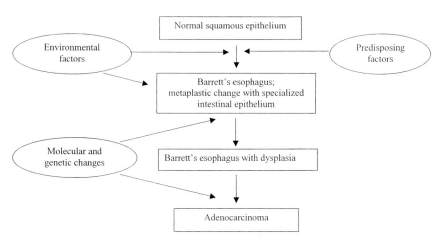

Figure 20–1. Multistep carcinogenesis in the development and progression of Barrett's esophagus to adenocarcinoma.

Acid and pepsin are believed to be important in causing mucosal injury, and animal studies have suggested that gastric acid and conjugated bile acids act synergistically to cause mucosal damage (Vaezi and Richter, 1995). Human studies have shown that bile reflux parallels acid reflux and increases with the severity of GERD, reaching a peak in Barrett's esophagus (Vaezi and Richter, 1995; Richter, 2000). The incidence of duodenogastroesophageal reflux increases significantly with the severity of reflux disease; the incidence is greatest in patients with Barrett's esophagus and similar to that in patients with partial gastrectomy (Champion et al, 1994). Pulses of acid reflux stimulate cell proliferation and may be important in carcinogenesis in Barrett's esophagus (Fitzgerald et al, 1996). Aggressive acid-suppression therapy decreases both acid and bile reflux and may eliminate the synergism between these 2 factors (Richter, 2000).

Evidence suggests that infection with *H. pylori* may protect some patients from developing GERD and its complications, such as Barrett's esophagus (Falk, 1999). The proposed mechanism is that *H. pylori* reduces gastric acid production and therefore reduces the likelihood of acid damage in the esophagus. Pulses of acid refluxed into the esophagus have been shown to increase cell proliferation and the expression of cyclooxygenase-2 in Barrett's epithelium (Shirvani et al, 2000). In one study, 251 patients with GERD and short-segment or long-segment Barrett's esophagus were evaluated for the presence of *H. pylori* by biopsy and serology. It was concluded that patients with Barrett's esophagus were less likely to have *H. pylori* infection than were patients with GERD alone and that certain strains of *H. pylori* may be protective against the formation of short-segment and long-segment Barrett's esophagus and associated malignant complications (Vaezi et al, 2000). Other studies have shown that intestinal metaplasia detected at a normal-appearing gastroesophageal junction may be associated with intestinal metaplasia of the stomach and infection with *H. pylori*, whereas intestinal metaplasia in the esophagus is associated with GERD and not *H. pylori* (Falk, 1999).

SURVEILLANCE OF BARRETT'S ESOPHAGUS

Barrett's esophagus is usually discovered during endoscopic evaluation of patients who have symptoms caused by GERD or esophageal cancer. Studies suggest that in the general population, however, more than 90% of cases of Barrett's esophagus are not recognized, and many patients with the condition have few or no symptoms of GERD (Spechler, 1994). It is important to risk-stratify patients with GERD symptoms to determine who should undergo diagnostic upper endoscopy to effectively screen for Barrett's esophagus. Guidelines recommend that patients with longstanding GERD symptoms, especially but not exclusively white men over 50 years of age, undergo endoscopy at least once to screen for

Barrett's esophagus (Sampliner, 2002). If Barrett's esophagus is not identified at the initial endoscopy, then further evaluation is not needed. Screening for Barrett's esophagus, however, remains a controversial issue.

Adenocarcinoma develops in Barrett's esophagus by a multistep process in which specialized metaplasia progresses to dysplasia, then to early adenocarcinoma, and eventually to invasive disease. However, it is important to stress that most patients with Barrett's esophagus never experience progression to dysplasia or cancer; progression is not inevitable. Although this sequence has been well characterized, the timing of both the development of dysplasia and the subsequent transition to carcinoma remains unknown. The most significant predictor of the risk of malignancy in patients with Barrett's esophagus is the presence of dysplasia. Patients with Barrett's esophagus should undergo surveillance with regular endoscopy and biopsy at intervals determined by the grade of dysplasia (Table 20–1). Updated guidelines of the American College of Gastroenterology recommend that surveillance endoscopy intervals be lengthened if no evidence of dysplasia is found within Barrett's epithelium on 2 consecutive endoscopies with biopsy. If this circumstance, a 3-year surveillance interval is recommended (Sampliner, 2002). The optimal number of biopsies has not been determined but clearly depends on the length of the metaplastic segment. So far, the standard biopsy protocol for patients with Barrett's esophagus is as described earlier in the chapter—biopsy in 4 quadrants every 2 cm along the length of abnormal-appearing mucosa (Sampliner, 1998; Endlicher et al, 2001). Recommendations in the setting of high-grade dysplasia are discussed in the next section.

The rationale for surveillance in patients with Barrett's esophagus is an increased risk of esophageal adenocarcinoma and the poor prognosis of this cancer. However, definitive data supporting surveillance endoscopy in patients with Barrett's esophagus are lacking, and some controversy

Table 20–1. **Recommended Surveillance Intervals for Barrett's Esophagus With and Without Dysplasia**

Dysplasia	Documentation	Follow-up Endoscopy Interval
None	Two EGDs with biopsy	Every 3 years
Low grade	Highest grade on repeat biopsy	Every year until no dysplasia
High grade	Repeat EGD with biopsy to rule out cancer or document high-grade dysplasia; expert pathologist confirmation	Multifocal—intervention Mucosal irregularity—EMR

Abbreviations: EGD, esophagogastroduodenoscopy; EMR, endoscopic mucosal resection.
Adapted from Sampliner, 2002.

exists. Several studies suggest that esophageal adenocarcinomas detected by surveillance measures are earlier-stage and associated with more favorable survival than cancers detected at the time of diagnosis of Barrett's esophagus (Streitz et al, 1993; Peters et al, 1994; vanSandick et al, 1998; Corley et al, 2002). However, a cohort study of patients with Barrett's esophagus who did not undergo surveillance demonstrated that esophageal cancer was an uncommon cause of death, accounting for only 2.5% of deaths (n = 155) with a mean follow-up time of 9 years (VanderBurgh et al, 1996). In addition, a smaller study found that 9% of patients with Barrett's esophagus died of esophageal cancer (Ell et al, 2000).

Neither acid-suppression therapy nor antireflux surgery can reliably eliminate the malignant potential of established Barrett's metaplasia of the esophagus (Lagergren et al, 1999). Therefore, close endoscopic surveillance with biopsies in patients with this condition is considered to be the standard of care (Sampliner, 2002). The cost of such a surveillance program, however, is considerable and must be balanced against the true cancer burden of Barrett's esophagus. Many believe that the initial estimates were exaggerated and that the actual cancer burden may not warrant a national screening and surveillance program, especially given that the incidence of esophageal adenocarcinoma in 2001 was 15 times less than the incidence of colorectal, lung, or breast cancer (Richter and Falk, 1996; Arguedas and Eloubeidi, 2001; Falk, 2002). Cost-effectiveness analyses have been performed to estimate the economic impact and benefit of various surveillance programs (Inadomi et al, 2003). Studies have used different outcomes, including life-years gained, quality-adjusted life-years gained, and cases of cancer, and have shown that cost-effectiveness varies significantly because it is sensitive to the prevalence of Barrett's esophagus and the incidence of esophageal adenocarcinoma (Arguedas and Eloubeidi, 2001). In the United States, it is estimated that a population-wide surveillance program could result in a total cost of $289.9 million U.S. dollars (Arguedas and Eloubeidi, 2001). The outpatient management of Barrett's esophagus is estimated to cost $1,241 U.S. dollars per year per patient, with medication use alone accounting for over half of the total cost (Arguedas and Eloubeidi, 2001).

Dysplasia and Cancer

Dysplasia can occur in metaplastic Barrett's epithelium and is a neoplastic change. At present, dysplasia is the best indicator of cancer risk in patients with Barrett's esophagus. The grading of dysplasia in Barrett's esophagus is based on the system used for ulcerative colitis (Riddell et al, 1983). Interobserver variability in the recognition, grading, and reproducibility of detection of dysplasia in Barrett's esophagus is problematic

(Reid et al, 1988; Montgomery et al, 2001). The finding of dysplasia of any grade warrants repeat endoscopy with intensive biopsy of the area of dysplasia to exclude coexisting carcinoma (Sampliner, 2002).

Dysplasia is graded as indefinite, low-grade, high-grade, or intramucosal carcinoma and is believed to reflect a stepwise progression that culminates in invasive adenocarcinoma. The interval between steps is extremely variable—some patients with high-grade dysplasia never develop cancer, and many patients with low-grade dysplasia never develop high-grade dysplasia. The grade of dysplasia found determines the recommended surveillance interval. Updated recommendations are shown in Table 20–1 (Sampliner, 2002). When low-grade dysplasia is detected at follow-up endoscopy with concentrated biopsies in the area of dysplasia, annual endoscopy is recommended. Once low-grade dysplasia is identified, aggressive antisecretory therapy with a proton-pump inhibitor should be started.

The finding of high-grade dysplasia necessitates repeat endoscopy with particular attention to any mucosal lesion. An intensive biopsy protocol using therapeutic endoscopy and jumbo forceps is recommended. An expert pathologist should confirm the presence of high-grade dysplasia. The extent of high-grade dysplasia is also important. High-grade dysplasia is defined as focal when associated cytologic or architectural changes are limited to a single focus of 5 or fewer crypts and as diffuse when more than 5 crypts are involved in a single biopsy specimen or if high-grade dysplasia involves more than 1 biopsy fragment (Sampliner, 2002). Diffuse high-grade dysplasia is associated with a 3.7-fold increase in the risk of esophageal cancer compared with the risk in patients with focal high-grade dysplasia (Buttar et al, 2001b). Patients with focal high-grade dysplasia are less likely to have cancer during the first year after diagnosis or on subsequent follow-up than are patients with diffuse high-grade dysplasia (Buttar et al, 2001b). This observation highlights the importance of sending samples of high-grade dysplasia to experienced gastrointestinal pathologists specializing in such specimens. If uncertainty about the diagnosis cannot be resolved by expert pathology re-review, then repeat endoscopy with biopsy should be performed promptly. Updated guidelines suggest that patients with high-grade dysplasia (with 5 or fewer crypts) may be followed up with a 3-month surveillance interval. Patients with confirmed high-grade dysplasia within Barrett's esophagus have the highest risk for the development of esophageal adenocarcinoma if concurrent adenocarcinoma does not already exist. Detection of high-grade dysplasia is important because a significant proportion of patients with this condition will develop adenocarcinoma over a 5-year period. In patients with high-grade dysplasia within Barrett's esophagus referred for esophagectomy, adenocarcinoma is found in approximately 11% to 43% of cases (Heitmiller et al, 1996; Cameron and Carpenter, 1997; Tseng et al, 2003).

Available data suggest that in some patients, high-grade dysplasia actually regresses or persists and does not develop into cancer, suggesting a less aggressive approach for management (Rabinovitch et al, 2001; Schnell et al, 2001). Some cohort studies have shown that high-grade dysplasia may remain stagnant without further progression, especially if potent acid-suppression therapy is employed (Cooper et al, 1998). At the least, rigorous systematic surveillance in patients with high-grade dysplasia should involve repeat endoscopy every 3 months, with the distance between biopsies reduced to every 1 cm, as this has been shown to most consistently detect early cancers arising in high-grade dysplasia (Reid et al, 2000a). Management decisions in cases of high-grade dysplasia can be complex and challenging, particularly in patients with comorbid disease who are poor candidates for surgery. The role of endoscopic mucosal ablative therapies is discussed below. Chromoendoscopy and endoscopic fluorescence are being evaluated to improve recognition of Barrett's esophagus and, especially, to enhance detection of neoplastic lesions (Canto et al, 1996, 2000; Sharma et al, 2001a). Esophagectomy is regarded as the most definitive therapy for confirmed diffuse high-grade dysplasia and should be offered to patients deemed to be appropriate candidates for surgery (Sharma, 2001b). Outcomes of esophagectomy appear best at institutions that perform a high volume of such surgeries. Patient age and comorbid conditions also need to be weighed when deciding on the appropriate management strategy. The type of resection is based on the length of the Barrett's segment (Rusch et al, 1994).

Biomarkers

Adenocarcinoma develops in Barrett's esophagus by a multistep process in which specialized metaplasia progresses to dysplasia, then to early adenocarcinoma, and eventually to invasive disease (Figure 20–1). A variety of epithelial biomarker studies have been performed in Barrett's esophagus to identify key cellular and molecular markers that may provide valuable data on the risk of disease progression and cancer development. Markers of cancer risk, including changes in DNA content, have been identified, but these abnormalities have yet to be validated in multicenter studies with routine follow-up. Therefore, none of these potential biomarkers have yet been incorporated into routine patient care. Once and if such markers are validated, their use in clinical practice will have the potential to permit stratification of patients by risk and to enable a more individualized and perhaps more selective approach to endoscopic surveillance. Furthermore, an increased understanding of the genetic and cellular mechanisms leading to cancer development might allow earlier diagnosis and provide an opportunity to eliminate high-risk lesions before adenocarcinoma develops.

Dysplasia

Detection of dysplasia relies on extensive tissue sampling at endoscopy with random biopsies. Other techniques using cytology brushings of the esophageal mucosa have been tried but have been shown not to be as sensitive or specific as histologic sampling (Wang et al, 1997). Tissue biopsies, however, can be problematic because they have poor predictive values for indefinite and low-grade dysplasia and yield inconsistent results for high-grade dysplasia between different pathologists (Reid et al, 1988; Montgomery et al, 2001). Even with extensive biopsy regimens, it may be impossible to differentiate between high-grade dysplasia and invasive adenocarcinoma (Clark et al, 1996). Therefore, dysplasia alone is not an ideal marker for selecting patients at high risk for adenocarcinoma (Ertan and Younes, 2000). Alternatives need to be found to either supplement the histologic findings or to take the place of biopsies for risk stratification.

Aneuploidy

Abnormal DNA content as determined by DNA ploidy analysis has been extensively evaluated in single-institution studies in patients with Barrett's esophagus. Aneuploidy is an important chromosomal change that occurs during carcinogenesis and can predict histologic progression (Barrett et al, 1999; Reid et al, 2001). The prevalence of aneuploid cell populations increases with histologic progression from Barrett's metaplasia to low-grade dysplasia to high-grade dysplasia and finally cancer (Haggitt, 1994). Aneuploidy can be detected in more than 90% to 95% of esophageal adenocarcinomas. Furthermore, an aneuploid fraction greater than 6% can be used to distinguish between low-grade and high-grade dysplasia. Flow cytometric abnormalities in endoscopic biopsy specimens can therefore identify patients with a higher risk of progression to high-grade dysplasia or adenocarcinoma before histologic evidence of such is detected (Robaszkiewicz et al, 1991). In 322 patients with Barrett's epithelium, the relative risk of cancer development was significantly greater in patients with tetraploid or aneuploid DNA content than in patients without such abnormalities (Reid et al, 2000b). Flow cytometric results have also been combined with histologic determination of dysplasia in an attempt to improve predictive ability by defining low-risk and high-risk patient subsets (Reid et al, 2000b). Within aneuploid populations are subpopulations of cells with *p53* mutations, which are more frequently found in high-grade dysplasia and cancer.

Molecular Alterations

Loss of heterozygosity at 17p is a mechanism of *p53* inactivation that enables this tumor-suppressor gene to function as an oncogene. A single-center study (Reid et al, 2001) showed that in patients with Barrett's esophagus, allelic loss at chromosome 17p (site of *p53*) identified patients at increased risk for progression to adenocarcinoma. In 269 Barrett's patients with 17p loss of heterozygosity, the 3-year cumulative incidence of cancer was 38%, versus 3.3% in patients with two 17p alleles (Reid et al, 2001). Wu et al (1998) determined the prevalence of 17p and 18q chromosomal losses in Barrett's mucosa and in the dysplasia-to-adenocarcinoma sequence. 17p allelic loss occurred in 14% of cases of Barrett's mucosa, 42% of low-grade dysplasias, 79% of high-grade dysplasias, and 75% of adenocarcinomas; allelic loss of 18q was found in 32%, 42%, 73%, and 69%, respectively. Esophageal adenocarcinomas with allelic loss of both 17p and 18q were associated with worse survival than cancers with no or one allelic loss ($P = .002$) (Wu et al, 1998).

p53 mutations can be detected in dysplastic Barrett's epithelium before invasive cancer develops and are associated with an increased risk for progression to high-grade dysplasia as well as esophageal adenocarcinoma (Reid et al, 2001). While these mutations develop in diploid cell populations, the same *p53* mutations are also found in aneuploid cell populations in high-grade dysplasia, in esophageal cancer, and in multiple aneuploid cell populations within cancer (Neshat et al, 1994). These data suggest that *p53* may be a predictor of progression in Barrett's epithelium and may be useful for risk assessment (Ortiz-Hidalgo et al, 1998; Reid et al, 2001). Recent studies have shown that p53 protein accumulation, as determined by immunohistochemistry, can be detected in low-grade dysplasia as well as high-grade dysplasia within Barrett's epithelium, although the degree of expression is greatest with high-grade dysplasia (Ertan and Younes, 2000). Frequent overexpression of the p53 protein has also been reported in Barrett's adenocarcinomas (Neshat et al, 1994). While detection of p53 expression is suggestive of mutation, false-positive staining does occur, as shown by comparison with gene sequencing. p53 positivity has the potential to be combined with a panel of other biomarkers for use in risk assessment.

Chromosome p16 allelic loss has been detected in metaplastic Barrett's epithelium, providing cells with the ability to undergo clonal expansion and creating a field defect in which other abnormalities can arise that can lead to esophageal adenocarcinoma (Wong et al, 2001). Other genetic alterations may hold promise in risk-stratifying patients. In this regard, an increase in the frequency of chromosome 7q33–q35 loss between low-grade dysplasia and high-grade dysplasia, as determined by comparative genomic hybridization, suggests that this marker may be useful as a diagnostic tool (Riegman et al, 2002). Of note, microsatellite instability due to defective DNA mismatch repair is rare in Barrett's esophagus and esophageal adenocarcinoma (Wu et al, 1998; Kulke et al, 2001).

Proliferative Activity

Intestinalized epithelium in long-segment Barrett's esophagus shows increased proliferative activity and a statistically significant increase in the mean crypt proliferative index and mean crypt proliferation zone (Gillen et al, 1994; Hong et al, 1995). Intestinalized epithelium in the distal esophagus and gastroesophageal junction shows similar increases in proliferative activity, suggesting a similar process with an increased risk of carcinogenesis (Gulizia et al, 1999). Acid exposure increases proliferation and decreases apoptosis, implicating acid exposure in the metaplasia-dysplasia-adenocarcinoma sequence in Barrett's esophagus (Souza et al, 2002).

Cyclooxygenase-2

Recently, expression of the cyclooxygenase-2 (COX-2) enzyme has been detected in Barrett's esophagus and esophageal adenocarcinoma (Wilson et al, 1998; Zimmerman et al, 1999; Shirvani et al, 2000). In one report, the level of COX-2 expression was 3 times higher in Barrett's esophagus than in normal control samples, and after therapy with a selective COX-2 inhibitor, the levels of COX-2 and prostaglandin E2 were significantly decreased (Kaur et al, 2002). The constitutive COX-1 and inducible COX-2 isoforms regulate the synthesis of prostaglandins from arachidonic acid. COX-2 is induced by cytokines, growth factors, and tumor promoters, and studies indicate that COX-2 can protect cells from apoptosis, stimulate angiogenesis, and influence tumor cell invasiveness and metastatic potential (reviewed in Sinicrope et al, 2004). The synthesis of prostaglandins and other mediators of inflammation may be involved in the progression to neoplasia via mucosal injury. COX-2 is a target of nonsteroidal anti-inflammatory drugs (NSAIDs), including selective COX-2 inhibitors, which displayed chemopreventive effects in an animal model of Barrett's esophagus (Buttar et al, 2002b).

MANAGEMENT

Once Barrett's esophagus is diagnosed, the goals of therapy include the control of symptoms of GERD and the maintenance of healed esophageal mucosa. Other treatment objectives include the regression or removal of Barrett's-type tissue and the secondary prevention of adenocarcinoma in patients with known Barrett's esophagus.

Medical and Surgical Therapies

A critical question is whether regression of Barrett's esophagus occurs in response to medical or surgical therapy. The natural history of Barrett's esophagus can be altered by the use of medical therapies and by endoscopic surveillance with periodic biopsies (Sampliner, 2000). Regression is defined as a decrease in the length and surface area of Barrett's esophagus, along with the emergence of islands of squamous epithelium in the Barrett's segment. The extent of regression is difficult to assess because intestinal metaplasia may underlie the islands of squamous re-epithelialization, a situation called pseudo-regression (Sampliner, 2000). Biopsy is useful in ruling out progression to dysplasia or adenocarcinoma; however, complete regression of the lesion cannot be definitively proven by this technique. In long-term clinical studies, consistent acid-suppression therapy with proton-pump inhibitors decreases cell proliferation and increases differentiation in Barrett's esophagus, but the clinical importance of such effects is not clear.

Proton-pump inhibitors have become the predominant medical therapy for Barrett's esophagus because of their potent acid-suppressing effects and favorable safety profile (Falk, 2001). Proton-pump-inhibitor therapy in patients with Barrett's esophagus can in some cases cause an increase in squamous islands in the Barrett's esophagus segment, but data are insufficient to support the concept of complete regression of Barrett's esophagus (Sampliner, 2000; Castell, 2001). Patients who are appropriate candidates for surgery may elect antireflux surgery. Fundoplication effectively controls reflux symptoms in most patients, but Barrett's metaplastic epithelium generally persists (Haag et al, 1999). Conflicting data exist as to whether effective antireflux surgery can slow the occurrence and progression of Barrett's esophagus (Lagergren et al, 1999; Klaus and Hinder, 2001). Progression of Barrett's esophagus to high-grade dysplasia and carcinoma has been shown to be less common after antireflux surgery than during medical therapy (Klaus and Hinder, 2000). In contrast, a Swedish study found no difference between surgical and medical therapies in this situation. However, and more importantly, few patients with Barrett's esophagus show complete regression after medical or surgical therapy alone. Until more accurate and effective therapeutic modalities become available or molecular markers are developed or validated that can predict in whom cancer will develop, esophagectomy must be considered the standard means of managing Barrett's esophagus with high-grade dysplasia.

Endoscopic Ablative Techniques

Failure of conventional treatments has led to the emergence of newer endoscopic mucosal ablation techniques in combination with acid-suppression therapy (Sharma, 2001a). The aim of these new treatment options is to literally remove the metaplastic columnar epithelium. High-dose acid-suppression therapy is started immediately after ablation, with the premise that the new epithelium will be squamous and devoid of intestinal metaplasia. At present, 3 techniques have been evaluated: endoscopic thermal ablation, endoscopic mucosal resection, and photodynamic therapy. To date, however, the impact of endoscopic ablative therapy on neoplastic progression in Barrett's esophagus has not been defined.

The goal is to replace the specialized esophageal mucosa with normal squamous mucosa. Ablation of the Barrett's metaplastic epithelium has the potential in theory to remove its malignant potential. The major concern is that columnar epithelium may persist under the newly formed squamous epithelium and retain its malignant potential (Grade et al, 1999). This may occur because the depth of ablation was insufficient or because the esophageal stem cells have been irreversibly altered. Following ablative therapy, it is critical that antisecretory therapy with high-dose proton-pump inhibitors be employed immediately as this has been shown to reduce the likelihood of recurrence of columnar epithelium (Overholt, 2000a). Such therapy most likely provides an environment that allows the esophageal progenitor cells to develop into squamous mucosa (Overholt, 2000a).

Important issues for further investigation include the optimal depth of ablation; other considerations include the safety, feasibility, and cost of this treatment. Mucosal ablative techniques are best suited for patients who are poor candidates for surgery and patients treated in the setting of a clinical trial. Factors involved in patient selection for these techniques include the degree of dysplasia, the extent of disease, and patient age (Pacifico and Wang, 2002).

Endoscopic Thermal Ablation

Thermal ablative techniques include multipolar coagulation, argon-plasma coagulation, Nd:YAG laser therapy, and argon laser therapy. Photodynamic therapy and Nd:YAG laser therapy are used for neoplastic lesions, whereas argon-plasma coagulation and multipolar coagulation have been used successfully in nondysplastic Barrett's mucosa. These therapies have been shown to result in reversal of Barrett's epithelium to varying degrees, but a decrease in adenocarcinoma risk has not been established with any of them (Wang and Sampliner, 2001). Thus, long-term control of neoplastic risk has not been demonstrated, and in most studies some intestinal mucosa persists beneath new squamous mucosa. Further investigation is needed to determine which patients are most likely to benefit from such therapy and which therapies are most effective.

Endoscopic Mucosal Resection

Endoscopic mucosal resection has been used in the treatment of superficial squamous cell cancers and gastric malignancies. Attention has now moved to high-grade Barrett's esophagus and early esophageal adenocarcinoma. Endoscopic ultrasonography is necessary to determine the feasibility of endoscopic mucosal resection. Only lesions classified as T0 or T1N0, involving only the mucosa and muscularis mucosae but not the submucosa, can potentially be treated with this technique. Endoscopic mucosal resection has also been used for removing areas of high-grade dysplasia in an attempt to avoid esophagectomy. Endoscopic mucosal resection remains an investigative strategy, and studies have yet to show whether endoscopic mucosal resection in the esophagus is an effective and safe procedure for Barrett's esophagus (Sampliner, 2003). A recent study found that endoscopic mucosal resection was very effective at removing T1 esophageal cancers en bloc, with 97% of all patients having no residual cancer detectable at pathology review after surgery (May et al, 2003).

Photodynamic Therapy

Photodynamic therapy is a technique for the nonsurgical treatment of patients with dysplasia within Barrett's esophagus. The primary end point for photodynamic therapy is eradication of dysplasia. The effectiveness of photodynamic therapy varies with the photosensitizer used and the wavelength of light applied to activate the drug. Given the success of esophageal resection, the use of photodynamic therapy should be reserved for patients who are not candidates for surgery (Overholt, 2000b) or investigational protocols. Complications of photodynamic therapy include esophageal stricturing, and side effects of the photosensitizer are not trivial; these factors must be considered in the decision-making process and be weighed against any potential benefit (May et al, 2002).

Photodynamic therapy seems to control high-grade dysplasia within Barrett's esophagus in about 80% of cases. Long-term results are not available, but the preliminary results are promising (Wang, 2000; Wang and Sampliner, 2001). However, high-grade dysplasia has been detected several months after completion of photodynamic therapy. This most likely indicates that genetic abnormalities persisted even though there was initial histologic downgrading. Therefore, documentation of histologic removal of dysplasia alone may be an inadequate end point for photodynamic therapy in Barrett's esophagus (Krishnadath et al, 2000). This suggests that since the genetic abnormalities remain, the epithelium still harbors the potential to develop high-grade dysplasia or adenocarcinoma despite histologic improvement (Krishnadath et al, 2000).

Combined Endoscopic Mucosal Resection and Photodynamic Therapy

Endoscopic mucosal resection and photodynamic therapy can also be used together in selected circumstances to treat patients with early-stage esophageal cancers (May et al, 2003). In a study of 17 patients, combined endoscopic mucosal resection and photodynamic therapy appeared to remove the superficial cancer and eliminate the remaining mucosa at risk for cancer development (Buttar et al, 2001a). In a more recent study of 103 patients, photodynamic therapy with supplemental Nd:YAG photoablation and continuous therapy with an acid-suppressing agent was found to reduce the length of Barrett's esophagus, eliminate high-grade dysplasia, and potentially reduce the risk of progression to adenocarcinoma (Overholt et al, 2003).

Chemoprevention

In addition to the therapeutic interventions mentioned above, pharmaceutical agents may prevent neoplastic development or progression in Barrett's epithelium. In case-control studies (Farrow et al, 1998; Langman et al, 2000) and in a recent meta-analysis (Corley et al, 2003), NSAIDs were found to reduce the incidence of esophageal adenocarcinoma. These data suggest that NSAIDs may be effective chemopreventive agents in patients with Barrett's esophagus. In this regard, a selective COX-2 inhibitor was shown to inhibit the proliferation of cultured Barrett's esophageal epithelial cells, and cell proliferation was restored by exogenous prostaglandins (Buttar et al, 2002a). A COX-2 inhibitor also increased apoptosis in Barrett's-associated adenocarcinoma cells that expressed COX-2 (Souza et al, 2000). In an animal model of Barrett's esophagus, non-selective COX (sulindac) and selective COX-2 (MF-tricyclic) inhibitors significantly reduced the incidence of esophageal cancer relative to controls, and these drugs showed an equivalent chemopreventive effect (Buttar et al, 2002b). These findings provide further evidence that NSAIDs may be effective chemopreventive agents against Barrett's esophagus, resulting in a decreased incidence of esophageal cancer in humans. A clinical trial evaluating a selective COX-2 inhibitor is ongoing in patients with Barrett's esophagus and mucosal dysplasia.

Another agent that has been evaluated in a limited number of patients with Barrett's esophagus is difluoromethylornithine (DFMO). DFMO is an inhibitor of ornithine decarboxylase that regulates the rate-limiting enzyme in the synthesis of mucosal polyamines. Polyamines are known to regulate cellular proliferation and differentiation (Garewal et al, 1992). DFMO is a potent inhibitor of epithelial carcinogenesis in a variety of animal model systems. Furthermore, DFMO has been shown to inhibit the growth of Barrett's epithelium–derived cell lines, suggesting a role for this compound in the treatment of this disease (Garewal et al, 1988). Gerner et al (1994) performed a biomarker modulation trial to evaluate the effect of oral DFMO on polyamine levels in 8 patients with Barrett's esophagus. DFMO was shown to decrease polyamine levels, particularly levels of spermidine, in Barrett's epithelium. Studies have yet to be done to determine whether this decrease in polyamine levels has an effect on neoplastic development virgule progression in Barrett's epithelia. Chemoprevention is a field in its infancy, and future studies of existing and new agents are likely to provide important insights into the difficult problem of interrupting the process of carcinogenesis in Barrett's epithelium. What is being learned from prevention studies in other epithelial premalignant conditions is already being applied to the esophagus.

KEY PRACTICE POINTS

- Barrett's esophagus is a metaplastic change that can occur in the normal squamous epithelium of the esophagus.

- Barrett's esophagus is a premalignant condition that can progress through a multistep process into adenocarcinoma.

- GERD is an established risk factor for Barrett's esophagus.

- The recommended frequency of surveillance endoscopy depends on the degree of dysplasia within the Barrett's segment.

- If high-grade dysplasia is detected, esophagectomy should be offered. Endoscopic ablative therapies remain investigational but are an alternative for selected patients, especially in the setting of a clinical trial.

- Esophagectomy is the only known method to reliably remove all Barrett's epithelium and thereby eliminate neoplastic potential.

ACKNOWLEDGMENT

The authors wish to express their appreciation to Yvonne Romero, MD, for her careful review of the manuscript.

SUGGESTED READINGS

Arguedas MR, Eloubeidi MA. Barrett's oesophagus: a review of costs of the illness. *Pharmacoeconomics* 2001;19:1003–1011.

Barrett MT, Sanchez CA, Prevo LJ, et al. Evolution of neoplastic cell lineages in Barrett oesophagus. *Nat Genet* 1999;22:106–109.

Benipal P, Garewal HS, Sampliner RE, et al. Short segment Barrett's esophagus: relationship of age with extent of intestinal metaplasia. *Am J Gastroenterol* 2001; 96:3084–3088.

Blot WJ, Devesa SS, Kneller RW, Fraumeni JF Jr. Rising incidence of adenocarcinoma of the esophagus and gastric cardia. *JAMA* 1991;265:1287–1289.

Buttar NS, Wang KK, Anderson MA, et al. The effect of selective cyclooxygenase-2 inhibition in Barrett's esophagus epithelium: an in vitro study. *J Natl Cancer Inst* 2002a;94:422–429.

Buttar NS, Wang KK, Leontovich O, et al. Chemoprevention of esophageal adenocarcinoma by COX-2 inhibitors in an animal model of Barrett's esophagus. *Gastroenterology* 2002b;122:1101–1112.

Buttar NS, Wang KK, Lutzke LS, Krishnadath KK, Anderson MA. Combined endoscopic mucosal resection and photodynamic therapy for esophageal neoplasia within Barrett's esophagus. *Gastrointest Endosc* 2001a;54:682–688.

Buttar NS, Wang KK, Sebo TJ, et al. Extent of high-grade dysplasia in Barrett's esophagus correlates with risk of adenocarcinoma. *Gastroenterology* 2001b;120: 1630–1639.

Cameron AJ. Barrett's esophagus: prevalence and size of hiatal hernia. *Am J Gastroenterol* 1999;94:2054–2059.

Cameron AJ, Carpenter HA. Barrett's esophagus, high-grade dysplasia, and early adenocarcinoma: a pathological study. *Am J Gastroenterol* 1997;92:586–591.

Cameron AJ, Lagergren J, Henriksson C, et al. Gastroesophageal reflux disease in monozygotic and dizygotic twins. *Gastroenterology* 2002a;122:55–59.

Cameron AJ, Lomboy CT. Barrett's esophagus: age, prevalence, and extent of columnar epithelium. *Gastroenterology* 1992;103:1241–1245.

Cameron AJ, Lomboy CT, Pera M, Carpenter HA. Adenocarcinoma of the esophagogastric junction and Barrett's esophagus. *Gastroenterology* 1995;109:1541– 1546.

Cameron AJ, Souto EO, Smyrk TC. Small adenocarcinomas of the esophagogastric junction: association with intestinal metaplasia and dysplasia. *Am J Gastroenterol* 2002b;97:1375–1380.

Cameron AJ, Zinsmeister AR, Ballard DJ, Carney JA. Prevalence of columnar-lined (Barrett's) esophagus. Comparison of population-based clinical and autopsy findings. *Gastroenterology* 1990;99:918–922.

Canto MI, Setrakian S, Petras RE, et al. Methylene blue selectively stains intestinal metaplasia in Barrett's esophagus. *Gastrointest Endosc* 1996;44:1–7.

Canto MI, Setrakian S, Willis J, et al. Methylene blue directed biopsies improve detection of intestinal metaplasia and dysplasia in Barrett's esophagus. *Gastrointest Endosc* 2000;51:560–568.

Castell DO. Aggressive acid control: minimizing progression of Barrett's esophagus. *Am J Manag Care* 2001;7:S15–S18.

Chalasani N, Wo JM, Hunter JG, et al. Significance of intestinal metaplasia in different areas of esophagus including esophagogastric junction. *Dig Dis Res* 1997;42:603–607.

Champion G, Richter JE, Vaezi MF, Singh S, Alexander R. Duodenogastroesophageal reflux: relationship to pH and importance in Barrett's esophagus. *Gastroenterology* 1994;107:747–754.

Chow WC, Finkle WD, McLaughlin JK, Frankl H, Ziel HK. The relation of gastroesophageal reflux disease and its treatment to adenocarcinomas of the esophagus and gastric cardia. *JAMA* 1995;274:474–477.

Clark GW, Ireland AP, DeMeester TR. Dysplasia in Barrett's esophagus: diagnosis, surveillance and treatment. *Dig Dis* 1996;14:213–227.

Clark GW, Smyrk TC, Budiles P, et al. Barrett's metaplasia the source of adenocarcinomas of the cardia? *Arch Surg* 1994;129:609–614.

Conio M, Cameron AJ, Romero Y, et al. Secular trends in the epidemiology and outcome of Barrett's esophagus in Olmsted County, Minnesota. *Gut* 2001;48: 304–309.

Cooper BT, Neumann CS, Cox MA, Iqbal TH. Continuous treatment with omeprazole 20 mg daily for up to 6 years in Barrett's oesophagus. *Aliment Pharmacol Ther* 1998;12:893–897.

Corley DA, Kerlikowske K, Verma R, Buffler P. Protective association of aspirin/NSAIDs and esophageal cancer: a systematic review and meta-analysis. *Gastroenterology* 2003;124:47–56.

Corley DA, Levin TR, Habel LA, Weiss NS, Buffler PA. Surveillance and survival in Barrett's adenocarcinomas: a population-based study. *Gastroenterology* 2002; 122:633–640.

Cossentino MJ, Wong RK. Barrett's esophagus and risk of esophageal adenocarcinoma. *Semin Gastrointest Dis* 2003;14:128–135.

DeVault KR. Epidemiology and significance of Barrett's esophagus. *Dig Dis* 2000; 18:195–202.

Devesa SS, Blot WJ, Fraumeni JF Jr. Changing patterns in the incidence of esophageal and gastric carcinoma in the United States. *Cancer* 1998;83:2049–2053.

Drewitz DJ, Sampliner RE, Garewal HS. The incidence of adenocarcinoma in Barrett's esophagus: a prospective study of 170 patients followed 4.8 years. *Am J Gastroenterol* 1997;92:212–215.

Eckardt VF, Kanzler G, Bernhard G. Life expectancy and cancer risk in patients with Barrett's esophagus: a prospective controlled investigation. *Am J Med* 2001; 111:33–37.

Ell C, May A, Gossner L, et al. Endoscopic mucosal resection of early cancer and high-grade dysplasia in Barrett's esophagus. *Gastroenterology* 2000;118:670–677.

Endlicher E, Knuchel R, Messmann H. [Surveillance of patients with Barrett's esophagus]. *Z Gastroenterol* 2001;39:593–600.

Ertan A, Younes M. Barrett's esophagus. *Dig Dis Sci* 2000;45:1670–1673.

Falk GW. Barrett's esophagus. *Gastroenterology* 2002;122:1569–1591.

Falk GW. Gastroesophageal reflux disease and Barrett's esophagus. *Endoscopy* 2001;33:109–118.

Falk GW. Reflux disease and Barrett's esophagus. *Endoscopy* 1999;31:9–16.

Farrow D, Vaughn T, Hansen P, et al. Use of aspirin and other nonsteroidal anti-inflammatory drugs and risk of esophageal and gastric cancer. *Cancer Epidemiol Biomarkers Prev* 1998;7:49–102.

Fitzgerald RC, Omary MB, Triadafilopoulos G. Dynamic effects of acid on Barrett's esophagus. An ex vivo proliferation and differentiation model. *J Clin Invest* 1996;98:2120–2128.

Gadour M, Ayoola EA. Barrett's esophagus: a review. *Trop Gastroenterol* 2002;23: 157–161.

Garewal HS, Gerner EW, Sampliner RE, Roe D. Ornithine decarboxylase and polyamine levels in columnar upper gastrointestinal mucosae in patients with Barrett's esophagus. *Cancer Res* 1988;48:3288–3291.

Garewal HS, Sampliner RE, Fennerty MB. Chemopreventive studies in Barrett's esophagus: a model premalignant lesion for esophageal adenocarcinoma. *J Natl Cancer Inst Monogr* 1992:51–54.

Gerner EW, Garewal HS, Emerson SS, Sampliner RE. Gastrointestinal tissue polyamine contents of patients with Barrett's esophagus treated with alpha-difluoromethylornithine. *Cancer Epidemiol Biomarkers Prev* 1994;3:325–330.

Giard RW, Coebergh JW, Ouwendijk RJ. [Revision needed of follow-up policy for Barrett's esophagus]. *Ned Tijdschr Geneeskd* 2002;146:150–154.

Gillen P, McDermott M, Grehan D, Hourihane DO, Hennessy TP. Proliferating cell nuclear antigen in the assessment of Barrett's mucosa. *Br J Surg* 1994;81:1766–1768.

Grade AJ, Shah IA, Medlin SM, Ramirez FC. The efficacy and safety of argon plasma coagulation therapy in Barrett's esophagus. *Gastrointest Endosc* 1999; 50:18–22.

Gulizia JM, Wang H, Antonioli D, et al. Proliferative characteristics of intestinalized mucosa in the distal esophagus and gastroesophageal junction (short-segment Barrett's esophagus): a case control study. *Hum Pathol* 1999;30: 412–418.

Haag S, Nandurkar S, Talley N. Regression of Barrett's esophagus: the role of acid suppression, surgery and ablative methods. *Gastrointest Endosc* 1999;50:229–240.

Haggitt RC. Barrett's esophagus, dysplasia, and adenocarcinoma. *Hum Pathol* 1994; 25:982–993.

Haggitt RC, Reid BJ, Rabinovitch PS, Rubin CE. Barrett's esophagus. Correlation between mucin histochemistry, flow cytometry, and histologic diagnosis for predicting increased cancer risk. *Am J Pathol* 1988;131:53–61.

Haggitt RC, Tryzelaar J, Ellis FH, et al. Adenocarcinoma complicating columnar epithelial lined (Barrett's) esophagus. *Am J Clin Pathol* 1978;70:1–5.

Heitmiller RF, Redmond M, Hamilton SR. Barrett's esophagus with high-grade dysplasia. An indication for prophylactic esophagectomy. *Ann Surg* 1996;224: 66–71.

Hong MK, Laskin WB, Herman BE, et al. Expansion of the Ki-67 proliferative compartment correlates with degree of dysplasia of Barrett's esophagus. *Cancer* 1995;75:423–429.

Inadomi JM, Sampliner R, Lagergren J, et al. Screening and surveillance for Barrett esophagus in high-risk groups: a cost-utility analysis. *Ann Intern Med* 2003;138: 176–186.

Kaur BS, Khamnehei N, Iravani M, et al. Rofecoxib inhibits cyclooxygenase 2 expression and activity and reduces cell proliferation in Barrett's esophagus. *Gastroenterology* 2002;123:60–67.

Khan S, Do KA, Kuhnert P, et al. Diagnostic value of p53 immunohistochemistry in Barrett's esophagus: an endoscopic study. *Pathology* 1998;30:136–140.

Klaus A, Hinder RA. Indications for antireflux surgery in Barrett's. *Semin Laparosc Surg* 2001;8:234–239.

Klaus A, Hinder RA. Medical therapy versus antireflux surgery in Barrett's esophagus: what is the best therapeutic approach? *Dig Dis* 2000;18:224–231.

Krishnadath KK, Wang KK, Taniguchi K, et al. Persistent genetic abnormalities in Barrett's esophagus after photodynamic therapy. *Gastroenterology* 2000;119:624–630.

Kulke MH, Thakore KS, Thomas G, et al. Microsatellite instability and hMLH1/hMSH2 expression in Barrett esophagus-associated adenocarcinoma. *Cancer* 2001;91:1451–1457.

Lagergren J, Bergstrom R, Lindgren A, Nyren O. Symptomatic gastroesophageal reflux as a risk factor for esophageal adenocarcinoma. *N Engl J Med* 1999; 340:825–831.

Langman M, Cheng K, Gilman E, et al. Effect of anti-inflammatory drugs on overall risk of common cancer: case control study in general practice research database. *BMJ* 2000;320:1642–1646.

Leung WK, Sung JJ. Review article: intestinal metaplasia and gastric carcinogenesis. *Aliment Pharmacol Ther* 2002;16:1209–1216.

May A, Gossner L, Behrens A, et al. A prospective randomized trial of two different endoscopic resection techniques for early stage cancer of the esophagus. *Gastrointest Endosc* 2003;58:167–175.

May A, Gossner L, Pech O, et al. Local endoscopic therapy for intraepithelial high-grade neoplasia and early adenocarcinoma in Barrett's oesophagus: acute-phase and intermediate results of a new treatment approach. *Eur J Gastroenterol Hepatol* 2002;14:1085–1091.

Montgomery E, Bronner MP, Goldblum JR, et al. Reproducibility of the diagnosis of dysplasia in Barrett's esophagus: a reaffirmation. *Hum Pathol* 2001;32:368–378.

Morales TG, Sampliner RE, Bhattacharyya A. Intestinal metaplasia of the gastric cardia. *Am J Gastroenterol* 1997;92:414–418.

Neshat K, Sanchez CA, Galipeau PC, et al. p53 mutations in Barrett's adenocarcinoma and high-grade dysplasia. *Gastroenterology* 1994;106:1589–1595.

Ormsby AH, Goldblum JR, Rice TW, Richter JE, Gramlich TL. The utility of cyto-keratin subsets in distinguishing Barrett's-related oesophageal adenocarcinoma from gastric adenocarcinoma. *Histopathology* 2001;38:307–311.

Ortiz-Hidalgo C, De La Vega G, Aguirre-Garcia J. The histopathology and biologic prognostic factors of Barrett's esophagus: a review. *J Clin Gastroenterol* 1998;26: 324–333.

Overholt BF. Acid suppression and reepithelialization after ablation of Barrett's esophagus. *Dig Dis* 2000a;18:232–239.

Overholt BF. Evaluating treatments of Barrett's esophagus that shows high-grade dysplasia. *Am J Manag Care* 2000b;6:S903–S908.

Overholt BF, Panjehpour M, Halberg DL. Photodynamic therapy for Barrett's esophagus with dysplasia and/or early stage carcinoma: long-term results. *Gastrointest Endosc* 2003;58:183–188.

Pacifico RJ, Wang KK. Role of mucosal ablative therapy in the treatment of the columnar-lined esophagus. *Chest Surg Clin N Am* 2002;12:185–203.

Paraf F, Flejou JF, Pignon JP, et al. Surgical pathology of adenocarcinoma arising in Barrett's esophagus. *Am J Surg Pathol* 1995;19:183–191.

Pera M, Cameron AJ, Trastek VF, Carpenter HA, Zinsmeister AR. Increasing incidence of adenocarcinoma of the esophagus and esophagogastric junction. *Gastroenterology* 1993;104:510–513.

Peters JH, Clark GWB, Ireland AP, et al. Outcome of adenocarcinoma arising in Barrett's esophagus in endoscopically surveyed and nonsurveyed patients. *J Thorac Cardiovasc Surg* 1994;108:811–822.

Rabinovitch PS, Longton G, Blount PL, Levine DS, Reid BJ. Predictors of progression in Barrett's esophagus III: baseline flow cytometric variables. *Am J Gastroenterol* 2001;96:3071–3083.

Reid BJ. Barrett's esophagus and esophageal adenocarcinoma. *Gastroenterol Clin North Am* 1991;20:817–834.

Reid BJ, Blount PL, Feng Z, Levine DS. Optimizing endoscopic biopsy detection of early cancers in Barrett's high-grade dysplasia. *Am J Gastroenterol* 2000a;95: 3089–3096.

Reid BJ, Haggitt RC, Rubin CE, et al. Observer variation in the diagnosis of dysplasia in Barrett's esophagus. *Hum Pathol* 1988;19:166–178.

Reid B, Levine D, Longton G, et al. Predictors of progression to cancer in Barrett's esophagus: baseline histology and flow cytometry identify low and high risk patient subsets. *Am J Gastroenterol* 2000b;95:1669–1679.

Reid BJ, Prevo LJ, Galipeau PC, et al. Predictors of progression in Barrett's esophagus II: baseline 17p (p53) loss of heterozygosity identifies a patient subset at increased risk for neoplastic progression. *Am J Gastroenterol* 2001;96:2839–2848.

Richter JE. Importance of bile reflux in Barrett's esophagus. *Dig Dis* 2000;18:208–216.

Richter JE, Falk GW. Barrett's esophagus and adenocarcinoma. The need for a consensus conference. *J Clin Gastroenterol* 1996;23:88–90.

Riddell RH, Goldman H, Ransohoff DE, et al. Dysplasia in inflammatory bowel disease. *Hum Pathol* 1983;14:931–968.

Riegman PH, Burgart LJ, Wang KK, et al. Allelic imbalance of 7q32.3–q36.1 during tumorigenesis in Barrett's esophagus. *Cancer Res* 2002;62:1531–1533.

Robaszkiewicz M, Hardy E, Volant A, et al. [Flow cytometric analysis of cellular DNA content in Barrett's esophagus. A study of 66 cases]. *Gastroenterol Clin Biol* 1991;15:703–710.

Romero Y, Cameron AJ, Locke GR 3rd, et al. Familial aggregation of gastro-esophageal reflux in patients with Barrett's esophagus and esophageal adenocarcinoma. *Gastroenterology* 1997;113:1449–1456.

Rosenberg JC, Budey H, Edwards RC, et al. Analysis of adenocarcinoma in Barrett's esophagus utilizing a staging system. *Cancer* 1985;55:1353–1360.

Rugge M, Russo V, Busatto G, et al. The phenotype of gastric mucosa coexisting with Barrett's oesophagus. *J Clin Pathol* 2001;54:456–460.

Rusch VW, Levine DS, Haggitt R, Reid BJ. The management of high grade dysplasia and early cancer in Barrett's esophagus. A multidisciplinary problem. *Cancer* 1994;74:1225–1229.

Sampliner RE. Practice guidelines on the diagnosis, surveillance, and therapy of Barrett's esophagus. *Am J Gastroenterol* 1998;93:1028–1032.

Sampliner RE. Prevention of adenocarcinoma by reversing Barrett's esophagus with mucosal ablation. *World J Surg* 2003;27:1026–1029.

Sampliner RE. Reduction of acid exposure and regression of Barrett's esophagus. *Dig Dis* 2000;18:203–207.

Sampliner RE. Updated guidelines for the diagnosis, surveillance, and therapy of Barrett's esophagus. *Am J Gastroenterol* 2002;97:1888–1895.

Schnell TG, Sontag SJ, Chejfec G, et al. Long-term nonsurgical management of Barrett's esophagus with high grade dysplasia. *Gastroenterology* 2001;120:1607–1619.

Sharma P. An update on strategies for eradication of Barrett's mucosa. *Am J Med* 2001b;111 Suppl 8A:147S–152S.

Sharma P. Controversies in Barrett's esophagus: management of high grade dysplasia. *Semin Gastrointest Dis* 2001a;12:26–32.

Sharma P, Topalovski M, Mayo MS, Weston AP. Methylene blue chromoendoscopy for detection of short segment Barrett's esophagus. *Gastrointest Endosc* 2001;54:289–293.

Shirvani V, Ouatu-Lascar R, Kaur B, et al. Cyclooxygenase-2 expression in Barrett's esophagus and adenocarcinoma. Ex vivo induction by bile salts and acid exposure. *Gastroenterology* 2000;118:487–496.

Sinicrope FA, Gill S. Role of cylcooxygenase-2 in colorectal cancer. *Cancer Metastasis Rev* 2004;23:63–75.

Skinner DB, Walther BC, Riddell RH, et al. Barrett's esophagus. Comparison of benign and malignant cases. *Ann Surg* 1983;198:554–565.

Smith RRL, Hamilton SR, Boitnott JK, et al. The spectrum of carcinoma arising in Barrett's esophagus. *Am J Surg Pathol* 1984;8:563–573.

Souza RF, Shewmake K, Beer DG, Cryer B, Spechler SJ. Selective inhibition of cyclooxygenase-2 suppresses growth and induces apoptosis in human esophageal adenocarcinoma cells. *Cancer Res* 2000;60:5767–5772.

Souza RF, Shewmake K, Terada LS, Spechler SJ. Acid exposure activates the mitogen-activated protein kinase pathways in Barrett's esophagus. *Gastroenterology* 2002;122:299–307.

Spechler SJ. Barrett's esophagus. *Gastroenterologist* 1994;2:273–284.

Spechler SJ. Screening and surveillance for complications related to gastroesophageal reflux disease. *Am J Med* 2001;111 Suppl 8A:130S–136S.

Spechler SJ. Short and ultrashort Barrett's esophagus—what does it mean? *Semin Gastrointest Dis* 1997;8:59–67.

Spechler SJ, Zeroogian JM, Antonioli DA. Prevalence of metaplasia at the gastroesophageal junction. *Lancet* 1994;92:414–418.

Streitz JM, Andrews CW, Ellis FH. Endoscopic surveillance of Barrett's esophagus. *J Thorac Cardiovasc Surg* 1993;105:383–388.

Tseng EE, Wu TT, Yeo CJ, Heitmiller RF. Barrett's esophagus with high grade dysplasia: surgical results and long-term outcome—an update. *J Gastrointest Surg* 2003;7:164–170.

Vaezi MF, Falk GW, Peek RM, et al. CagA-positive strains of Helicobacter pylori may protect against Barrett's esophagus. *Am J Gastroenterol* 2000;95:2206–2211.

Vaezi MF, Richter JE. Synergism of acid and duodenogastroesophageal reflux in complicated Barrett's esophagus. *Surgery* 1995;117:699–704.

VanderBurgh A, Dees J, Hop WCI, et al. Oesophageal cancer is an uncommon cause of death in patients with Barrett's oesophagus. *Gut* 1996;139:5–8.

vanSandick J, vanLanschot J, Kuiken B, et al. Impact of endoscopic biopsy surveillance of Barrett's oesophagus on pathological stage and clinical outcome of Barrett's carcinoma. *Gut* 1998;43:216–222.

Vizcaino AP, Moreno V, Lambert R, Parkin DM. Time trends incidence of both major histologic types of esophageal carcinomas in selected countries, 1973–1995. *Int J Cancer* 2002;99:860–868.

Wang HH, Sovie S, Zeroogian JM, et al. Value of cytology in detecting intestinal metaplasia and associated dysplasia at the gastroesophageal junction. *Hum Pathol* 1997;28:465–471.

Wang KK. Photodynamic therapy of Barrett's esophagus. *Gastrointest Endosc Clin N Am* 2000;10:409–419.

Wang KK, Sampliner RE. Mucosal ablation therapy of Barrett esophagus. *Mayo Clin Proc* 2001;76:433–437.

Wilson K, Fu S, Ramanujam K, et al. Increased expression of inducible nitric oxide synthase and cyclooxygenase-2 in Barrett's esophagus and associated adenocarcinoma. *Cancer Res* 1998;58:2929–2934.

Wong DJ, Paulson TG, Prevo LJ, et al. p16(INK4a) lesions are common, early abnormalities that undergo clonal expansion in Barrett's metaplastic epithelium. *Cancer Res* 2001;61:8284–8289.

Wu TT, Watanabe T, Heitmiller R, et al. Genetic alterations in Barrett esophagus and adenocarcinomas of the esophagus and esophagogastric junction region. *Am J Pathol* 1998;153:287–294.

Zimmerman K, Sarbia M, Weber A, et al. Cyclooxygenase-2 expression in human esophageal carcinoma. *Cancer Res* 1999;59:198–204.

Zwas F, Shields HM, Doos WG, et al. Scanning electron microscopy of Barrett's epithelial and its correlation with light microscopy and mucin stains. *Gastroenterology* 1986;90:1932–1941.

INDEX